Contrast-Enhanced Clinical Magnetic Resonance Imaging

Contrast-Enhanced Clinical Magnetic Resonance Imaging

Val M. Runge, editor

Rosenbaum Professor of Diagnostic Radiology
University of Kentucky

The University Press of Kentucky

Portions of chapters 1, 2, 3, 4, and 6 are reprinted in revised form, with permission, from *Topics in Magnetic Resonance Imaging*, vol. 7, no. 3, Summer 1995.

The authors and publisher have exerted every effort to ensure that drug selection and dosage set forth in this text are in accord with current recommendations and practice at the time of publication. However, in view of ongoing research, changes in government regulations, and the constant flow of information relating to drug use and drug reactions, the reader is urged to check the package insert for each drug for any change in indications and dosage and for added warnings and precautions. This is particularly important when the recommended agent is a new or infrequently employed drug.

Published 1997 by The University Press of Kentucky

Scholarly publisher for the Commonwealth, serving Bellarmine College, Berea College, Centre College of Kentucky, Eastern Kentucky University, The Filson Club, Georgetown College, Kentucky Historical Society, Kentucky State University, Morehead State University, Murray State University, Northern Kentucky University, Transylvania University, University of Kentucky, University of Louisville, and Western Kentucky University.

Editorial and Sales Offices: The University Press of Kentucky
663 South Limestone Street, Lexington, Kentucky 40508-4008

01 00 99 98 97 5 4 3 2 1

Library of Congress Cataloging-in-Publication Data

Contrast-enhanced clinical magnetic resonance imaging / Val M. Runge, editor
p. cm.
Includes bibliographical references and index.
ISBN 0-8131-1944-8 (cloth : alk. paper)
1. Magnetic resonance imaging. 2. Contrast media. I. Runge, Val M.
[DNLM: 1. Magnetic Resonance Imaging—methods. 2. Contrast Media.
3. Neoplasms—diagnosis. WN 185 C759 1996]
RC78.7.N83C664 1996
616.07'548—dc20
DNLM/DLC
for Library of Congress 96-16767

This book is printed on recycled, acid-free paper meeting the requirements of the American National Standard for Permanence of Paper for Printed Library Materials.

Manufactured in the United States of America

To my two daughters, Valerie and Sadie
and my wife, B. J.
with all my love

CONTENTS

Preface

Dedicated research involving magnetic resonance (MR) contrast media has spanned the last fifteen years. Pharmaceutical development in this field has offered opportunities not matched by x-ray-based modalities, given in particular the lower dose required for image enhancement. Three agents (ProHance, Magnevist, and Omniscan) are currently approved by the US Food and Drug Administration for clinical use. All are extracellular in distribution, with renal excretion. Development of more tissue-specific contrast media has also been possible. Clinical trials of hepatobiliary gadolinium chelates, for example Gd BOPTA, are currently underway. Despite the newness of the field, contrast use plays a dominant role in clinical imaging, and in particular in studies of the head and spine.

The explosive growth in contrast media development and the modality itself has been unparalleled in the history of diagnostic imaging. Although development still continues, it is now possible, because of the large clinical experience, to summarize current applications.

This textbook presents an overview of basic principles, summarizes applications in the head, spine and body, and discusses safety, new applications, and new agents. Common applications of contrast media in MR clinical practice are illustrated using case material. The use of ProHance and other gadolinium chelates in head MR approaches the levels of use of iodinated agents in computed tomography (CT). Application of contrast media in MR imaging of the spine is also very common. Improved sensitivity and specificity for both intradural and extradural diseases have been demonstrated. Body imaging represents the largest area for potential growth in the near future. First pass dynamic studies and routine image acquisition during suspended respiration, both recent technologic advances, will no doubt enhance the use of contrast media both in and outside the central nervous system.

This textbook is intended for physicians, technologists, and basic scientists. Covered in depth is the current clinical use of contrast media in MR. Most applications provide improved lesion detection or characterization, although physiologic and biochemical data are now also available using new imaging techniques and newer agents. The patient material presented provides the reader with an understanding of clinical applications, ensuring informed use of MR contrast media and appropriate image interpretation.

Contributors

J. Randy Jinkins, M.D., FACR
Director of Neuroradiology, Department of Radiology, University of Texas Health Science Center
San Antonio, Texas

Lawrence R. Muroff, M.D., FACR
Clinical Professor of Radiology, University of Florida and University of South Florida Colleges of Medicine

Kevin L. Nelson, M.D.
Chairman, Department of Radiology, Clarkson Hospital
Omaha, Nebraska

Val M. Runge, M.D.
Rosenbaum Professor of Diagnostic Radiology, University of Kentucky
Lexington, Kentucky

John W. Wells, R.T.
Research Associate, University of Kentucky
Lexington, Kentucky

Chapter 1

Principles of MR Contrast

Kevin L. Nelson, M.D. and Val M. Runge, M.D.

Introduction

In just over a decade, magnetic resonance (MR) has become the imaging modality of choice for the study of central nervous system disease, with additional broad applications in the abdomen, pelvis and musculoskeletal system. Concurrent development of contrast media, now in widespread use, has aided the rapid expansion of this field and improved clinical efficacy. Magnetic resonance imaging offers high spatial resolution and soft tissue contrast, with sensitivity to contrast media greater than that of x-ray computed tomography (CT). First pass brain studies now make possible the assessment of regional cerebral blood volume, with high spatial and temporal resolution. New hardware developments, together with advances in contrast media design, continue to drive expansion of contrast media applications, building upon the large base of current clinical use.

Because MR provides excellent soft tissue contrast on unenhanced images, it was initially speculated that there would be no need for a contrast agent. However, in the early 1980s it became apparent that contrast enhancement could substantially improve sensitivity and specificity in both the brain and spine. For example, brain metastases that are unaccompanied by vasogenic edema could easily be visualized following contrast enhancement, due to disruption of the blood-brain barrier.[1] Small extraaxial tumors, such as meningiomas and acoustic neuromas, were also noted to be well visualized following gadolinium chelate administration, yet often unrecognized on pre-contrast scans. With the use of contrast enhancement, lesion conspicuity was dramatically increased.[2] As the benefits of paramagnetic contrast agents became more obvious, their use increased exponentially. Today, contrast agents are commonly employed in many indications for clinical MR imaging.

This chapter is intended to serve as a review of the basic principles responsible for the generation of image contrast in clinical MR. Contrast agent design requirements, mechanisms of MR image contrast, and relaxivity theory will be reviewed, in addition to clinical applications.

Contrast Agent Design Requirements

Certain criteria need to be met in the design of a MR contrast agent.[3,4] The first and foremost of these criteria is the ability to alter the parameters responsible for image contrast. MR is unique in that there are multiple parameters responsible for signal intensity. The contrast agent must be efficient in its ability to influence these parameters at low concentration, in order to minimize dose and potential toxicity.

Second, the contrast agent should possess some tissue specificity in vivo so that it is delivered to a tissue or organ in a higher concentration than to other areas in the body. Additionally, once delivered to the desired tissue or organ, it must remain localized for a reasonable period of time so that imaging can be performed.

Third, the contrast agent must be substantially cleared from the targeted tissue or organ in a reasonable period of time, usually several hours following imaging, in order to minimize potential effects from chronic toxicity. The contrast agent must also be excreted from the body, usually by renal or hepatobiliary routes.

Fourth, the contrast agent must have low toxicity and be stable in vivo, while being administered in doses that can affect the MR relaxation parameters sufficiently to result in visible contrast enhancement. The dose levels of the contrast agent required to meet these criteria must be evaluated for potential mutagenicity, teratogenicity, carcinogenicity, and immunogenicity.

Finally, the contrast agent must possess a suitable shelf life for storage. It must remain stable in vitro for a reasonable period of time while being stored. A shelf life of months, and preferably years, is desirable.

MR Contrast Mechanisms

In conventional radiography and computed tomography (CT), image contrast is generated by differential attenuation of the x-ray beam by the tissues of the body. The degree of attenuation is directly related to the mass absorption coefficient of the tissue being imaged, or, more specifically, the electron density and the effective atomic number of the tissue. Therefore, in conventional radiography and computed tomography, the mechanism for contrast enhancement involves manipulation of the mass absorption coefficient alone. The use of a contrast agent with a high mass absorption coefficient, for example any of the iodinated agents, results in attenuation of the x-ray beam to a greater degree, thereby producing contrast enhancement.

Compared with conventional radiography and CT, the mechanisms responsible for contrast enhancement in MR are not singular, but multiparametric. The large inherent differences of signal intensity between various tissues are what makes MR unique compared to other imaging modalities used in radiology today. Additionally, the appropriate selection of operator-dependent imaging parameters is critical so that these signal intensity differences can be exploited to optimize MR image contrast.

The parameters that determine MR signal intensity and contrast are many.[5] The first of these, and easiest to understand, is spin density. Spin density refers to the fraction of protons that exists in the voxel of tissue being imaged and determines the maximum potential MR signal intensity that can be realized from that volume of tissue. Most protons in tissue are water protons. These far outweigh in number the protons that are associated with organic compounds in tissue. Since the in vivo water content of tissue cannot easily be altered by a contrast agent, compounds which effect spin density have received little attention.

Another common parameter exploited in generation of MR contrast is relaxivity. There are two relaxivity parameters that are unique to each tissue — T1 and T2. Longitudinal or spin-lattice relaxation time, known as T1, refers to the amount of time it takes for the tissue magnetization to return to its equilibrium state in the longitudinal direction of the main magnetic field following excitation with a radio frequency (RF) pulse. The excess energy that is absorbed by the magnetic spins from the RF pulse is transferred back to the environment or lattice during the relaxation process. The second relaxivity property of tissue is transverse or spin-spin relaxation, referred to as T2 relaxation. In this relaxation process, the excess energy deposited in the tissue by the RF pulse is transferred between the magnetic spins. This transferred energy results in loss of spin phase coherency in the transverse plane and spin dephasing.

Contrast agent enhancement that is based upon alteration of these two relaxivity parameters can be categorized according to the relative change it imparts upon either T1 or T2.[6,7,8] A contrast agent that predominantly affects T1 relaxation is referred to as a positive relaxation agent. This is because the enhanced shortening of T1 relaxation results in increased signal intensity on a T1-weighted image. By comparison, a contrast agent that predominantly affects T2 relaxation is considered a negative relaxation agent. This is because reducing T2 results in decreased signal intensity on a T2-weighted image.

Another determinate of signal intensity in the MR image is magnetic susceptibility. Susceptibility describes the ability of a substance to become magnetized in an external magnetic field.[9] There are four categories of magnetic susceptibility. Most organic compounds are diamagnetic substances and have a small, negative magnetic susceptibility when placed in an external magnetic field. Paramagnetic substances have a net positive magnetic susceptibility, while superparamagnetic and ferromagnetic materials have very large net positive susceptibilities. Diamagnetic susceptibility has a negligible effect in clinical MR and, therefore, diamagnetic substances are of little interest as contrast agents.

Paramagnetic substances afford the greatest flexibility in contrast agent design and have, therefore, received the greatest attention in contrast media development. The presence of a paramagnetic ion can strongly influence the relaxation properties of nearby protons, leading to changes in tissue contrast. Paramagnetic contrast agents are predominantly used as positive T1 relaxation contrast agents, with little effect seen on T2 relaxation, and then only at high concentrations. The positive net magnetic susceptibility of a paramagnetic ion actually has little influence as an actual enhancement mechanism in conventional MR.

By comparison, the large net magnetic susceptibility of superparamagnetic and ferromagnetic compounds more directly influences tissue contrast, with little effect on relaxation per se. Superparamagnetic substances are individual particles that are large enough to be a domain. When these particles are exposed to an external magnetic field, they align with the field, resulting in a large net positive magnetization. When removed from the magnetic field, they return to random orientations and lose their net positive magnetization. By comparison, ferromagnetic compounds are large collections of interacting domains in a crystalline matrix. They exhibit an extremely large net positive magnetization in an external magnetic field, and maintain this when removed from the field. Both superparamagnetic and ferromagnetic compounds have received substantial attention in regard to their application as clinical MR contrast agents. These agents function as negative contrast agents since their large net positive magnetic moments induce spin dephasing in tissue, with resultant signal loss.

The final two parameters that provide image contrast in MR are diffusion and perfusion. The intensity of the MR signal is based on the magnitude of the bulk magnetization lying in the transverse plane. It is maximal when all the transverse spins are in phase coherence. Movement or diffusion of bulk water between tissues in a random motion leads to spin dephasing and loss of phase coherence in the transverse plane. This subsequently results in the loss of MR signal intensity. Similarly, perfusion of blood in the microcirculation of the tissue being imaged also contributes to spin dephasing, and a decrease in the intensity of the MR signal. In this manner, different degrees of diffusion and perfusion within tissue contribute to contrast in the MR image. The use of a relaxivity or susceptibility contrast agent to manipulate diffusion coefficients, and thus function as a contrast agent, has received limited attention to date. However, the presence of a susceptibility agent in the blood pool can cause large changes in signal intensity. This approach is being actively investigated as a means of contrast enhancement, specifically for the measurement of regional cerebral blood volume.

Relaxivity Theory

Nearly all the attention in development of MR contrast agents has focused upon the use of paramagnetic compounds. The most commonly employed paramagnetic ion is the gadolinium ion, which is complexed with various ligands (such as DTPA and HP-DO3A) which act as chelating agents. While an extensive review of relaxivity theory is beyond the scope of this chapter, a basic conceptional understanding is necessary in order to appreciate the physics involved in paramagnetic contrast agent enhancement.

The presence of unpaired electrons in the paramagnetic ion is a mandatory component in order to affect a change in the T1 and T2 relaxation rates of water protons.[10,11] The magnetic dipole moment created by the unpaired electrons can thereby enhance the relaxation rates of water protons, either by direct interaction with the water protons or by its local magnetic field influence. The relaxivity contributions of a paramagnetic ion are highly dependent on its spin state. If S denotes the spin quantum number of the total electron spin of the paramagnetic ion, then the relaxation rate is proportional to $S*(S+1)$. Therefore, a paramagnetic ion with the highest spin quantum number is desirable. The gadolinium ion (Gd^{+3}) of the lanthanide metal group has a high spin quantum number of 7/2, making it a desirable relaxivity contrast agent. Other ions that have received attention as potential MR contrast agents include Fe^{+3}, Dy^{+3}, and Mn^{+3} (all with $S=5/2$). Although a high spin quantum number is theoretically desirable, it is not the only factor that determines whether a MR contrast agent will be efficacious.

The interactions that occur between a paramagnetic contrast agent and protons of water molecules can be classified into two categories. Inner sphere relaxation refers to the formation of a coordinate covalent molecular bond between a water molecule and the primary or intercoordination sphere of the paramagnetic ion. A chemical exchange occurs between the water molecule and the paramagnetic ion in this interaction, which leads to enhanced relaxation of the water protons based upon the magnetic influences and the efficiency of chemical exchange. It follows that the more water molecules that can bind with the paramagnetic ion, the greater its influence upon relaxation enhancement. Therefore, the shorter the residence time of the water molecule with the paramagnetic ion, the greater the relaxation enhancement effect will be, due to the ability of the paramagnetic ion to interact with other water molecules. In contrast agent design a rapid exchange (10^6 sec^{-1}) between water molecules and the paramagnetic ion is a desirable feature since it allows for greater relaxation enhancement. However, this factor is important only up to the point where the exchange contributes as a correlation time.

Outer sphere relaxation is a more complex concept. It does not involve a direct bonding or chemical exchange mechanism. It is the result of the relative rotational and translational diffusion of water molecules and the paramagnetic ion. Basically stated, the more water molecules that can approach the paramagnetic ion and interact with its dipole, the greater will be the relaxivity influence of the paramagnetic ion. The more the paramagnetic ion can move through space, the greater will be its ability to interact with other water protons. Additionally, the closer the water protons can approach the paramagnetic ion, the more efficient the relaxation enhancement will be. This interaction of the dipole moments of the paramagnetic ion and the water molecules in the environment has been termed a dipole-dipole relaxation process. Inner sphere relaxation for Gd^{3+} is also a dipolar process ("through space"), as Gd^{3+} has no scalar relaxation ("through bond").

These factors are critical in contrast agent design. For example, if the paramagnetic ion is complexed with a ligand such as DTPA, the molecular complex will rotate slower and translate slower in space. This will not allow as many water proton-paramagnetic ion interactions to occur, thereby limiting the relaxation effect. Also, by complexing the paramagnetic ion, there will be increased distance between the water proton dipole and the paramagnetic ion dipole, decreasing the paramagnetic ion's relaxation enhancement effect.

The Solomon-Bloembergen-Morgan equation is a mathematical expression that describes the relaxation of water protons in the presence of a paramagnetic ion species.[12] This equation is utilized as a predictor of relaxation efficiency of a paramagnetic ion species in contrast agent design. The Solomon-Bloembergen-Morgan equation can be thought of in two terms. The first component, the dipole-dipole term, expresses a distance factor between interacting species. In one dimension, this is a statement of the inverse square law in that the magnitude of the paramagnetic effect is related to the reciprocal of the square of the distance (d^{-2}). In three dimensions, this becomes d^{-6} expressed as r^{-6} (r = radius). The dipole-dipole component is critically affected by the distance factor. Simply stated, the more closely a water molecule approachs the paramagnetic ion species, the more efficient will be the relaxation enhancement effect. Since the dipole-dipole component is critically affected by distance, it is important in contrast agent design to use carrier ligands that minimize this effect. Some of the carrier ligands, however, may be quite large. These ligands cause an undesirable effect from the standpoint of relaxation enhancement. Use of chelates is required because of the high toxicity of paramagnetic ions, such as gadolinium, when free in the body. Large carrier ligands and their surrounding water molecules of hydration tend to displace free or bulk water molecules from the surrounding inner sphere of influence of the paramagnetic ion, decreasing proton relaxation enhancement effects. Of all factors, this has the largest negative impact.

The total correlation time (τ_c) between the two interacting species can be expressed mathematically for both dipole-dipole and scalar interactions as follows:

$$1/\tau_c = 1/\tau_r + 1/\tau_s + 1/\tau_m$$

where τ_c is the correlation time of interaction, τ_r is the correlation time of rotation, τ_s is the correlation time of electron relaxation, and τ_m is the correlation time of chemical exchange. The critical feature of this mathematical expression is that for any specific interaction, of the three components (τ_r, τ_s, and τ_m) comprising the total correlation time of interaction, the component that is of the smallest magnitude will be the most important in determining the total correlation time of interaction.

Correlation times are important in paramagnetic agent design. As an example, the larger the carrier ligand to which the paramagnetic ion is bound, the slower it will rotate and translate in space, thereby increasing the magnitude of τ_r. The total correlation time of interaction is thus increased in most instances of a large carrier ligand molecule, somewhat offsetting the distance factor for these large carrier ligands. Correlation times will always reflect the interaction possessing the shortest time characteristic or the fastest dynamic behavior of the paramagnetic contrast agent, providing that chemical exchange is fast enough (10^6 sec^{-1}).

Clinical Applications

This section deals with the application of MR pulse sequences for visualization of contrast media, building upon the knowledge of MR physics presented in the preceding paragraphs. As is now evident, the mechanisms responsible for MR image contrast are multiparametric, including relaxivity effects of T1 and T2, spin density, susceptibility, perfusion, and diffusion. Similar to the multiple intrinsic MR properties of the tissues themselves, the methods of measurement of these parameters in clinical MR imaging are multiple. The type of MR pulse sequence used to generate a clinical MR image and its associated parameters also profoundly affects the contrast that is visualized from the tissues.

The ultimate goal when optimizing MR scan technique for contrast agent visualization is to suppress the contrast from unchanged tissue parameters and accentuate the contrast based on the parameter that is altered by the contrast agent.[13] This requires knowledge of the mechanism of contrast agent enhancement, the MR pulse technique being employed to measure that parameter, and how the operator dependent parameters can be altered to optimize the enhancement of the contrast agent being used. What follows is a discussion of the MR pulse sequences that are commonly used in conjunction with clinical MR contrast agents and the issues that are related to the optimization of these protocols. While the scope of this discussion is limited, there are many extensive discussions in the literature.[3,5,11]

Conventional spin echo imaging has remained the mainstay of MR pulse sequences employed with contrast agents. This approach can provide images with T1, T2, and spin density information. In spin echo imaging (figure 1), a 90 degree RF pulse is followed by a 180 degree RF pulse, which generates a MR signal or echo at an operator-specified echo time (TE). This measurement is repeated at a repetition time (TR), which is also specified by the operator. In spin echo imaging, short TR and short TE times produce an image with T1-weighted contrast. Long TR and TE times produce images with T2-weighted contrast. During the same long TR interval used to produce a T2-weighted image, a second image can be obtained with a short or intermediate echo time (resulting in a second image with spin density or intermediate T2 weighting). One of the major disadvantages of conventional spin echo imaging when used to produce T2-weighted scans is the long imaging time. Imaging time is directly proportional to TR, which is long for a typical T2-weighted pulse sequence, usually two to three seconds.

A recent innovation is fast or turbo spin echo imaging, which permits T2-weighted scans to be acquired in a much reduced scan time. In this approach, multiple echoes are acquired with different phase encoding during each TR interval. Images with both proton density and T2-weighted information can be obtained in times from one-fourth to one-sixteenth that required for conventional spin echo techniques. Since the images generated from this approach are for multiple TE data measurements that are then averaged together for an effective TE image, the image contrast is somewhat different from a conventional spin echo sequence. For ex-

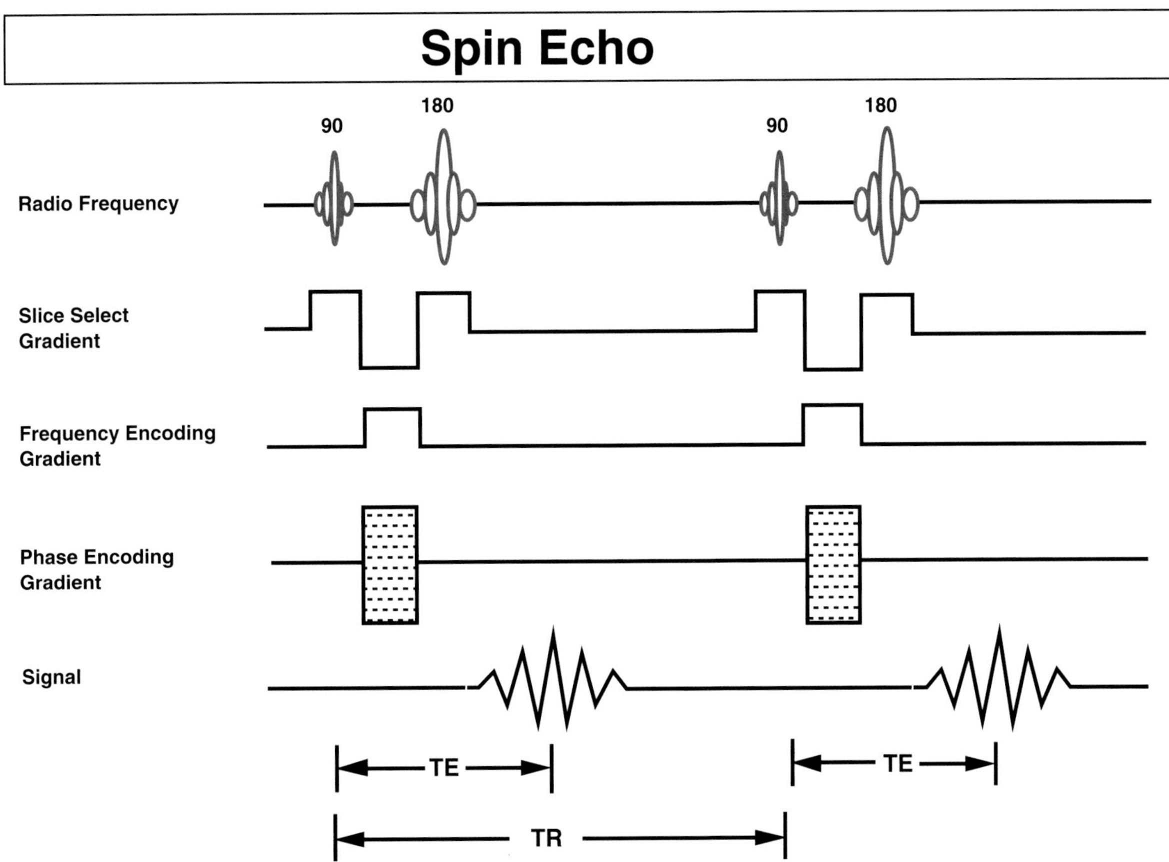

Figure 1. Pulse diagram for spin echo technique. This imaging approach continues to be the mainstay of clinical MR, particularly in the brain. A 90° radio frequency pulse is followed by a 180° radio frequency pulse, which generates a signal (echo) at time TE. This is repeated at intervals of TR. Spatial information within the slice is obtained by frequency and phase encoding, while the slice itself is specified by a third gradient (slice select).

ample, the MR signal from fat remains more intense on a T2-weighted image obtained with this pulse technique, reflecting the brighter signal fat produces on short TE images. Despite these and other minimal shortcomings of fast spin echo sequences, they have gained widespread popularity in clinical MR imaging of the brain and spine.

Another pulse technique that has gained popularity in neurologic applications is gradient echo imaging. This offers an alternate imaging approach with substantially reduced imaging time and RF power deposition. A gradient echo sequence differs from a spin echo sequence in that a 180 degree RF pulse is not employed. The initial RF pulse typically uses a flip angle of less than 90 degrees. Signal is then generated by manipulation of the gradient magnetic fields. By changing the operator dependent parameters of flip angle, TR and TE, image contrast with T1, $T2^*$ and spin density information can be generated. One of the major disadvantages of this technique is that susceptibility effects become prominent. This enhanced susceptibility effect can be exploited to advantage, however, in certain clinical situations. For example, the high magnetic susceptibility of blood degradation products, such as deoxyhemoglobin, results in increased conspicuity of hemorrhage on gradient echo scans.

Most of the contrast agents studied to date have been designed to affect relaxivity enhancement. This is because most of the intrinsic contrast in MR is dependent on T1 and T2 relaxation. While these contrast agents can be imaged with a variety of different MR techniques, including spin echo and gradient echo pulse sequences, it is paramount to choose appropriate imaging parameters in order to maximize visualization of the relaxation enhancement effect.

The gadolinium chelates, the major class of agents in use in clinical practice today, enhance T1 relaxivity and thereby result in visible contrast enhancement on T1-weighted pulse sequences with short TR and TE times. While these agents primarily affect T1 relaxation rates, producing positive contrast enhancement, their effect is biphasic in that at very high concentrations they can have T2 effects or negative contrast enhancement, even on T1-weighted pulse sequences (figure 2). In most clinical situations, the T2 effects have little contribution and the T1 effects are exploited to result in visible positive contrast enhancement. Their effects

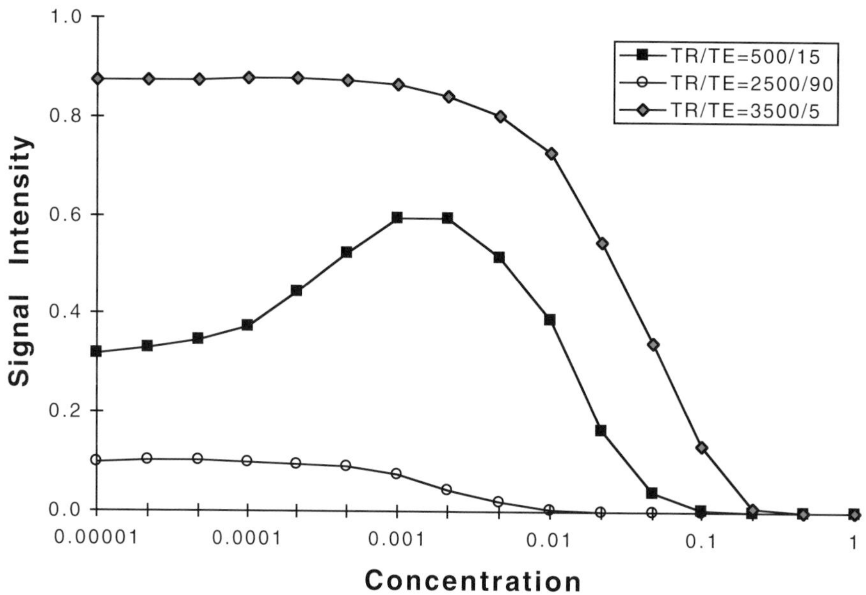

Figure 2. The dependence of contrast agent effect upon gadolinium chelate concentration and pulse technique. In MR, the effect of a gadolinium chelate upon signal intensity is nonlinear, with an additional dependency upon pulse technique. With T1-weighted spin echo techniques, an initial increase in signal intensity with concentration is observed. This results in positive lesion enhancement, forming the basis for most clinical applications in neuroimaging. With both proton density and T2-weighted spin echo techniques, little change is seen except at high concentrations, where signal intensity drops. The presence of the gadolinium ion enhances both the T1 and T2 relaxation of nearby water protons. This effect upon both T1 and T2, combined with the dependency of signal intensity on both parameters, leads to the complex relationship between concentration of the contrast agent and signal enhancement.

on proton density and T2-weighted images are generally not clinically relevant. The signal intensity decrease seen with increasing concentrations of a paramagnetic ion species, on the basis of T2 effects, is usually not seen at current doses (other than with hyperconcentration of these agents in the urine).

As previously noted, the positive T1 enhancement effects of the gadolinium contrast agents are well visualized on spin echo T1-weighted images. T1-weighted gradient echo imaging can also visualize the contrast enhancement effect of the gadolinium chelates. These techniques can be particularly useful when obtained in a volumetric fashion. A volumetric or 3-D acquisition permits image manipulation on a work station, with reconstruction of high resolution images in multiple planes, without the need for additional scans.

Currently in the United States, the Food and Drug Administration (FDA) has approved three MR contrast agents for general use, all of which use the gadolinium ion as the paramagnetic metal species. These agents are Gd HP-DO3A (gadoteridol or ProHance), Gd DTPA (gadopentetate dimeglumine or Magnevist), and Gd DTPA-BMA (gadodiamide or Omniscan), the first and last being non-ionic. These three parenteral paramagnetic compounds function as extracellular contrast agents. Following injection, they are distributed in the blood pool and extracellular fluid compartments of the body. All are rapidly excreted by glomerular filtration, with half lives between one to two hours. They act as positive T1 relaxation agents. In the central nervous system, these agents are not distributed within normal brain and spinal cord tissue, due to the presence of an intact blood-brain barrier. Slowly flowing venous structures (such as cortical veins and dural sinuses) will, however, demonstrate intense enhancement. When a pathologic process, such as a high grade tumor, results in disruption of the blood-brain barrier, administration of a gadolinium chelate produces positive contrast enhancement. This is best visualized on T1-weighted images, with little or no enhancement seen on proton density and T2-weighted images (figure 3). As has been extensively documented in the literature, contrast administration often proves very useful, increasing the conspicuity of diseases and providing physiologic information regarding the status of the blood-brain barrier. For diseases outside the CNS, lesion enhancement depends upon differential accumulation of the contrast agent between normal and abnormal tissue.

In the last few years, techniques using magnetization transfer (MT) have been introduced in clinical MR imaging.[14] The application of MT with spin echo imaging can

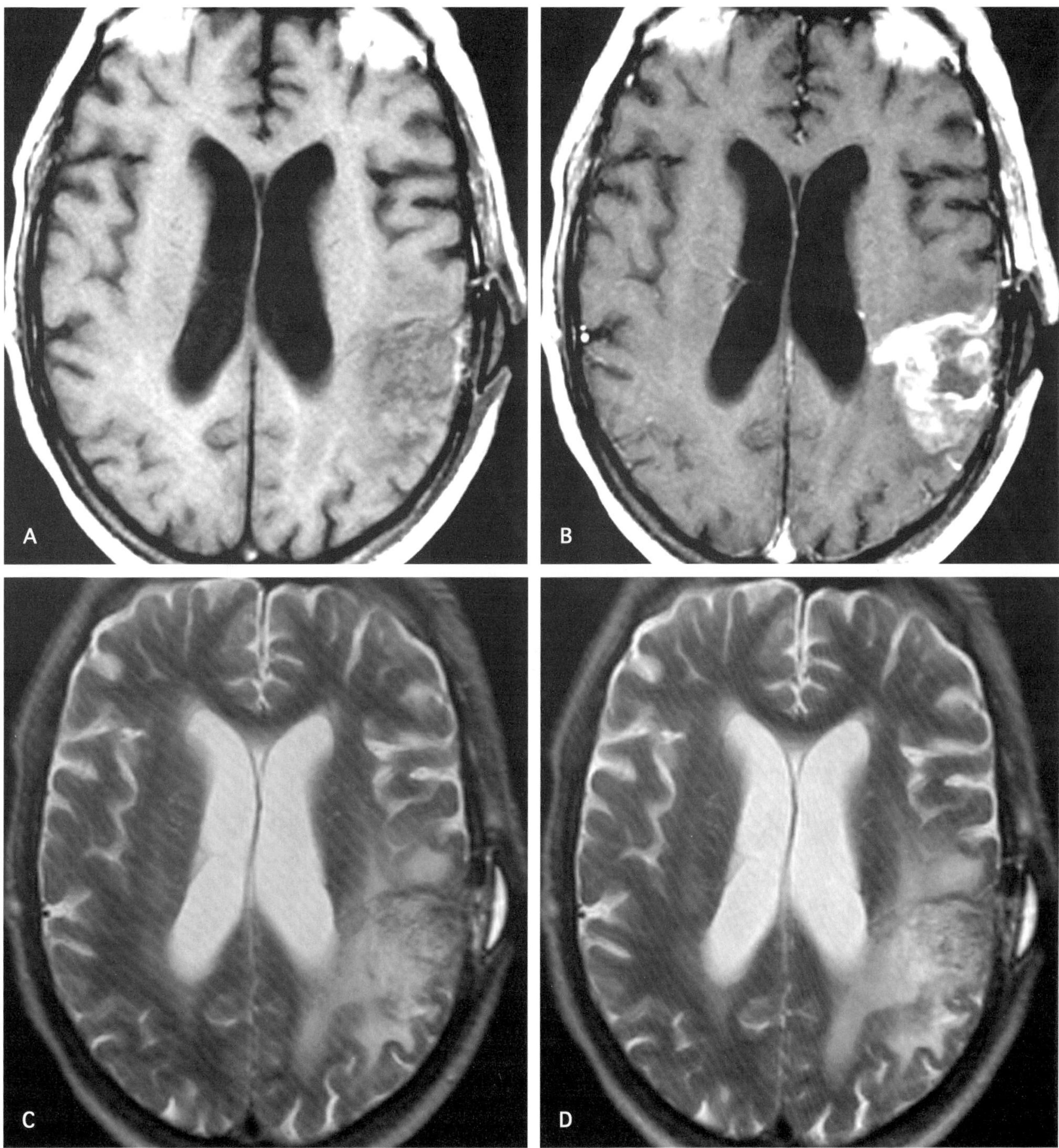

Figure 3. Lesion enhancement with a gadolinium chelate (Gd HP-DO3A or ProHance) on spin echo scans with both T1 and T2 weighting in a glioblastoma. (A) Pre- and (B) post-contrast T1-weighted scans are compared with (C) pre- and (D) post- contrast T2-weighted scans. On the T1-weighted scan post-contrast, positive lesion enhancement is noted in the region of blood-brain barrier disruption. Little change is seen in this region on the T2-weighted scan post-contrast.

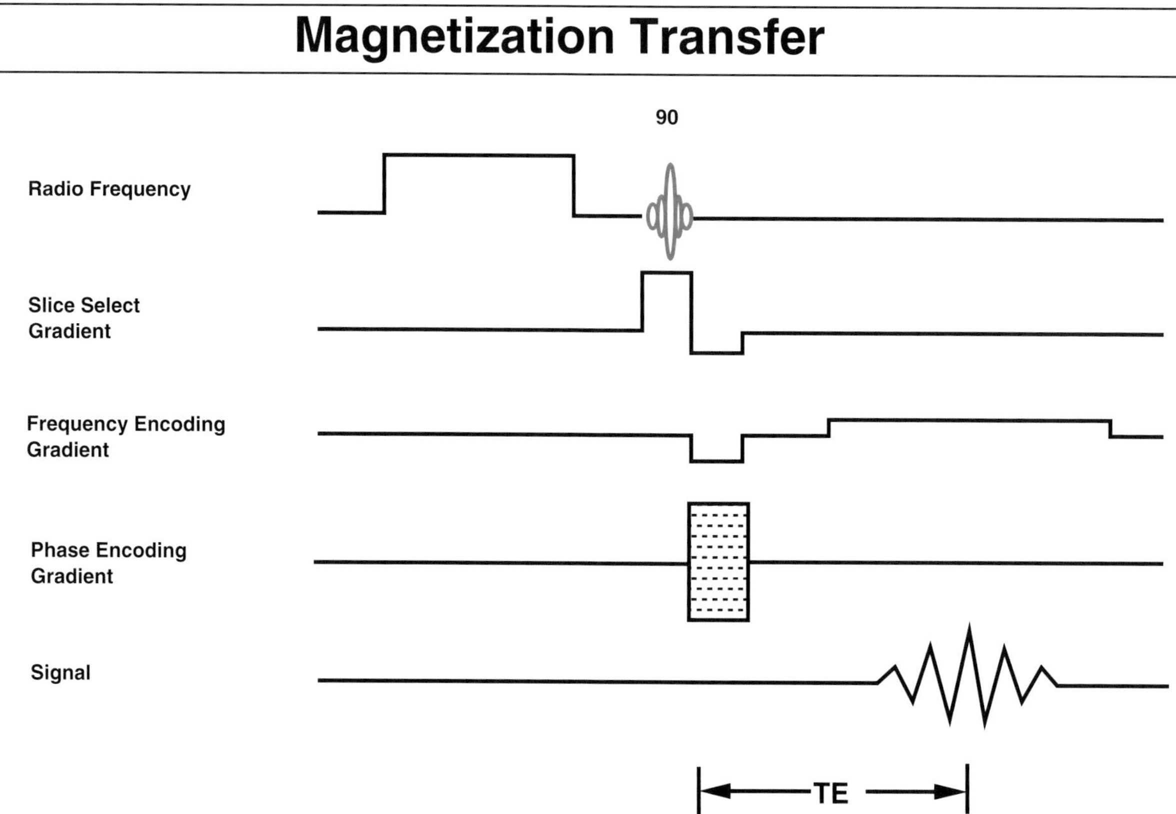

Figure 4. Pulse diagram for gradient echo technique with magnetization transfer (MT) suppression. MT provides an additional contrast mechanism to the previously described parameters of T1, T2, and proton density. In conventional MR techniques, the observed signal originates primarily from freely mobile hydrogen atoms (protons). Hydrogen atoms that are bound in complex molecular structures (the restricted hydrogen pool) are not imaged, due to their extremely short T2. By application of an additional radio frequency pulse, the restricted pool can be saturated, with magnetization then transferred to the freely mobile pool.

improve the enhancement effect produced by a gadolinium chelate in the brain. It is known that water protons in tissue exist in three distinctive pools. The protons in the free water pool exist in a narrow range of resonant frequencies and possess a long T2. It is these protons that account for most of the MR signal recorded in clinical MR imaging. The fat pool is isolated from the water pool and normally not present in the brain and spinal cord. The third pool of protons is the restricted pool. These protons represent structural or bound water protons that are associated with large molecules, such as phospholipids in the brain and spinal cord. These protons have a large range of resonant frequencies, and have an extremely short T2. Since the restricted pool of water protons decays so quickly during MR imaging (due to their short T2), it contributes little signal to the image. With the application of MT (figure 4), magnetization is transferred from the restricted hydrogen pool to the freely mobile hydrogen pool. The result is a shortening of T1, with lower overall available magnetization and signal intensity. In theory, enhancement with gadolinium chelates is not mediated by macromolecular interactions, and thus not suppressed by the application of MT.[15] Accordingly, MT pulses preferentially suppress the signal from background tissue, usually improving the conspicuity of gadolinium enhanced regions (figure 5).[16] This can lead to improved visualization of abnormal contrast enhancement at standard dose.

Contrast agents that principally affect T2 have received much less attention for application in clinical practice. In part, this has been related to the fact that T2-weighted spin echo images, necessary to visualize such contrast enhancement effects, require long TR times, resulting in long imaging times. Gradient echo pulse sequences can be used but again their sensitivity to bulk susceptibility artifacts limits usefulness. One of the more promising groups of parenteral T2 agents is the superparamagnetic contrast agents. These agents contain ferrite particles. Ferrites are crystalline oxides, of which magnetite (Fe_3O_4) in a particle size of 0.5 to 1.0 microns has been used most commonly. Ferrite particles in this size range are phagocytosed by macrophages of the reticuloendothelial system, with prominent uptake in normal liver and spleen parenchyma. In such tissue there is selective T2 shortening with profound signal loss. Since MR

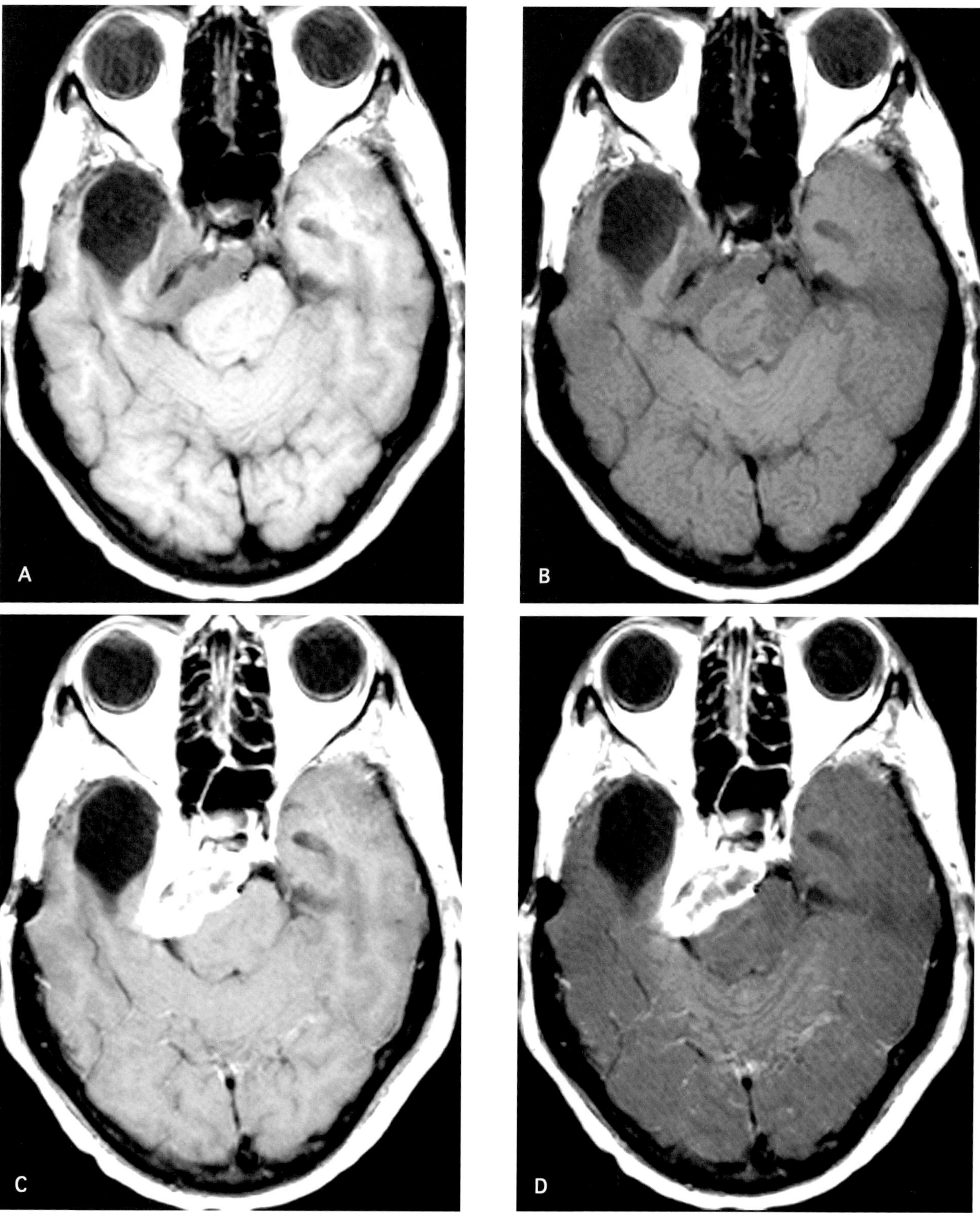

Figure 5. Lesion enhancement with a gadolinium chelate (Gd HP-DO3A or ProHance), comparing scans with and without magnetization transfer (MT) suppression in a meningioma. Pre-contrast scans, (A) without and (B) with MT suppression, and post-contrast scans, (C) without and (D) with MT suppression, are presented. MT suppression shortens the T1 of the freely mobile hydrogen pool and generally lowers the signal-to-noise ratio of the image, due to partial saturation of the mobile pool. MT suppression can, in certain instances, improve depiction of contrast enhancement, an effect synergistic with high dose contrast injection. In the example provided, however, to the naked eye lesion enhancement appears slightly greater on the post-contrast scan without MT suppression.

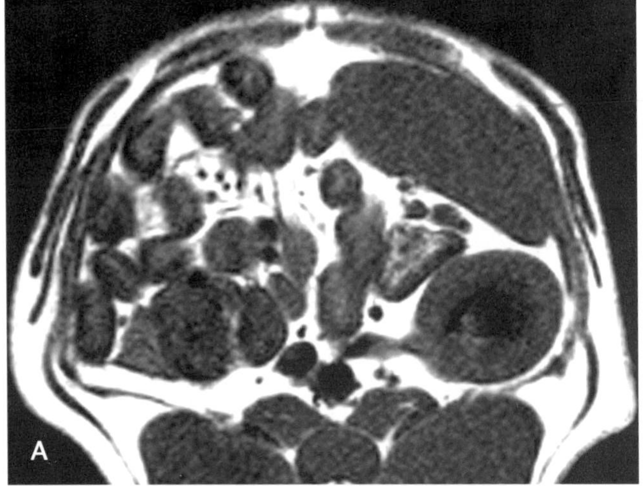

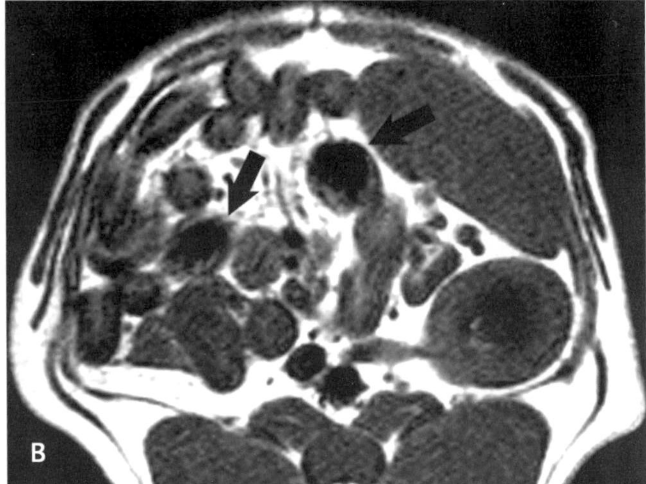

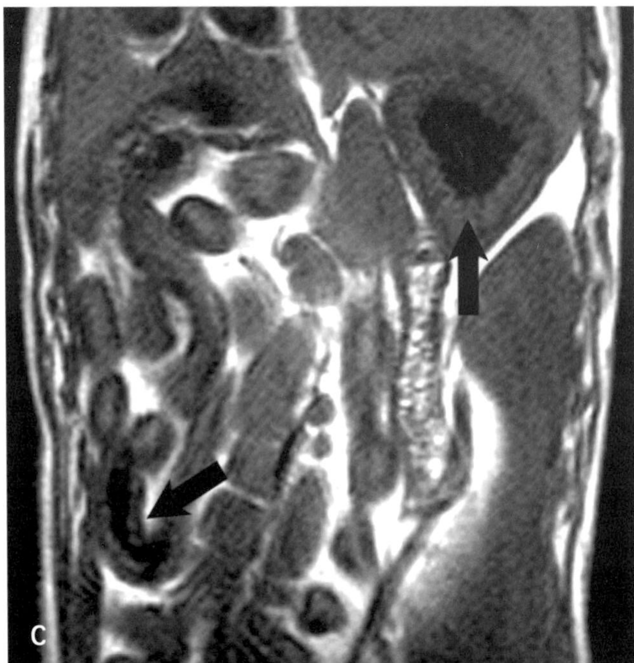

Figure 6. Negative enhancement of the stomach and small bowel, following oral contrast administration, by an agent (perfluorooctylbromide or PFOB) which affects proton density. (A) Pre-contrast axial and post-contrast (B) axial and (C) coronal T1-weighted scans are presented. Hydrogen atoms are replaced by halogen atoms in PFOB. The result is a material that appears black on all pulse sequences due to the lack of mobile protons. Prior to contrast administration (A), multiple small bowel loops are seen with intermediate signal intensity within the abdomen. The bowel wall is not well seen, and small intraluminal lesions cannot be excluded. On the (B) axial post-contrast scan, two loops containing the agent are identified (arrows). On the (C) coronal post-contrast scan, contrast agent is seen within the stomach and passing through a loop of distal small bowel (arrows).

signal intensity is decreased in normal liver and spleen, focal areas of replacement, such as metastatic disease, are seen as areas of higher signal intensity.[17] Ferrite particles exhibit a monophasic effect on signal intensity as progressively larger doses can only further reduce signal intensity until the level of background noise is reached.

One of the few compounds that has been investigated for use as a potential spin density contrast agent is perfluorooctylbromide. Perfluorobromides act as negative contrast enhancement agents with possible clinical utility for gastrointestinal tract imaging following oral administration (figure 6). A negative contrast agent is likely preferable as a bowel contrast agent since signal intensity loss does not cause motion artifacts. Artifacts due to peristalsis of bowel contents can be seen with positive contrast agents, such as the gadolinium chelates, when administered orally. Perfluorobromides did not fare well clinically when introduced in 1994, due to substantial side effects. Suspensions of iron particles, which also serve as negative contrast agents, may find greater acceptance.

Echo-planar imaging (EPI), which is currently undergoing investigation at a number of MR centers world-wide, promises to provide a further revolutionary change in clinical MR imaging. This ultrafast MR technique can provide high quality images in less than a second, which are free of motion artifact and provide almost unlimited proton density, T1- and T2- weighted contrast.[18] One of the primary advantages of EPI, when used in conjunction with contrast injection, is that it can provide information regarding physiologic parameters previously inaccessible to MR imaging. Tissue

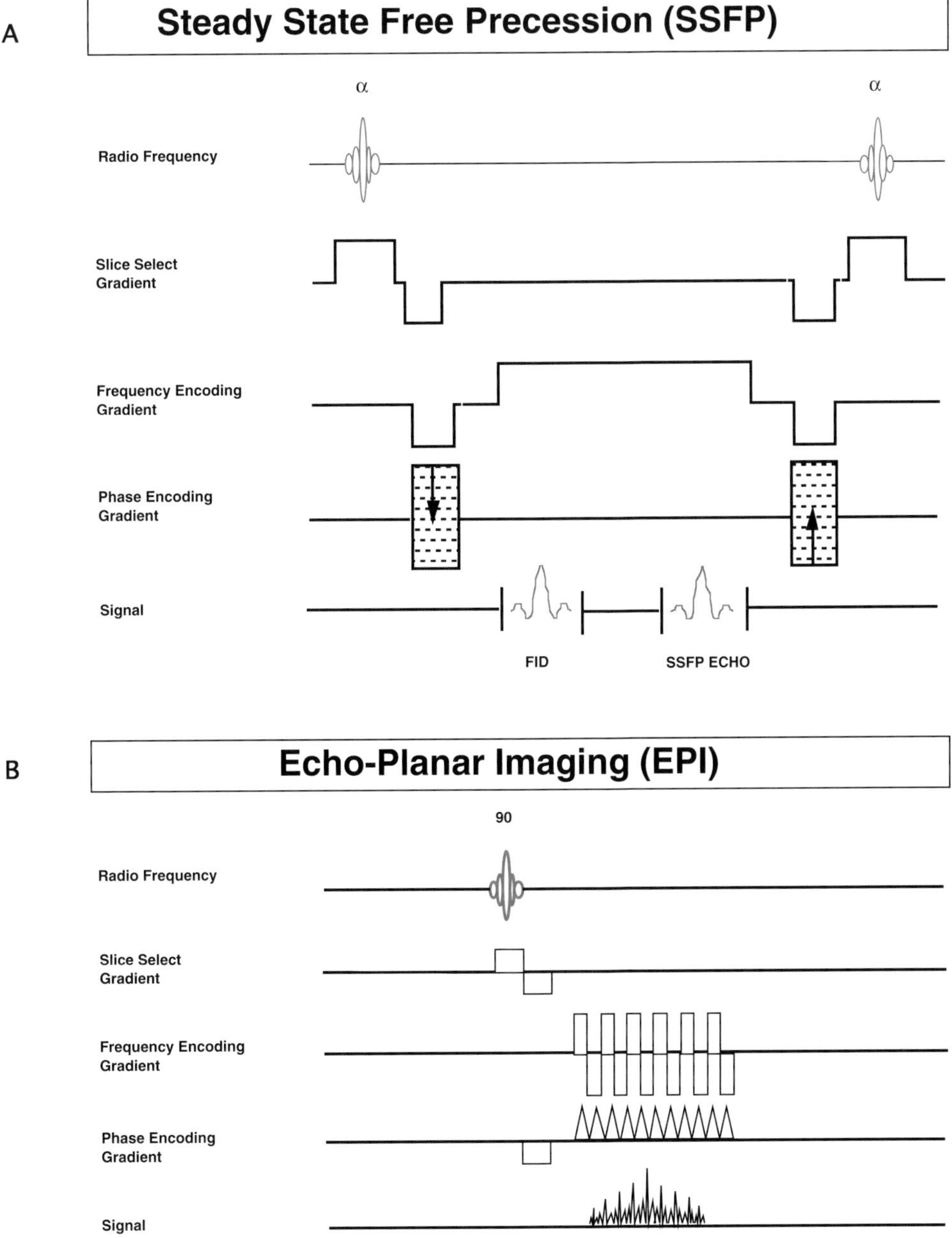

Figure 7. Pulse diagrams for (A) steady state free precession (SSFP) and (B) echo-planar techniques. Either pulse sequence can be employed to evaluate cerebral perfusion. In such an application, scans are repeated in a rapid dynamic fashion during intravenous bolus contrast administration, observing the first pass of the agent through the brain. SSFP is a gradient echo technique in which a very short TR is employed (A). In addition to the FID, a primary echo is generated with high sensitivity to T2 and susceptibility effects. Alternatively, if the frequency encoding (readout) gradient is very rapidly reversed, and each gradient echo individually phase encoded (B), then an entire image can be acquired from a single excitation. The latter approach forms the basis for echo-planar imaging. Higher sampling frequencies and more rapid gradient switching are required for echo-planar imaging, as compared to conventional imaging techniques.

perfusion and function can be assessed with high spatial resolution.[19] EPI has recently become commercially available, expanding further MR clinical utility in the hospital domain.

With the advent of ultrafast imaging techniques (figure 7), including both steady state free precession (SSFP) and EPI, the use of contrast agents in dynamic imaging has been investigated. With this approach, qualitative and quantitative physiologic information can be obtained. During controlled bolus injection of a susceptibility contrast agent, such as dysprosium or gadolinium HP-DO3A (figures 8 and 9),

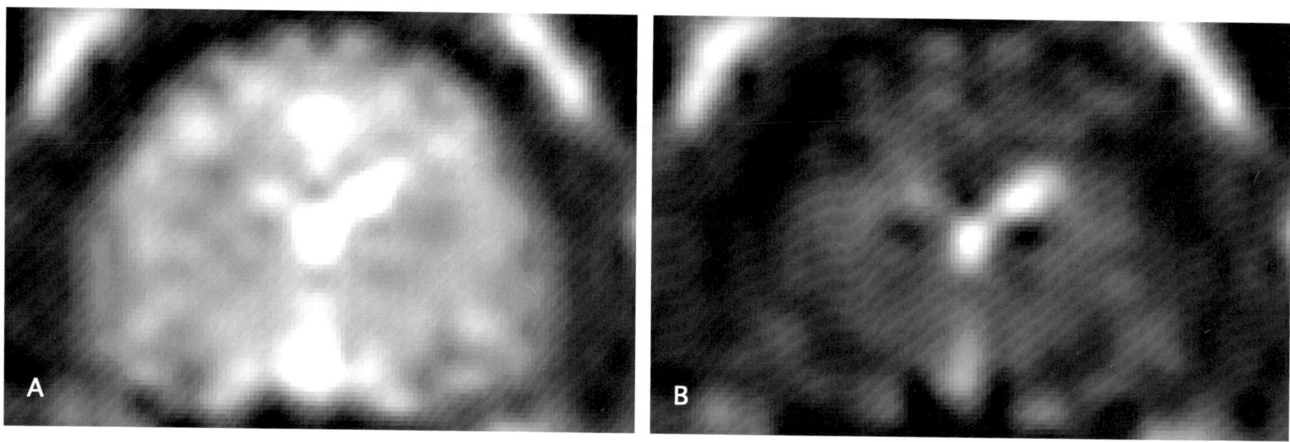

Figure 8. Assessment of cerebral perfusion by first pass, dynamic contrast enhanced imaging using a dysprosium chelate (Dy HP-DO3A, supplied by Bracco Diagnostics). Scans (A) prior to contrast injection and (B) at the peak of first pass are presented. Dysprosium has a negligible effect upon T1, and yet the highest susceptibility effect of the lanthanide metals (which include gadolinium). During the first pass of the agent through the brain, a decrease in tissue signal intensity is observed. This decrease is substantially greater in degree than observed with an equivalent gadolinium chelate injection (compare to figure 9). Use of a dysprosium chelate could thus lead to greater accuracy and higher sensitivity in the evaluation of cerebral perfusion. For example, the differentiation of gray and white matter at the peak of the bolus is greater using the dysprosium chelate. This reflects improved discrimination of tissues with higher (gray matter) as opposed to lower (white matter) blood volume.

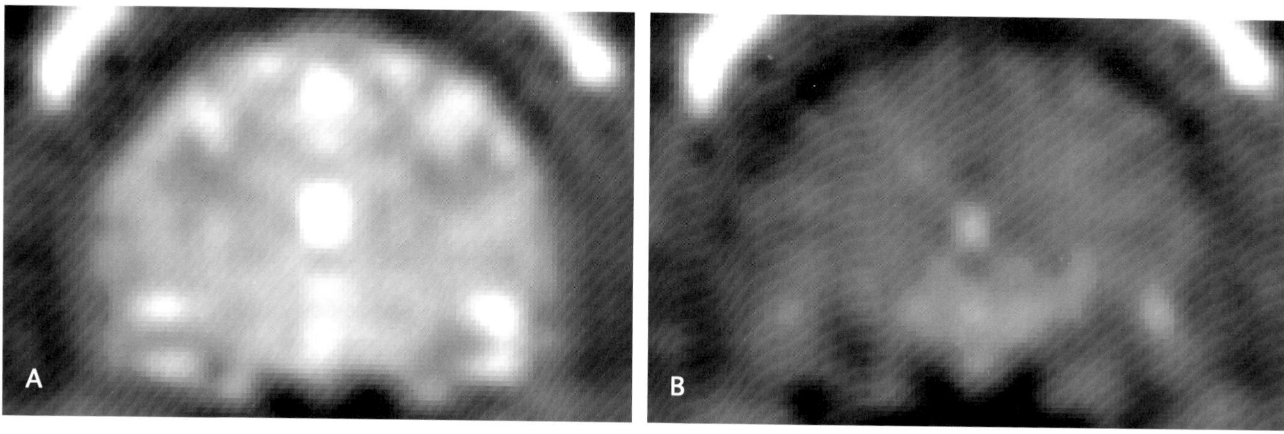

Figure 9. Assessment of cerebral perfusion by first pass, dynamic contrast enhanced imaging using a gadolinium chelate (Gd HP-DO3A or ProHance). Scans (A) prior to contrast injection and (B) at the peak of the first pass are presented. Following bolus IV contrast injection, a decrease in signal intensity is noted during the first pass of the contrast agent through the brain. Rather than observing the T1 effect of the agent, first pass studies rely upon observation of the combined T2 and susceptibility effects. The gadolinium ion enhances T2 relaxation, as well as T1, with the presence of contrast thus leading to a decrease in tissue signal intensity on T2-weighted scans.

ultrafast imaging techniques are applied with rapid sequential image acquisition. Decreases in brain signal intensity on these MR images are related to the presence of the susceptibility agent, which functions as a negative contrast agent. The change in intensity of the MR signal is directly related to the concentration of the contrast agent, thus yielding data on tissue perfusion. Dynamic ultrafast imaging with susceptibility agents promises to be an exciting new area of investigation, particularly in brain imaging for the evaluation of regional cerebral blood volume.

Conclusion

The mechanisms responsible for image contrast in MR are multiparametric, as are the methods used to measure them and produce a clinically useful MR image. MR contrast agent enhancement theory, design requirements, and principles of clinical application have been reviewed. Contrast media add a further dimension in the manipulation of inherent contrast in MR. Their application leads to improved sensitivity and specificity in clinical MR imaging.

References

1. Healy ME, Hesselink JR, Press GA, et al. Increased detection of intracranial metastases with Gd-DTPA. Radiology 1987;169:619-624.
2. Haughton VM, Rimm AA, Czervionke LF, et al. Sensitivity of Gd DTPA enhanced MR imaging of benign extraaxial tumors. Radiology 1988;166:829-833.
3. Nelson KL, Runge VM. Basic principles. In: Runge VM ed., Enhanced Magnetic Resonance Imaging. St. Louis, MO, C.V. Mosby, 1989.
4. Kirsch, JE. Basic principles of magnetic resonance contrast agents. Top Magn Reson Imaging 1991;3(2):1-18.
5. Wehrli FW. The basis of MR contrast. In: Atlas SW ed., Magnetic Resonance Imaging of the Brain and Spine. New York, NY, Raven Press, 1991.
6. Engelstad BL, Wolf GL. Contrast agents. In: Stark DD, Bradley WB, eds. Magnetic Resonance Imaging. St. Louis, MO, C.V. Mosby, 1988.
7. Lauffer RB. Principles of MR imaging contrast agents. In: Edelman RR, Hesselink JR, eds. Clinical Magnetic Resonance Imaging. Philadelphia, PA, WB Saunders, 1990.
8. Gore, JC. Contrast agents and relaxation effects. In: Atlas SW, ed. Magnetic Resonance Imaging of the Brain and Spine. New York, NY, Raven Press, 1991.
9. Saini S, Frankel RB, Stark DD, et al. Magnetism: a primer and review. AJR 1988;150:735-748.
10. Lauffer RB. Paramagnetic metal complexes as water proton relaxation agents for NMR imaging: theory and design. Chem Rev 1987;87:901-927.
11. Hendrick RE, Haacke EM. Basic physics of MR contrast agents and maximization of image contrast. J Magn Reson Imaging 1993;3:137-148.
12. Bloembergen N, Morgan L. Proton relaxation time in paramagnetic solutions: effect of electron spin relaxation. J Chem Phys 1961;34:842-850.
13. Davis PL, Parker DL, Nelson JA, et al. Interactions of paramagnetic contrast agents and the spin echo pulse sequence. Invest Radiol 1988;23:381-388.
14. Wolff SD, Balaban RS. Magnetization transfer contrast (MTC) and tissue water proton relaxation in vivo. Magn Res Med 1989;10:135-144.
15. Elster AD, Mathews VP, King JC, Hamilton CA. Improved detection of gadolinium enhancement using magnetization transfer imaging. Neuroimaging Clinics of North America 1994;4:185-92.
16. Boorstein JM, Wong KT, Grossman RI, et al. Metastatic lesions of the brain: imaging with magnetization transfer. Radiology 1994;191:799-803.
17. Stark DD, Weissleder R, Elizondo G, et al. Superparamagnetic iron oxide: clinical application as a contrast agent for MR imaging of the liver. Radiology 1988;168:247-302.
18. Schmitt F, Stehling MK, Lodebeck R, et al. Echo-planar imaging of the central nervous system at 1.0 T. J Magn Reson Imaging 1992;2:473-478.
19. LeBihan D, Breton E, Lallemand D, et al. MR imaging of intravoxel incoherent motions: application to diffusion and perfusion in neurologic disorders. Radiology 1986;161:401-407.

Chapter 2

Brain: Neoplastic Disease

Lawrence R. Muroff, M.D. and Val M. Runge, M.D.

Introduction

MR has evolved as the modality of choice in evaluating patients with actual or suspected brain tumors. It is noninvasive, has multiplanar capability, displays increased sensitivity to disease relative to other modalities, and employs no ionizing radiation. Cost, availability (in some locations and at some times), and decreased sensitivity to tumoral calcification and subtle bone erosion are limitations of MR relative to CT. However, these concerns are far outweighed by the ability of MR to provide rapid, accurate diagnoses of intracranial mass lesions.

MR contrast agents are used in about thirty percent of all central nervous system MR studies. However, contrast enhancement is utilized in virtually every MR procedure used to evaluate patients with actual or suspected neoplastic disease of the brain. MR contrast agents contain gadolinium, a paramagnetic metal ion that shortens the T1 of tissues in which it accumulates. While there is also a T2 shortening effect, it is of no clinical consequence in the concentrations routinely used for patient procedures. The gadolinium is chelated to ensure that the ion remains inert and is excreted rapidly and completely.[1]

At present, there are three FDA approved MR contrast agents. They are gadopentetate dimeglumine (Gd DTPA) known as Magnevist and distributed by Berlex, gadoteridol (Gd HP-DO3A) known as ProHance and distributed by Bracco Diagnostics, and gadodiamide (Gd DTPA-BMA) known as Omniscan and distributed by Sanofi-Winthrop.[2] All three agents are virtually identical in their ability to shorten T1 and thus enhance visualization of pathology.[3] These compounds are all extracellular contrast agents, which require blood-brain barrier breakdown for enhancement of intraaxial lesions. The agents are extremely safe, with mild reactions seen in less than three percent of patients injected. Safety, lesion detection, and cost are similar for the three different contrast media.

Chemically, MR contrast media differ in two basic ways. First, a contrast agent may be linear or macrocyclic. Second, the agent may be ionic or non-ionic. Macrocyclic chelates tend to hold the gadolinium ion more tightly than linear chelates.[4] More tightly bound gadolinium is associated with less free metal ion following injection. ProHance is macrocyclic, while Magnevist and Omniscan are both linear compounds. Of the two linear compounds, Magnevist binds gadolinium much more tightly than Omniscan. Theoretical considerations favor a more tightly bound gadolinium ion, with lower risk for heavy metal deposition in the body. However, no major adverse clinical effects have been ascribed at this time to the differences in gadolinium binding.

The clinical relevance of an ionic MR contrast agent versus one that is non-ionic is also unclear. Magnevist is an ionic compound, while ProHance and Omniscan are non-ionic. Non-ionic agents have a considerably lower osmolality and are less viscous than ionic agents. Thus, these non-ionic compounds are more readily administered via bolus injection through a small needle. Of potential clinical concern is the administration of large volumes of MR contrast. With large volume administration, non-ionic agents present a lower osmolar load to the extracellular spaces. Despite these differences, there does not appear to be a clinically relevant difference in the safety record of these agents. However, since the osmolality of these compounds is comparable to that of conventional radiographic contrast media, at high volume (high dose) administration, osmolality may be a clinical concern.

MR contrast agents are of major importance in the evaluation of patients with known or suspected central nervous system (CNS) neoplastic disease. Contrast enhanced MR can visualize lesions that would be seen only with difficulty (or not at all) without contrast use. Enhancement can better delineate the extent of neoplastic involvement. MR contrast permits visualization of lesions with greater clarity. Contrast enhanced MR imaging is also invaluable in establishing the presence of additional lesions in both primary and metastatic disease, as well as defining the existence and extent of meningeal pathology.

Normal Enhancement Patterns

For optimal image interpretation, it is important to be familiar with normal intracerebral anatomy and appreciate some technical aspects of imaging with MR contrast agents. The intracerebral circulation is unique. Glial cells line the small intracranial vessels, preventing the leakage of solutes that occurs through small vessels in other parts of the body. This phenomenon is referred to as the "blood-brain barrier." Because of this barrier there is little or no enhancement of normal brain tissue following intravenous administration of gadolinium MR contrast agents.[5] However, a few commonly visualized intracerebral structures do not have a blood-brain barrier. Thus, there is strong enhancement in the pituitary, the infundibulum, and the pineal following gadolinium chelate administration. Also, the mucosal surfaces of the nasopharynx and sinuses, slowly flowing blood, and the retinal choroid all show prominent contrast enhancement after the administration of a MR contrast agent. On occasion, normal meningeal enhancement may be demonstrated as a thin, discontinuous line of faint enhancement.[6] Also visualized will be the enhancement of superficial venous structures, although this may be both variable and asymmetric. Normally, there is little or no enhancement of gray matter, white matter, cerebrospinal fluid, muscle, fat, and cortical bone.

The timing of the scan after the administration of a gadolinium chelate can effect visualization of both pathologic and normal structures. While some pathologic processes may benefit from delayed imaging,[7] contrast enhancement of normal structures tends to diminish substantially after fifteen minutes post-injection. There does not appear to be a significant difference in either lesion visualization or safety whether the contrast is given in bolus form or by slow injection. Bolus studies can, however, provide additional information concerning lesion perfusion.

Primary Intracranial Neoplasms

Although most intracranial tumors occur in patients older than forty-five years, CNS tumors are the most common solid neoplasms of childhood, the second leading cancer related cause of death in children younger than fifteen years, and the third leading cancer related cause of death in adolescents and adults between the ages of fifteen and thirty-four years.[8] CNS tumors represent 1.5 percent of all new cancers and 2.2 percent of cancer deaths. About half of adult intracranial tumors are glial in origin, and approximately seventy percent of brain tumors in adults are supratentorial. Infratentorial lesions are more common in children.

Intracranial tumors produce symptoms primarily by two mechanisms: mass effect or infiltration with destruction of normal tissue. The term mass effect includes the impact of the tumor and surrounding vasogenic edema. Since the adult cranial vault cannot expand to accommodate increased intracranial pressure, these changes are particularly important to detect.[9]

Symptoms associated with brain tumors include headache, nausea and vomiting, personality changes, and slowing of psychomotor function. Although fewer than ten percent of patients presenting with seizures have a brain tumor as the cause of the seizure, seizures are a presenting symptom in approximately twenty percent of patients with supratentorial brain tumors. With rapidly growing, infiltrative, malignant gliomas, they are likely to take the form of focal motor or sensory seizures, although generalized seizures can also be seen.

Most primary CNS neoplasms are unifocal; however, these lesions tend to infiltrate for a considerable distance into normal surrounding CNS tissue. Their borders may be poorly demarcated even by CT or MR. MR is the method of choice for imaging most CNS tumors, because of its high sensitivity, multiplanar capability, and non-invasive nature. CT can supplement MR in brain tumor evaluation in cases where MR is contraindicated, when it is important to document calcification or acute hemorrhage, and when there are modeling changes within the calvarium.[10]

Grading of tumors can be difficult both from diagnostic imaging and from surgical biopsy. Gliomas may have a heterogeneity of tumor grades, and surgical biopsy may not include the more aggressive parts of the tumor. Tumor development is such that there may also be a significant change in the degree of malignancy over time.[11] Furthermore, it is important to understand that the histologic extension of an astrocytoma is invariably greater than the tumor extent demonstrated by imaging.[12] However, MR shows greater extent of tumor involvement than can be demonstrated by CT. Contrast enhancement, particularly triple dose, will also show greater extent of tumor than non-contrast studies.[13,14,15]

Imaging can help assess the aggressiveness of brain tumors. However, no modality can definitively establish the grade of malignancy present. Generally, the degree of contrast enhancement relates to tumor aggressiveness, but there are exceptions to this rule, making it less reliable than desired. Usually, an infiltrative rather than focal appearance is a sign of a more aggressive malignancy. Necrosis within a mass also is associated with higher tumor grade.

Astrocytoma/Glioblastoma

Gliomas represent almost half of all intracranial tumors. Most of these lesions are supratentorial in location, although in children an infratentorial location predominates. The peak incidence of supratentorial astrocytomas occurs in the fourth to fifth decade. They are most common in the frontal lobes, with relative sparing of the occipital lobes. Astrocytomas have a better prognosis in younger patients. Cerebral astrocytomas vary in degrees of aggressiveness ranging from the juvenile pilocytic astrocytoma to the glioblastoma multiforme. Slower growing (less aggressive) lesions are often referred to as low grade, while the more rapidly growing neoplasms are referred to as high grade. Except for juvenile pilocytic astrocytomas, subependymomas, and a limited number of astrocytomas that can be completely resected, even "benign" astrocytomas are highly lethal.

The most commonly used classification of astrocytomas is that established by Kernohan.[16] This classification has four grades, with grade one representing the least aggressive astrocytoma and grade four representing the highly anaplastic glioblastoma multiforme. The World Health Organization and the Radiation Treatment Oncology Group utilize a three category classification.[17] These categories are low grade astrocytoma, anaplastic astrocytoma, and glioblastoma multiforme.

The MR appearance of a low grade astrocytoma is that of a relatively homogeneous mass (figure 1). However, in a significant number of patients heterogeneous signal can be seen within the lesion. The presence of vasogenic edema correlates in a rough sense with the degree of malignancy. Edema is far more common in glioblastomas than in lower grade astrocytomas. Although contrast enhancement usually correlates with the degree of malignancy (figure 2), this correlation is not reliable. Approximately twenty percent of astrocytomas exhibit calcification. However this is usually not evident on MR. With lower grade astrocytomas, subarachnoid extension is rare. On the other hand, glioblastomas commonly disseminate through the subarachnoid space.

Glioblastomas are the most malignant of the glial neoplasms. Unfortunately, they comprise more than half of all adult glial tumors. The mean survival time of patients with these aggressive tumors is about six months from the date of discovery. Most cases are diagnosed in the fifth to sixth decades of life. Frontal lobe involvement is most common, and extension along the corpus callosum in a "butterfly" pattern is not infrequent. The MR appearance of a glioblastoma includes a mass lesion with irregular enhancement, prominent edema, and heterogeneity of signal (figure 3). These tumors may exhibit cystic and solid components, and hemorrhage is common. Typically, tumor margins are not well defined, an appearance that has been correlated with an aggressive, infiltrative lesion. Invariably the image presentation of a glioblastoma underestimates the microscopic extent of tumor. Contrast enhancement is extremely important in patient management. It can be particularly helpful in planning surgical biopsy, as enhancement correlates with tumor viability.

Pilocytic astrocytomas are the most common posterior fossa tumor in childhood. These tumors occur in the cerebellar vermis, and present with headache, nausea, vomiting, lethargy, and ataxia.[18] Pilocytic astrocytomas are usually encapsulated and are therefore more amenable to surgical removal. They can be totally cured in many patients and enjoy the best prognosis of all astrocytomas.[19]

The MR appearance of pilocytic astrocytoma is that of a cystic, heterogeneously enhancing, posterior fossa tumor (figure 4). These lesions are typically hypo- to isointense on T1-weighted images and hyperintense on T2-weighted images. There is usually little or no edema and hemorrhage is rare. Herniation of the cerebellar tonsils may be seen. With midline lesions, the fourth ventricle is invariably displaced anteriorly and may be obliterated.[20]

Oligodendroglioma

Oligodendrogliomas (figure 5) are relatively uncommon, accounting for about five percent of all primary gliomas.[21] These tumors peak in incidence in the fourth to fifth decades of life. They are most commonly located in the frontal lobes, however on occasion they can occur in the lateral or third ventricles. The typical MR appearance of an oligodendroglioma is that of a solid, well-demarcated lesion. Although these tumors can appear clinically similar to astrocytomas, they are distinguished from astrocytomas by a long antecedent history (averaging seven to eight years) and a relatively common association with seizures.[22]

Although ninety percent of oligodendrogliomas show histologic calcification and approximately seventy percent show sufficient calcification to be detected on computed tomography, this calcification may be difficult to see on MR imaging. Gradient echo imaging can be far more sensitive to the presence of calcifications than conventional spin echo imaging.[23] Computed tomography is also more sensitive than MR in demonstrating subtle calvarial modeling secondary to the slowly growing tumor. Enhancement is seen in about half of oligodendrogliomas. The enhanced appearance of these lesions is non-specific and does not aid in differential diagnosis. Hemorrhage is not uncommon, but vasogenic edema is rarely noted.

Ganglion Cell Tumors

Gangliogliomas (figure 6) are rare primary brain tumors that contain both neuronal and glial elements. Gangliocytomas are composed simply of neuronal elements, and can be differentiated only on histologic exam. These tumors are most common in children and young adults. The majority are supratentorial in location.[24] Ganglion cell tumors are slow

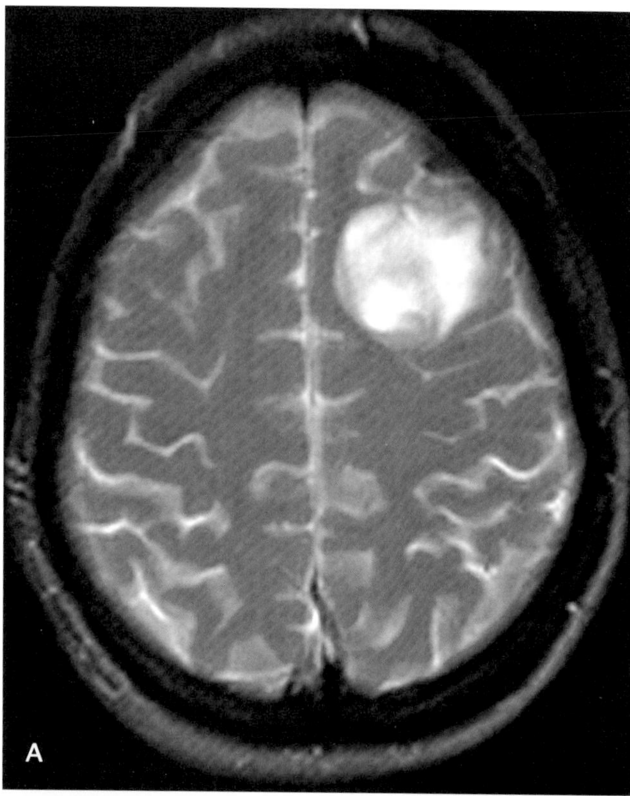

Figure 1. Low grade astrocytoma. On the pre-contrast (A) T2-weighted scan, a high signal intensity abnormality is demonstrated in the left frontal lobe. The lesion is low signal intensity on (B) the pre-contrast T1-weighted scan, and does not demonstrate abnormal enhancement on (C) the post-contrast scan. On MR, low grade astrocytomas appear well defined, without substantial mass effect. Unlike higher grade astrocytomas, these lesions do not enhance post-contrast. *(From Runge VM, Brack MA, Garneau RA, Kirsch JE. Magnetic resonance imaging of the brain. Philadelphia, JB Lippincott, 1994).*

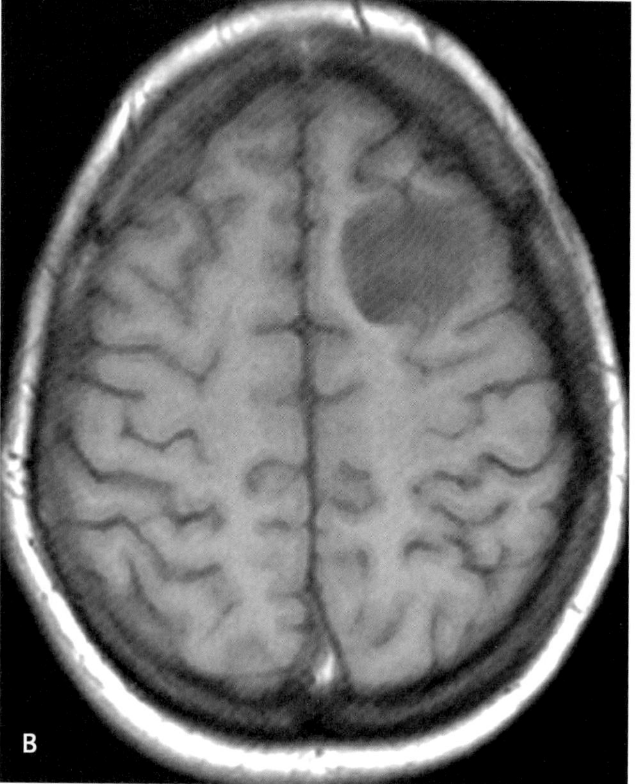

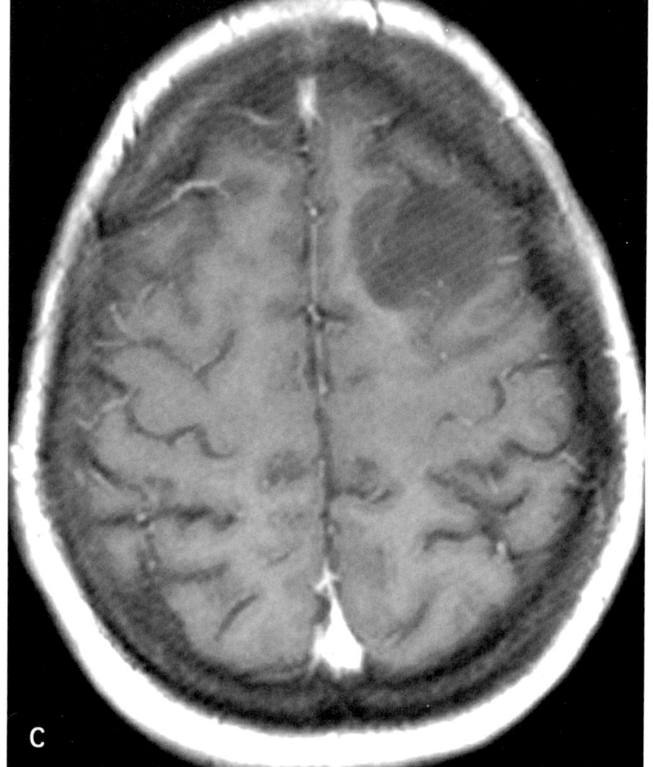

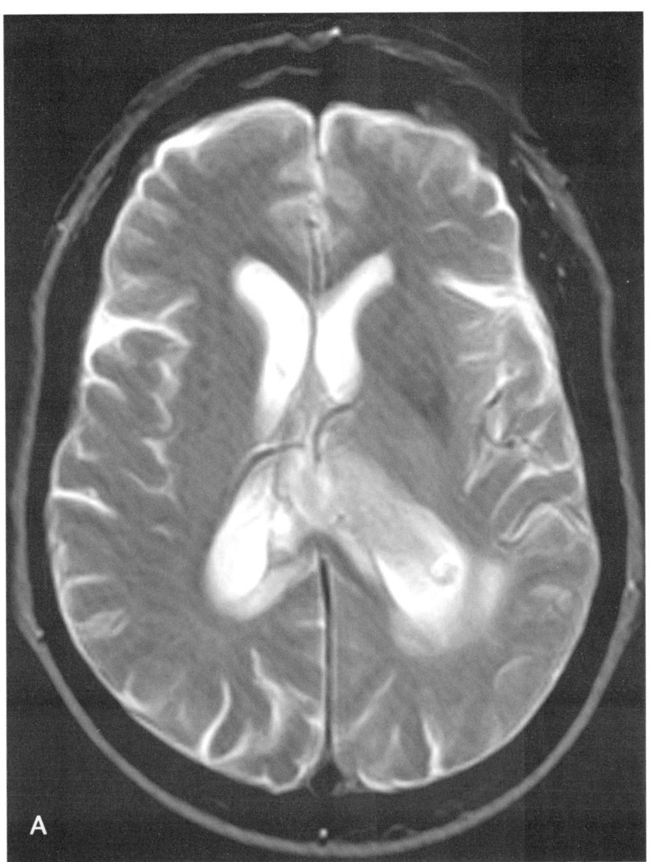

Figure 2. Anaplastic astrocytoma. On the pre-contrast (A) T2-weighted scan, a midline lesion with intermediate signal intensity is noted. There is subtle low signal intensity on (B) the pre-contrast T1-weighted scan. Neither scan well depicts the lesion itself or its margins. There is enhancement of the mass on (C) the post-contrast scan, which also demonstrates involvement of the splenium of the corpus callosum. On MR, anaplastic astrocytomas, as compared with low grade astrocytomas, tend to be less well defined, heterogeneous, with moderate mass effect, and may demonstrate contrast enhancement.

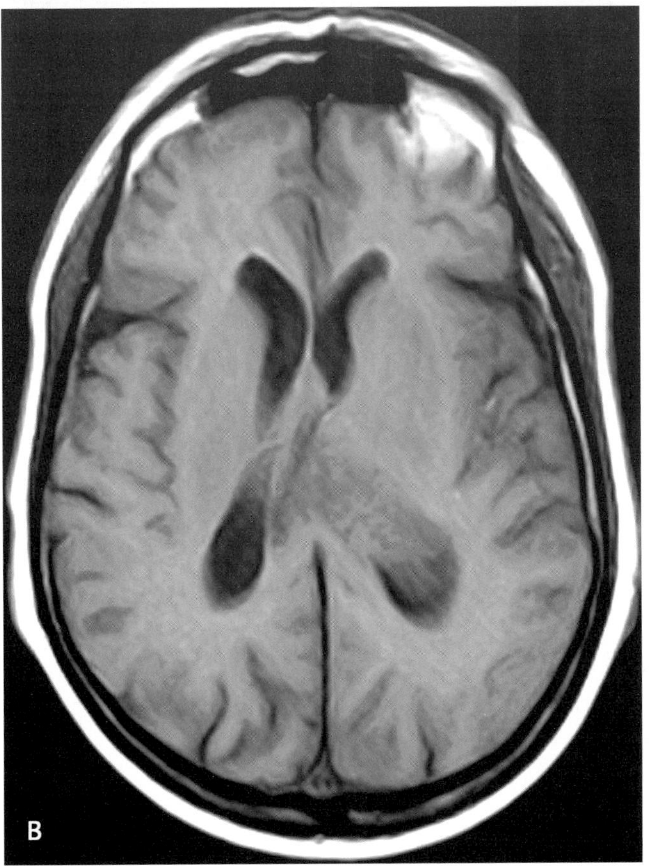

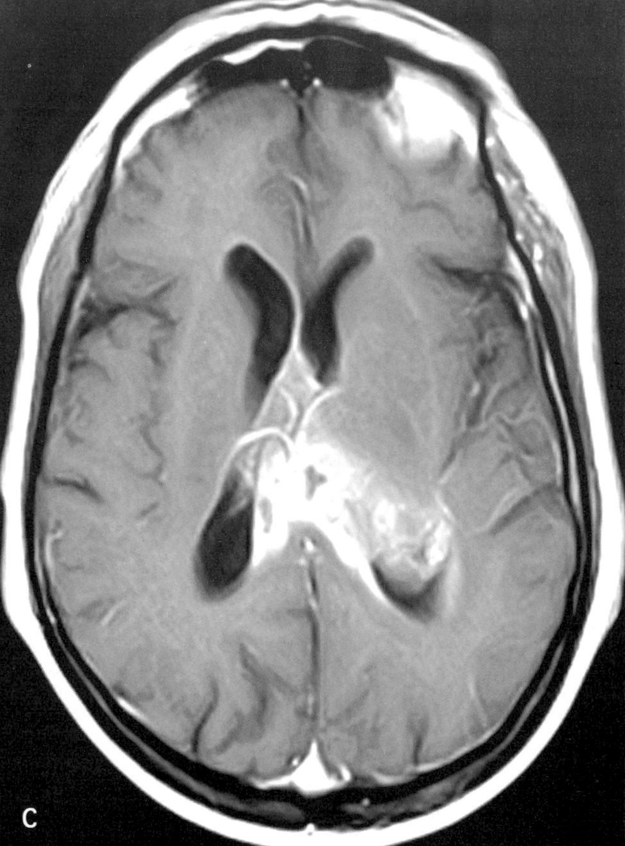

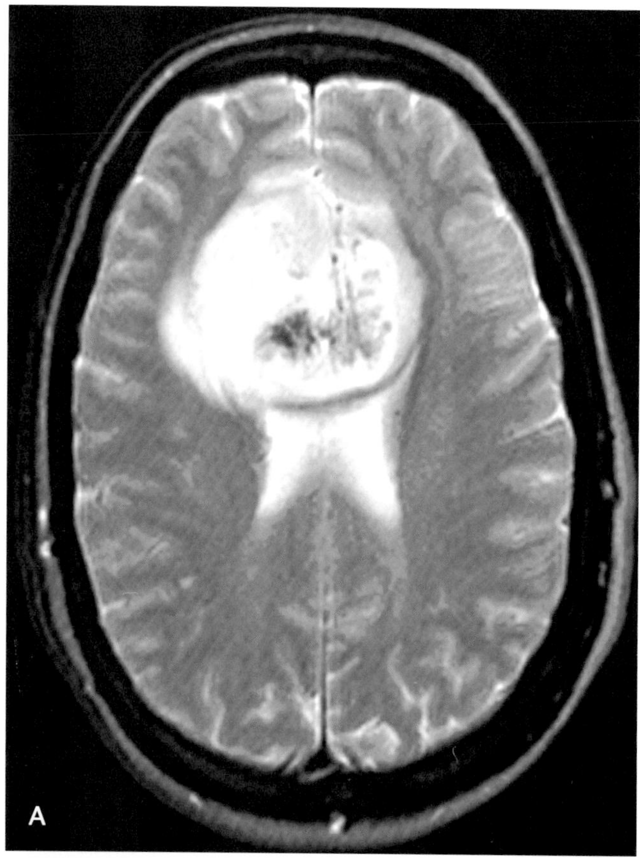

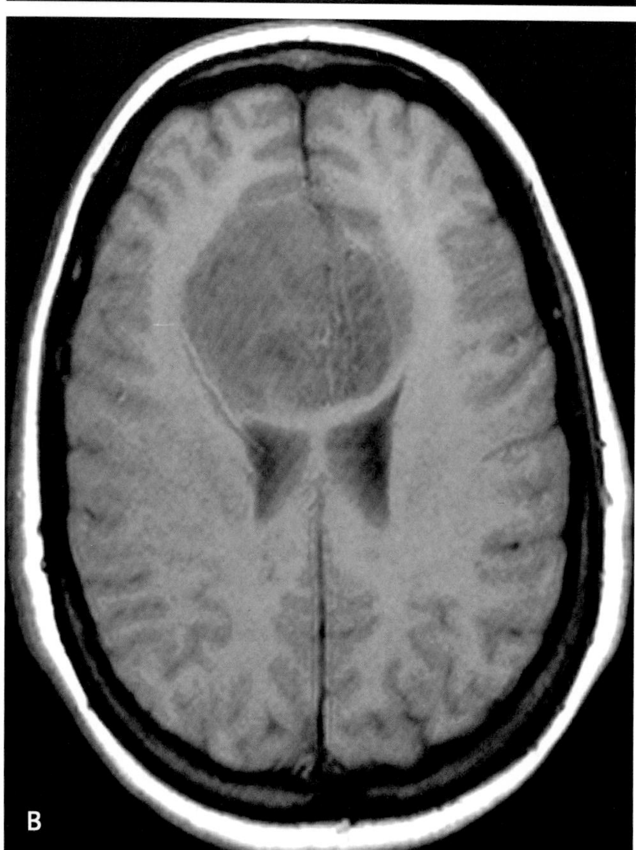

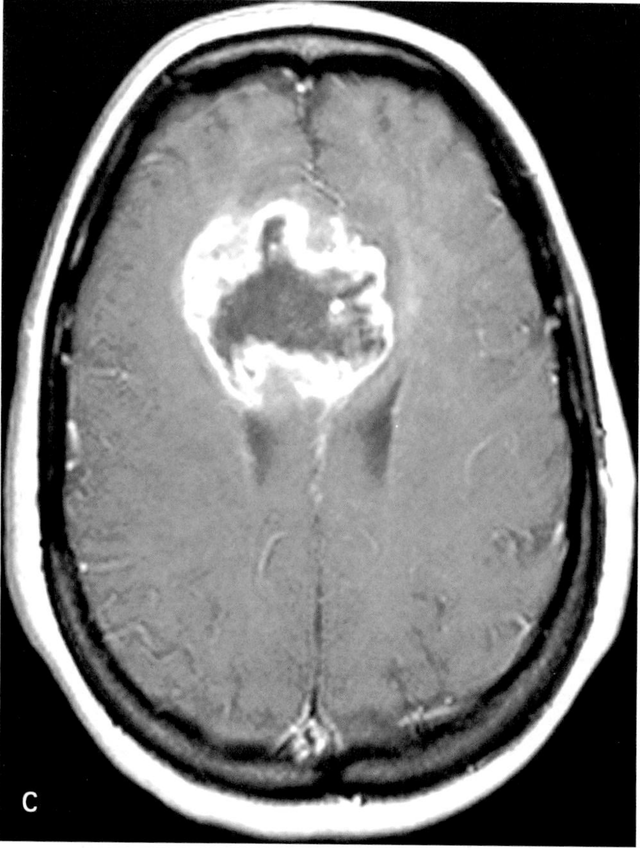

Figure 3. Glioblastoma multiforme. A large bifrontal lesion, with involvement of the genu of the corpus callosum, is noted on pre-contrast (A) T2 and (B) T1-weighted axial scans. (C) Following contrast administration, irregular ring enhancement is demonstrated. A nonenhancing central component is best seen post-contrast, corresponding to necrotic debris and fluid. Glioblastomas are highly malignant, widely infiltrative lesions, which grow along white matter tracts. A thick irregular enhancing ring with central necrosis is characteristic. Spread to the opposite hemisphere via the corpus callosum, producing a butterfly appearance, is not uncommon. *(From Runge VM, Brack MA, Garneau RA, Kirsch JE. Magnetic resonance imaging of the brain. Philadelphia, JB Lippincott, 1994).*

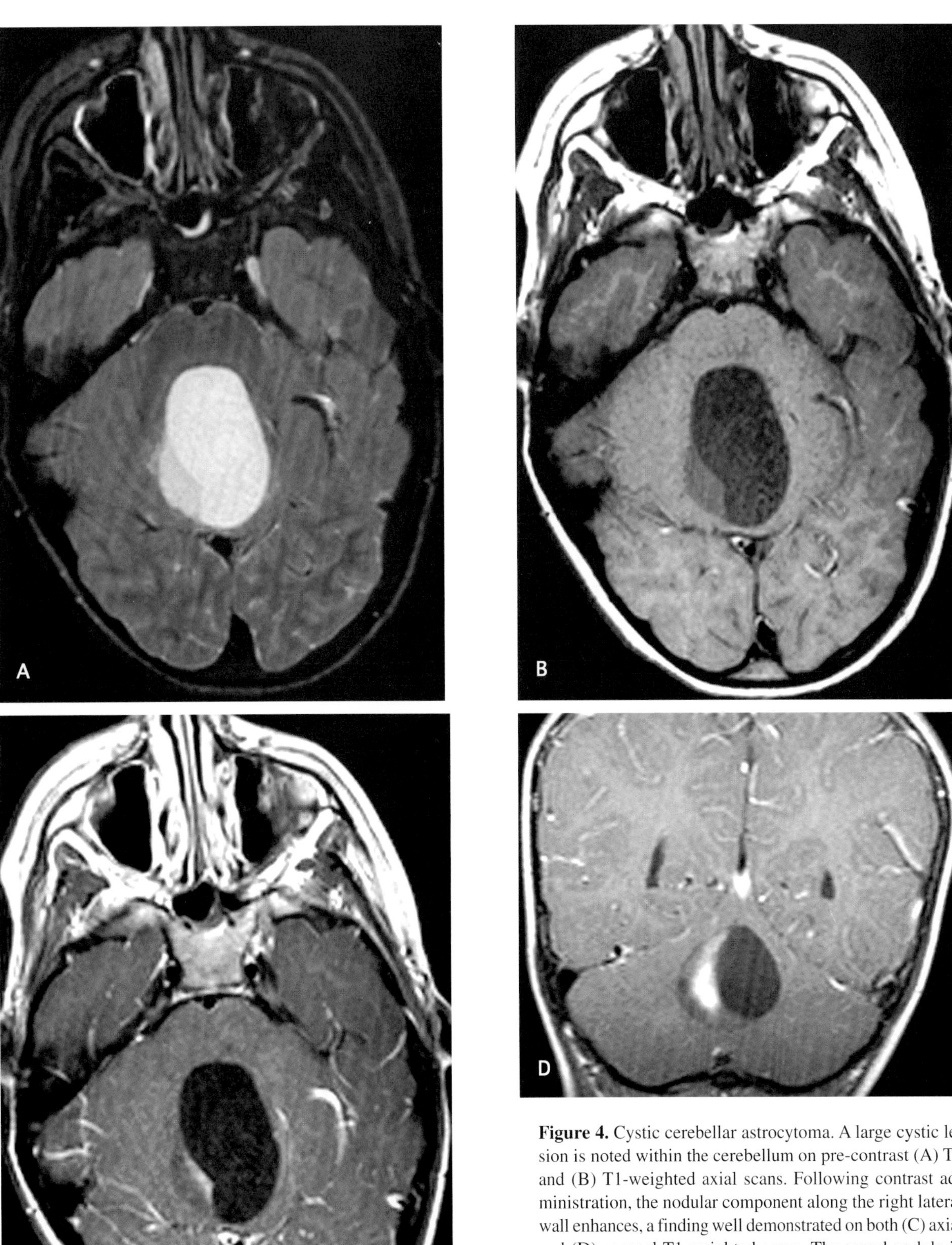

Figure 4. Cystic cerebellar astrocytoma. A large cystic lesion is noted within the cerebellum on pre-contrast (A) T2 and (B) T1-weighted axial scans. Following contrast administration, the nodular component along the right lateral wall enhances, a finding well demonstrated on both (C) axial and (D) coronal T1-weighted scans. The mural nodule in cystic astrocytomas, which is best demonstrated post-contrast, corresponds to neoplastic tissue. The cyst wall, which does not enhance, is non-neoplastic. *(From Runge VM, Brack MA, Garneau RA, Kirsch JE. Magnetic resonance imaging of the brain. Philadelphia, JB Lippincott, 1994).*

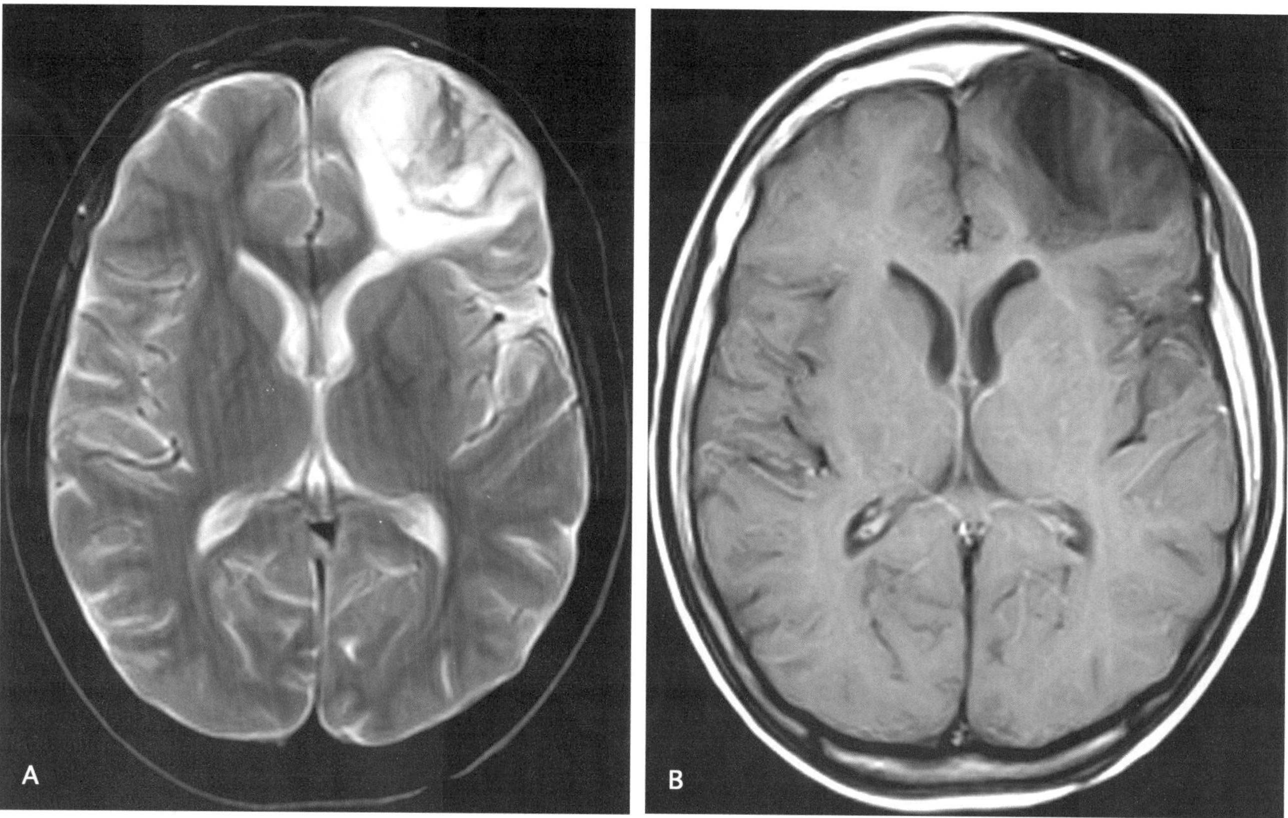

Figure 5. Oligodendroglioma. A large, hyperintense, frontal lobe lesion is noted on the pre-contrast (A) T2-weighted scan. The mass demonstrates moderate low signal intensity on the (B) T1-weighted scan. There was no abnormal contrast enhancement (scan not shown). Calvarial erosion, due to location and slow growth, is well evident on both scans. Enhancement is seen in about half of all oligodendrogliomas, typically being mild in degree and inhomogeneous.

growing and low grade, with a good prognosis. 60% are solid, and 40% predominantly cystic.

Brainstem Gliomas

Brainstem gliomas comprise about one-third of all childhood intracranial tumors.[25] In the adult most brainstem lesions are gliomas (figure 7), however their overall incidence in the adult population is low.[26] Brainstem gliomas can be lower grade neoplasms. However, anaplastic transformation with hemorrhage and necrosis can occur. Radiation is usually the treatment of choice, and therapy may be instituted without tissue diagnosis. Clinically, brainstem gliomas present either because of obstruction of the aqueduct or fourth ventricle, or as a result of cranial nerve palsies. Tectal gliomas (figure 8) present as bulbous masses, and can cause obstruction of the aqueduct at any point along its length. The bulbous nature serves to differentiate this tumor from benign aqueductal stenosis, which can present as a thin rim of periaqueductal hyperintensity on T2-weighted images.

The MR appearance of a brainstem glioma is that of a hypointense lesion on T1-weighted images, with increased signal intensity seen on proton density and T2-weighted sequences. Pontine swelling and fourth ventricular displacement are also seen. Contrast enhancement is variable, with lesions seen as either homogeneous or heterogeneous masses. Contrast enhanced MR can be valuable in the detection, delineation, and post-therapy evaluation of these tumors.

Ependymoma/Subependymoma

Ependymomas arise from ependymal cells that line the ventricles. On rare occasions, they can arise from ependymal cell rests within white matter and then present as intraaxial lesions. Intracranial ependymomas are generally a tumor of childhood. Usually they are located in the fourth ventricular region, although in adults they can be seen in the lateral and third ventricles. These tumors are well vascularized and enhance intensely with gadolinium chelates.[27] Ependymomas seed through the cerebrospinal fluid (CSF) space. Thus, they are difficult to contain and have a poor prognosis. Contrast enhanced MR imaging is essential to demonstrate CSF spread. Peak incidence is bimodal, with one peak seen at age three to five and a second peak noted in the late teens.

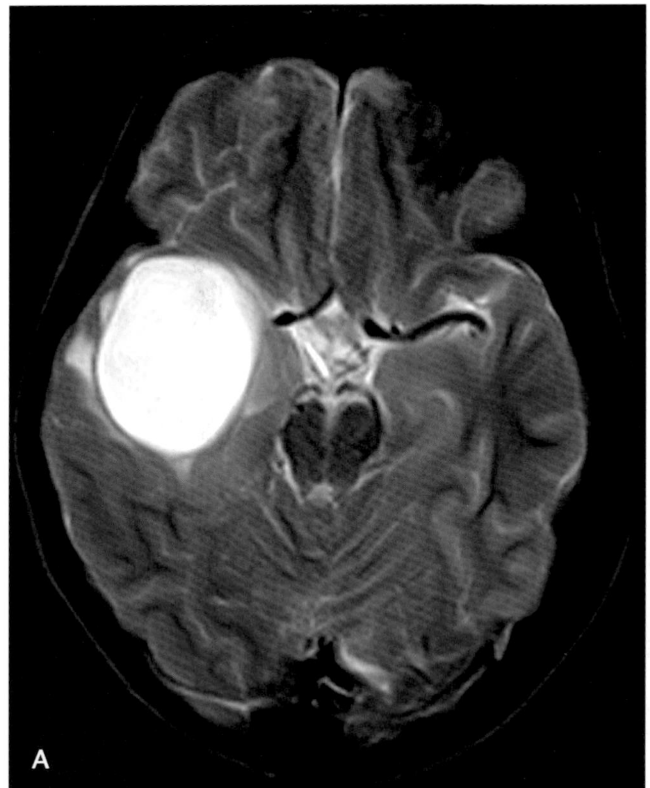

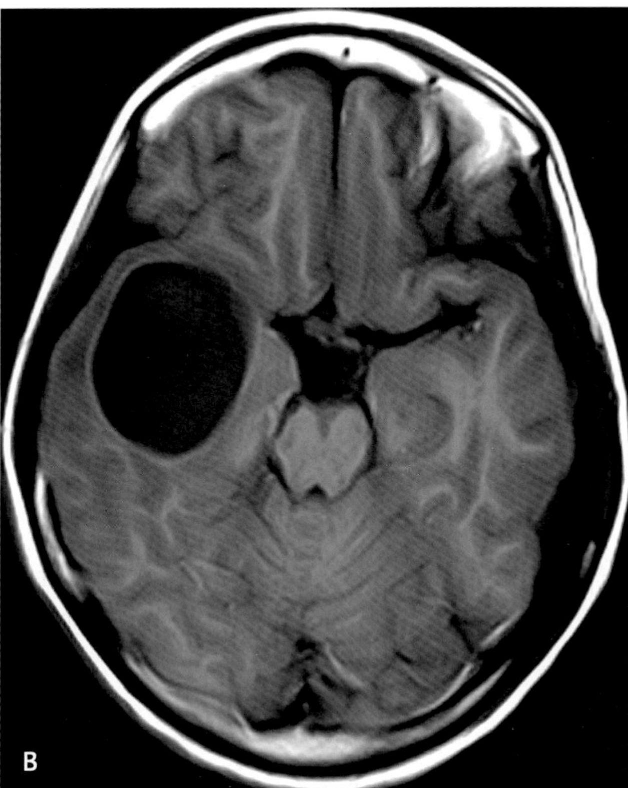

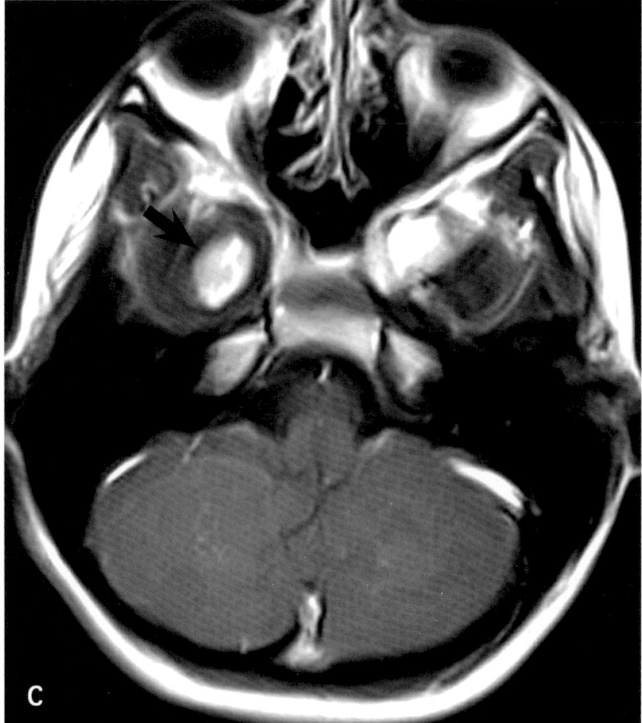

Figure 6. Ganglioglioma. A cystic abnormality is noted in the right temporal lobe on pre-contrast (A) T2 and (B) T1-weighted scans. (C) Post-contrast, on the lowest section through the temporal lobe, an enhancing tumor nodule (arrow) can be identified. Ganglion cell tumors represent a spectrum from gangliocytoma to ganglioglioma, with similar appearance and biologic behavior. Like cystic cerebellar astrocytomas, ganglion cell tumors are usually slow growing and low grade.

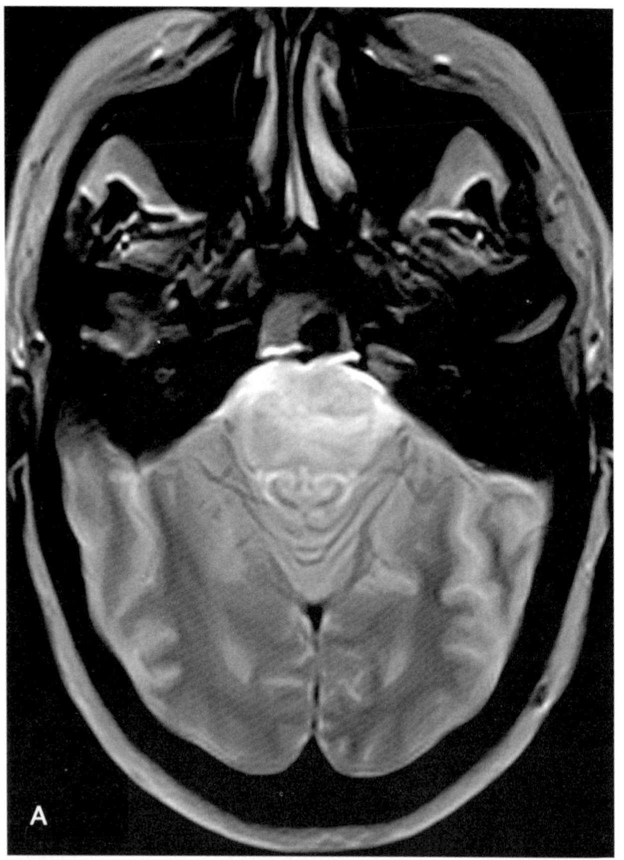

Figure 7. Pontine glioma. A subtle abnormality of the anterior pons is noted on pre-contrast (A) T2 and (B) T1-weighted scans. (C) Post-contrast, lesion enhancement permits ready identification. On histologic exam, brainstem (pontine) gliomas are pilocystic astrocytomas, but demonstrate a tendency to undergo anaplastic change. Exophytic extension and CSF seeding are common.

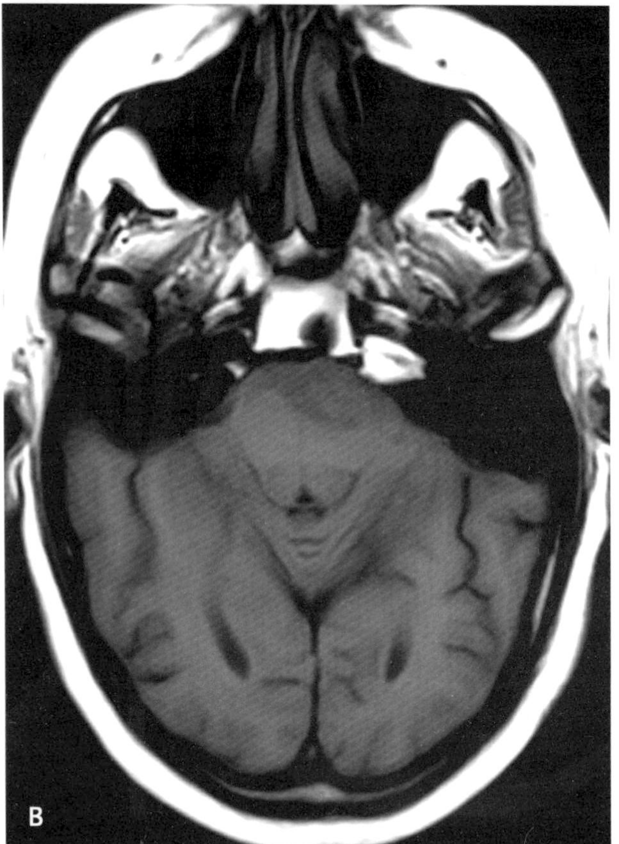

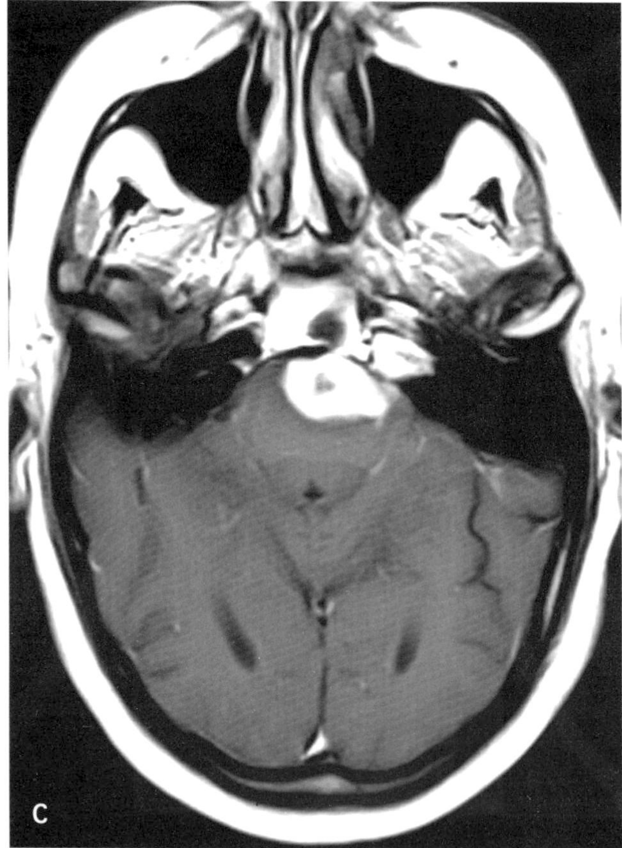

The MR appearance of ependymoma is variable. Lesions are hyperintense on T2-weighted images, and may appear well defined or irregular. These tumors may protrude into the ventricles, but more often grow toward the cortical surface. As discussed above, ependymomas show marked enhancement after gadolinium chelate administration.

Subependymomas are unusual tumors with prominent astrocytic components. They have a sharply demarcated, ovulated appearance, and are characterized by their slow growth and relatively noninvasive behavior. Subependymomas are most commonly seen in the fourth ventricular region; however, unlike ependymomas they less commonly cause hydrocephalus. Subependymomas do not generally invade adjacent brain tissue, and they tend not to recur if surgically removed.[28] Also, unlike ependymomas these tumors are typically seen in an older population (peak incidence in the sixth decade).

Medulloblastoma/PNET

The term "PNET" or primitive neuroectodermal tumor includes both medulloblastomas and ependymoblastomas. While these lesions are usually midline in the region of the cerebellar vermis in children, in adults a lateral hemispheric location is more common.[29,30]

Although medulloblastomas are rare in the adult,[31] they account for about twenty percent of all pediatric central nervous system tumors and about forty percent of all posterior fossa tumors in children. Typically, these tumors arise from poorly differentiated cells originating in the roof of the fourth ventricle. Medulloblastomas are rapidly growing tumors that can hemorrhage, although hemorrhage is more common in adult primitive neuroectodermal tumors. These tumors tend to seed through the CSF spaces of the brain and the spine. Patients with primitive neuroectodermal tumors usually have a poor prognosis. Similarly, supratentorial medulloblastomas (figure 9) tend to be aggressive and seed through the CSF spaces. Contrast enhanced MR can delineate the extent of these tumors and can be quite helpful in establishing CSF spread. Typically, these lesions are large and irregular in appearance, with contrast enhancement invariably noted. The midline posterior fossa location can suggest the diagnosis, however if supratentorial in location, the MR appearance is relatively non-specific. Although medulloblastomas may be difficult to differentiate from ependymomas, typically medulloblastomas distort the fourth ventricle while ependymomas enlarge the ventricle but maintain its shape.

Lymphoma

In the past, intracranial primary lymphoma was a relatively rare neoplasm. However, with the advent of the AIDS epidemic, this tumor is more commonly encountered. Lymphoma can also be seen in other immune suppressed patients, such as those who have received organ transplants.[32] In non-AIDS patients, lymphoma typically presents as a solid, well-circumscribed mass with homogeneous contrast enhancement.[33] Lymphoma in AIDS patients can be extremely variable in appearance. Enhancement may be ring-shaped and irregular (figure 10). The lesions may incite vasogenic edema and they may be multiple. Hemorrhage and cysts are unusual, although in AIDS patients lymphoma appears more aggressive and central necrosis is often noted. Lymphoma can spread by CSF seeding.[34] Involvement of the subarachnoid space is almost impossible to detect without contrast enhancement.

Areas of tumor location include the frontal and parietal lobes, the basal ganglia, the brainstem, and the hypothalamus. An infiltrating form of lymphoma may also be seen.[35] Lymphomas can involve the corpus callosum and spread across the midline, much like the pattern seen with glioblastoma multiforme. Lesions in immune compromised patients can mimic a variety of other entities, and lymphoma should always be considered in the differential diagnosis of intracranial lesion(s) seen in these patients.

In AIDS patients, the differentiation of CNS lymphoma from toxoplasmosis can be difficult. However, there are helpful imaging signs that can facilitate this differential. Lymphoma is commonly hyperdense on unenhanced CT scans, a characteristic not seen with toxoplasmosis. Similarly, subependymal spread noted on either CT or MR imaging is characteristic of lymphoma, but not of toxoplasmosis.[36] Both entities can present with either single or multiple lesions and both can have ring-shaped enhancement (particularly in patients with AIDS).

Choroid Plexus Papilloma

Choroid plexus papillomas are relatively rare tumors that can present either in childhood or later in life. Most cases are seen in the first decade of life. In children, these lesions are usually seen in the lateral ventricles, while in adults a fourth ventricular location is more common. These tumors do not invade through the ventricular wall, but may extend out of the fourth ventricle through the foramina of Luschka or Magendie.[37] Choroid plexus papillomas may be iso- to slightly hypo-intense to gray matter on T1-weighted images. On long TR images, the presence of calcification, hemorrhage, cyst formation, or tumor vascularity may result in a heterogeneous appearance.

Hydrocephalus is frequent and may be secondary to either overproduction of CSF or obstruction of CSF pathways. These lesions typically project from the choroid plexus, and if large, may expand the ventricle or cause CSF trapping. Choroid plexus papillomas may calcify heavily and may even ossify. Hemorrhage is not uncommon. These tu-

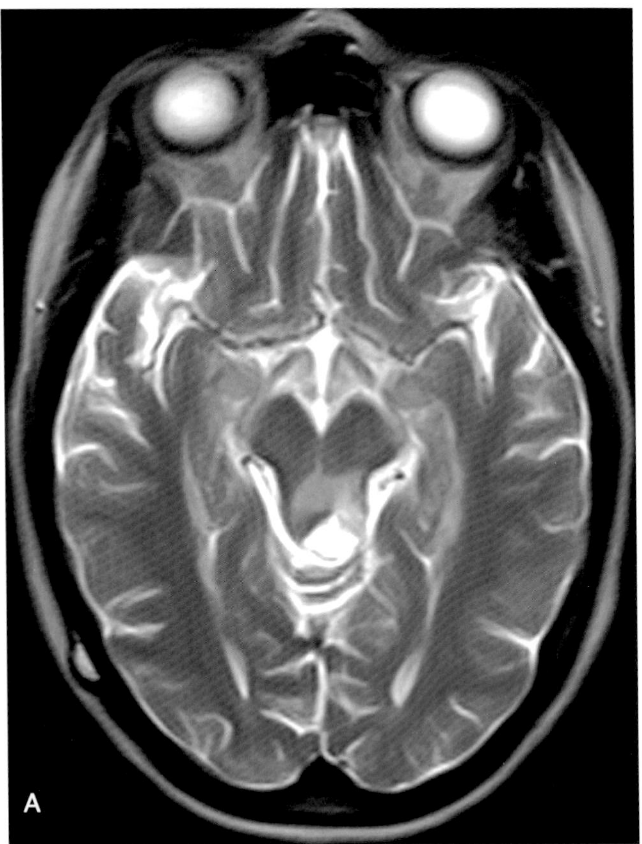

Figure 8. Tectal glioma. Abnormal tectal hyperintensity is noted on the pre-contrast (A) T2-weighted scan, with corresponding hypointensity on the (B) T1-weighted scan. (C) Post-contrast, there is prominent enhancement of this bulbous mass. (D) Sagittal and (E) coronal 1 mm reformatted images from a post-contrast 3D MP-RAGE exam better demonstrate the precise location of the lesion and the compression of adjacent structures, in particular the cerebral aqueduct.

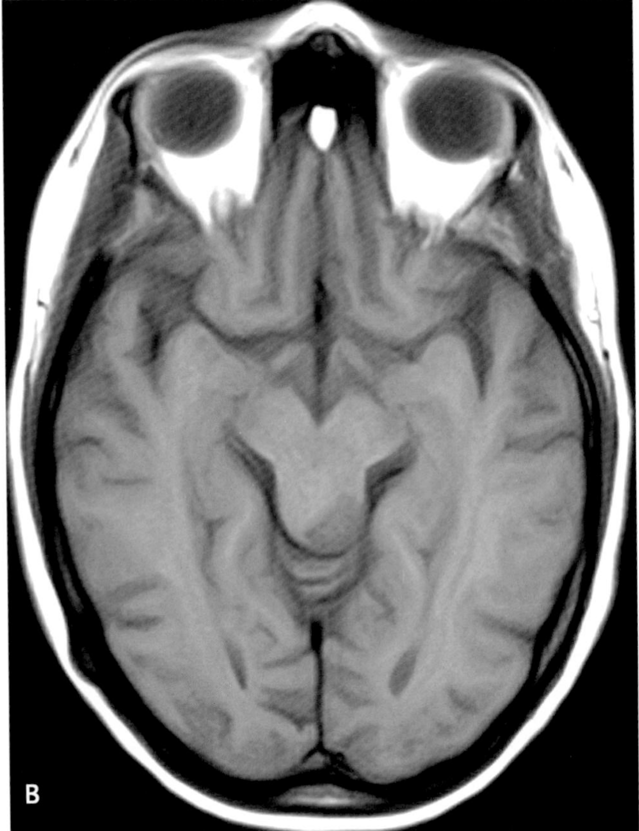

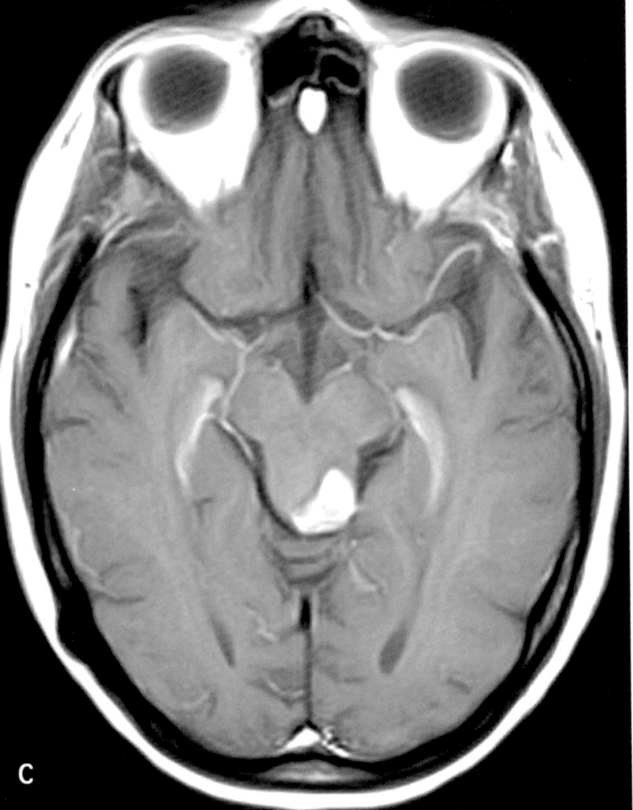

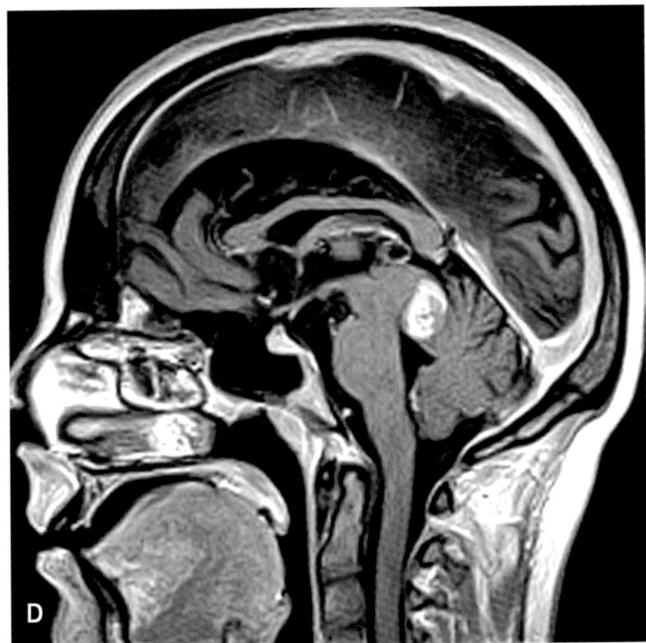

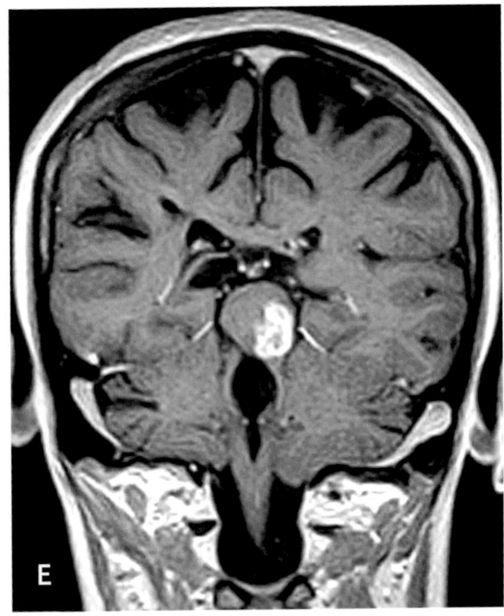

Figure 8. *Continued*

mors show marked contrast enhancement on either CT or MR. Because of signal changes seen from hemorrhage and calcification, this enhancement can be quite inhomogeneous.

Acoustic Neuroma

Acoustic schwannomas are the most common extraaxial neoplasm of the posterior fossa (figure 11). Although popularly called "acoustic neuromas," these lesions are invariably schwannomas. They present in the fifth and sixth decades of life. The MR appearance of acoustic schwannoma is variable. Small lesions can be isointense with normal brain tissue and quite difficult to identify without contrast administration (figure 12).[38] Acoustic schwannomas typically demonstrate intense enhancement. Contrast enhanced MR studies can also be quite helpful in diagnosing the presence of associated intracanalicular extension.

Since the detection of abnormalities on imaging studies relates to the contrast between the abnormality and surrounding normal structures, imaging of most intracranial pathology depends on differentiating the signal of the lesion from that of surrounding brain. Acoustic schwannomas represent an exception to this rule. These lesions are surrounded either by CSF or air. Thus, these lesions can be detected with half dose MR contrast administration (full dose is 0.1 mmol/kg). Thin slice, high resolution techniques are important for lesion detection, and the coronal plane can be helpful in delineating tumor extent. Differential diagnoses include cerebellopontine angle meningioma, metastases, and inflammatory processes.

Most often radiologists are faced with differentiating an acoustic schwannoma from a cerebellopontine angle meningioma. While this differentiation may, at times, be impossible, there are several factors that can help in differential diagnosis. First, acoustic schwannomas often cause flaring of the porus acusticus and extend into the internal auditory canal; meningiomas rarely do either, although they can cause associated hyperostosis of adjacent bone. Second, meningiomas are often associated with a "dural tail," while acoustic schwannomas are not. Finally, meningiomas usually make an obtuse angle with the petrous bone, while an acute angle is most often seen with acoustic schwannomas.

Contrast enhanced MR is less helpful in differentiating these two entities, although typically the enhancement of meningiomas is more homogeneous. This pattern of enhancement is relatively unreliable since most acoustic schwannomas show homogeneous enhancement as well. However, about a third will have an inhomogeneous pattern of enhancement. The major benefit of MR contrast use is to define the lesion and assess intracanalicular extension. As noted above, extension into the internal auditory canal is typical of an acoustic schwannoma.

Contrast enhanced MR imaging is essential to evaluate a patient appropriately after resection of an acoustic schwannoma.[39] However, it should be understood that a small percentage of post-operative patients can have a linear area of enhancement secondary to the presence of surgical reparative tissue. Thus, it is often prudent to utilize serial scanning in such patients. Post-operative change will remain stable or regress, while a schwannoma will grow slowly.

Schwannomas can develop in other intracranial nerves, although they most commonly occur in the eighth nerve. Lesions are seen, not infrequently, of the trigeminal, facial, and vagal nerves.

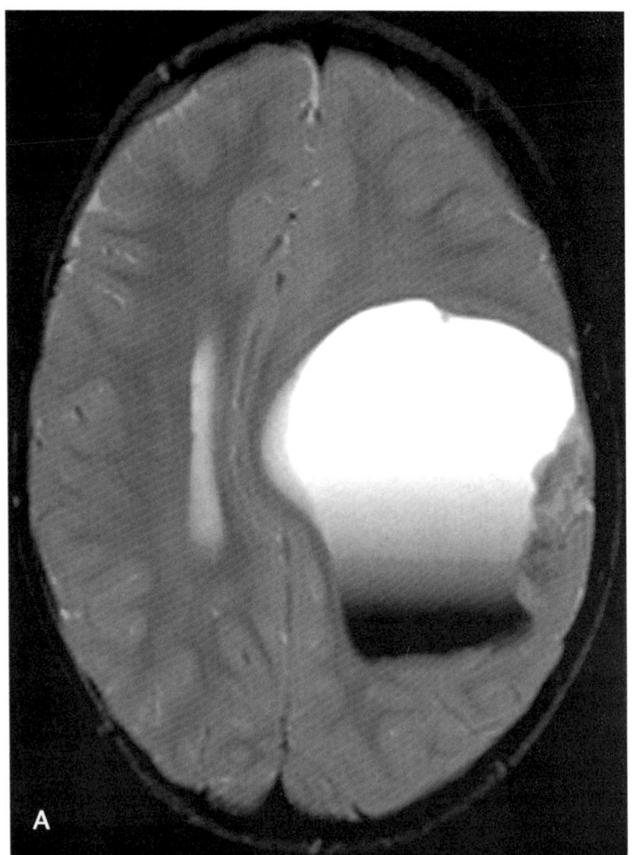

Figure 9. Primitive neuroectodermal tumor (PNET). A large cystic lesion is noted in the left frontal lobe on pre-contrast (A) T2 and (B) T1-weighted scans. Hemorrhage within the mass has caused the hyperintensity anteriorly on both T2 and T1-weighted scans, with layering and hypointensity posteriorly. (C) Following contrast administration, a large enhancing soft tissue component is noted along the lateral wall. The entire rim of the lesion also enhances. PNETs present as large, well-circumscribed lesions, with a predilection for the frontal and parietal lobes. Other common features include a large cystic component, with adjacent enhancing neoplastic tissue. *(From Runge VM, Brack MA, Garneau RA, Kirsch JE. Magnetic resonance imaging of the brain. Philadelphia, JB Lippincott, 1994).*

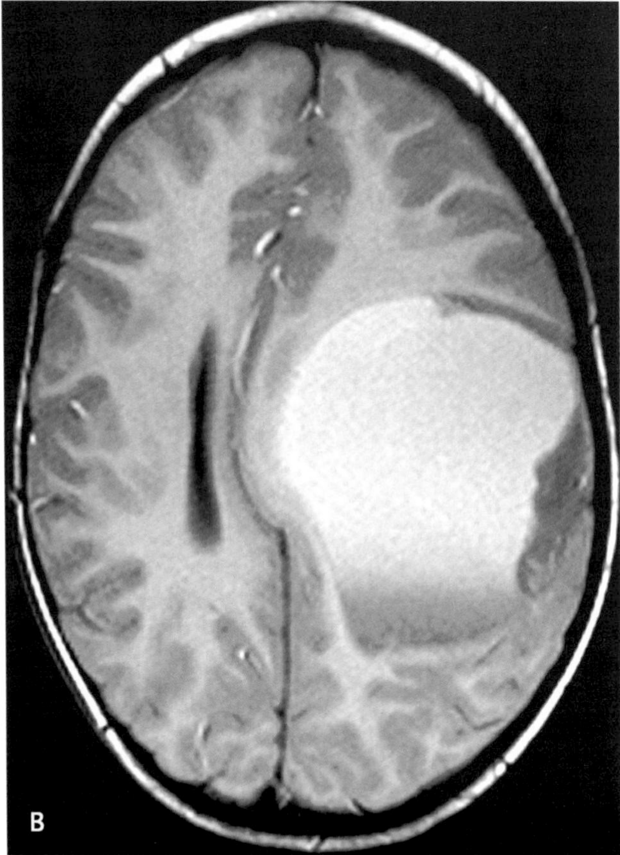

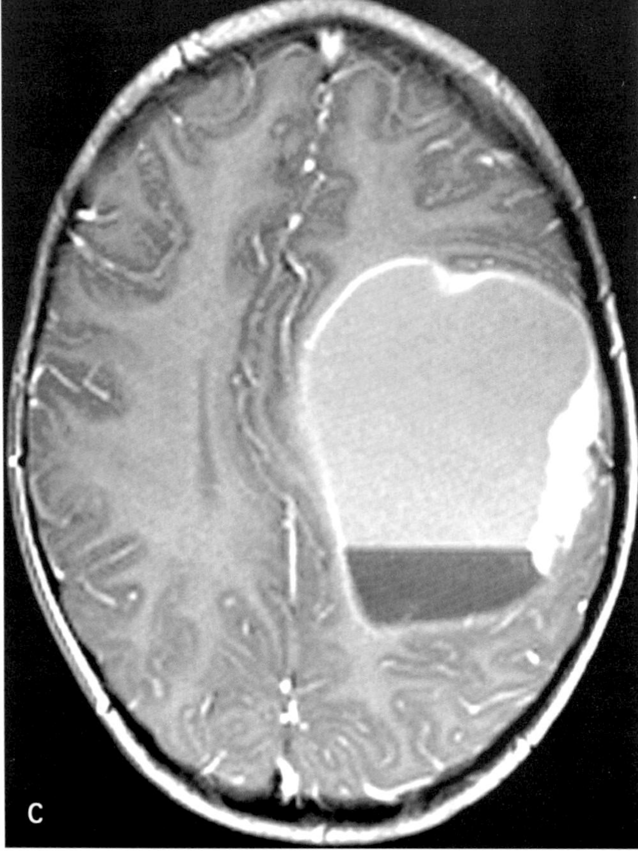

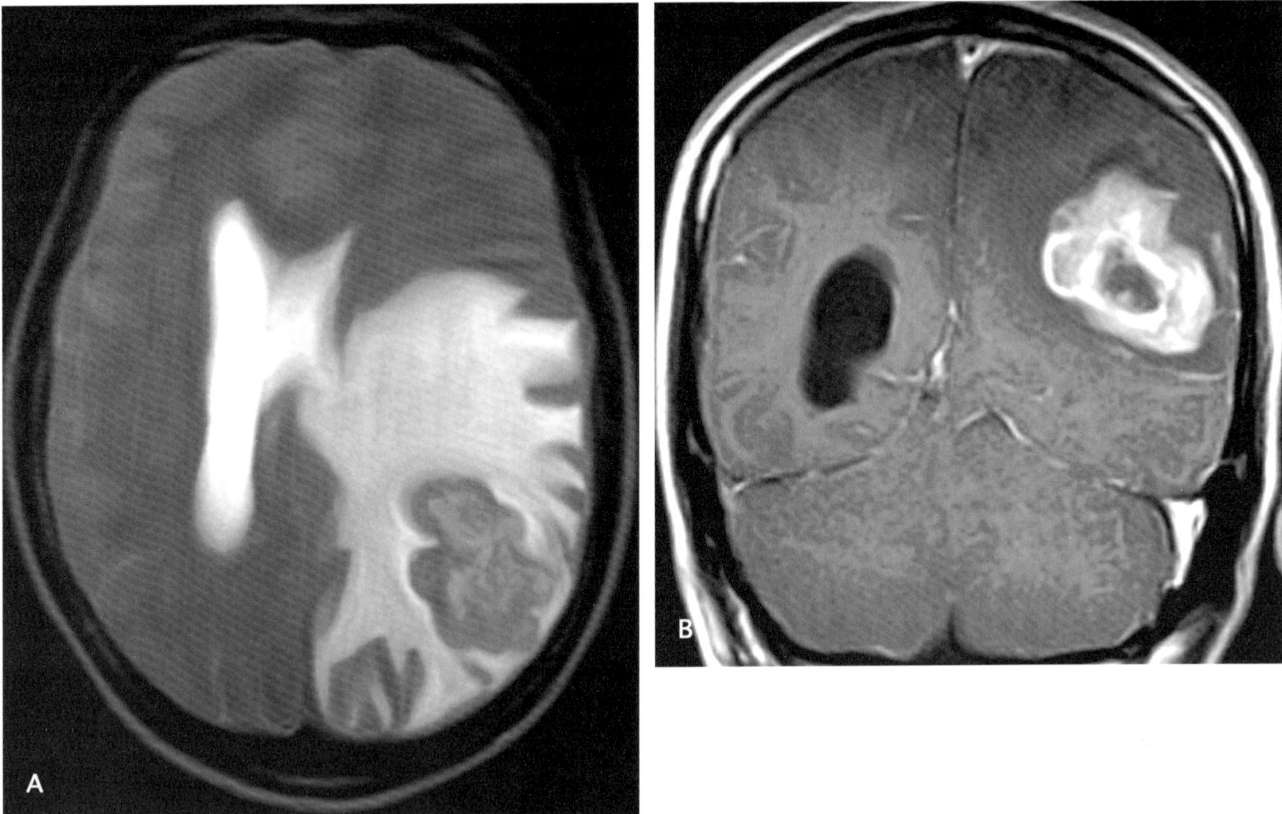

Figure 10. Lymphoma. A mass with intermediate signal intensity and extensive surrounding high signal intensity edema is noted on (A) the axial T2-weighted scan. (B) The post-contrast coronal T1-weighted scan demonstrates prominent peripheral enhancement, with central hypointensity. Prior to the advent of AIDS, the majority of cerebral lymphomas were primary in origin, with prominent homogeneous contrast enhancement. In AIDS, primary and secondary lymphomas occur with equal frequency, and enhancement is typically ring-like in nature with central lesion necrosis.

Hemangioblastoma

Hemangioblastomas comprise less than ten percent of posterior fossa tumors in adults. Yet, after metastases, these are the most common intraaxial neoplasms of the adult posterior fossa. Hemangioblastomas are usually located in the cerebellar midline. Most often they are peripheral in location, extending to the pia from which they derive their blood supply. The typical cerebellar hemangioblastoma is a well-circumscribed lesion with an enhancing nodule (figure 13). They act as benign lesions and are usually curable by surgery. Most lesions are cystic in appearance with an enhancing mural nodule, although solid tumors can exist, particularly in a supratentorial location. When not associated with von Hippel-Lindau disease, they are usually solitary lesions. Approximately half of patients with von Hippel-Lindau disease have hemangioblastomas. Conversely, about a quarter of patients with hemangioblastomas have von Hippel-Lindau disease.[40] Therefore, when an enhancing nodule is found in the cerebellum, it is imperative that the spinal cord also be evaluated with enhanced MR to search for additional hemangioblastomas. Associated findings in von Hippel-Lindau disease include retinal angiomas, renal cell carcinoma, and angiomatous lesions of various abdominal organs.[41]

Meningioma

Meningiomas are the most common primary intracranial tumor of nonglial origin. They comprise almost twenty percent of all intracranial tumors in adults. Most (approximately ninety percent) of meningiomas are supratentorial in location.[42] Less than ten percent of intracranial meningiomas are multiple, with multiplicity often associated with neurofibromatosis. Most commonly, meningiomas are seen in middle-aged females. These lesions are slow growing, expansile, and adherent to dural surfaces. Bony erosion and hyperostosis are common findings. Meningiomas are benign and curable when totally resected.

The MR appearance of a meningioma is different from that of other intracranial tumors. Meningiomas may remain isointense with adjacent normal brain on all pulse sequences.[43] For that reason, contrast enhanced studies are very

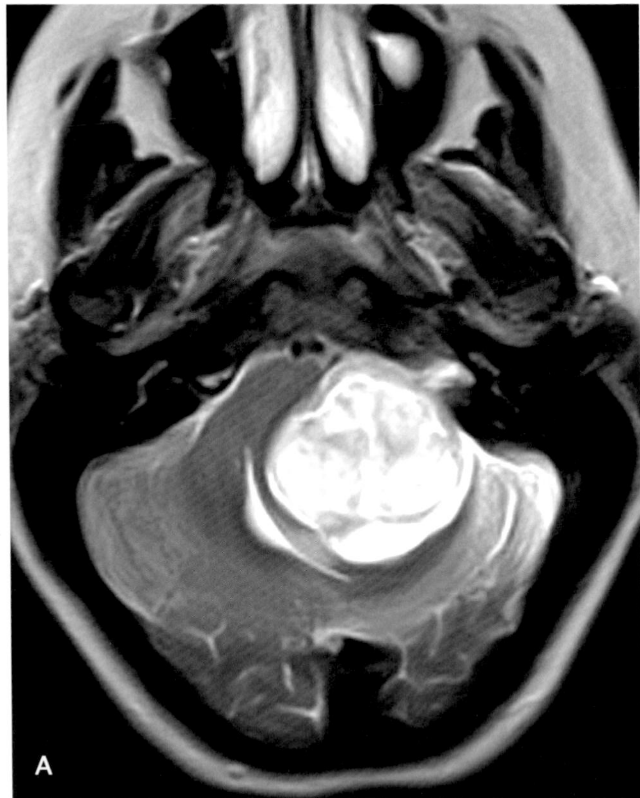

Figure 11. Acoustic neuroma. A large soft tissue mass is noted in the left cerebellopontine angle on pre-contrast (A) T2 and (B) T1-weighted scans. (C) Post-contrast, there is intense lesion enhancement, consistent with a vascular extraaxial mass. Enlargement of the internal auditory canal (IAC) by the mass, with extension into the canal, favors diagnosis of an acoustic neuroma. A meningioma, the other major consideration in differential diagnosis, is unlikely to cause enlargement of the IAC at its origin.

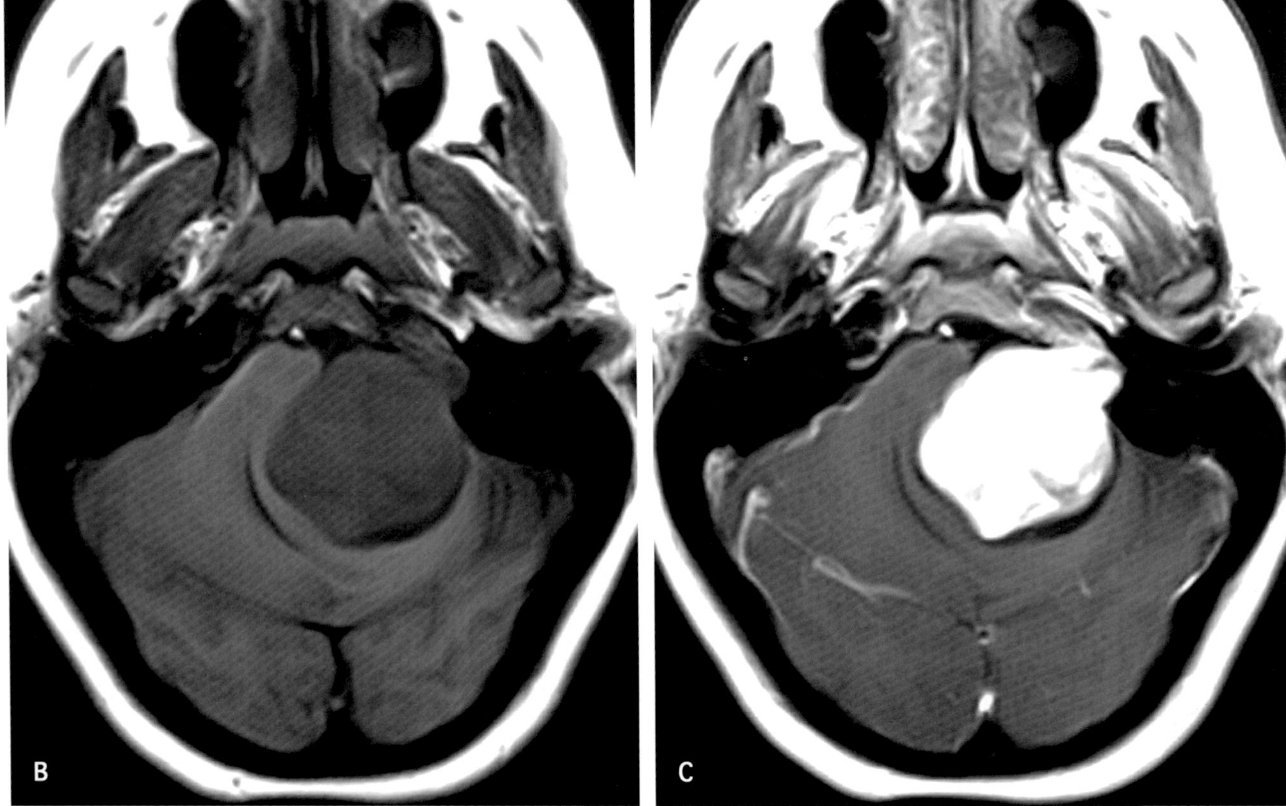

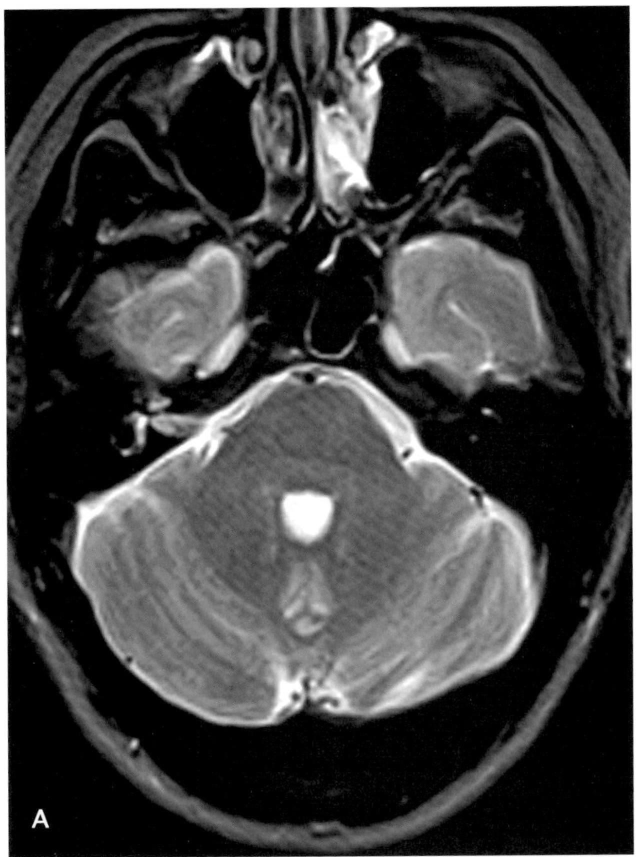

Figure 12. Intracanalicular acoustic neuroma. On pre-contrast (A) T2 and (B) T1-weighted scans, the question of a right-sided intracanalicular lesion is raised. (C) Post-contrast, there is intense lesion enhancement, permitting definitive diagnosis. The clinical presentation was that of right-sided sensorineural hearing loss. Other entities to be considered in differential diagnosis, on the basis of imaging alone, include facial (seventh) nerve tumor and inflammatory disease, although the latter should not result in a mass lesion.

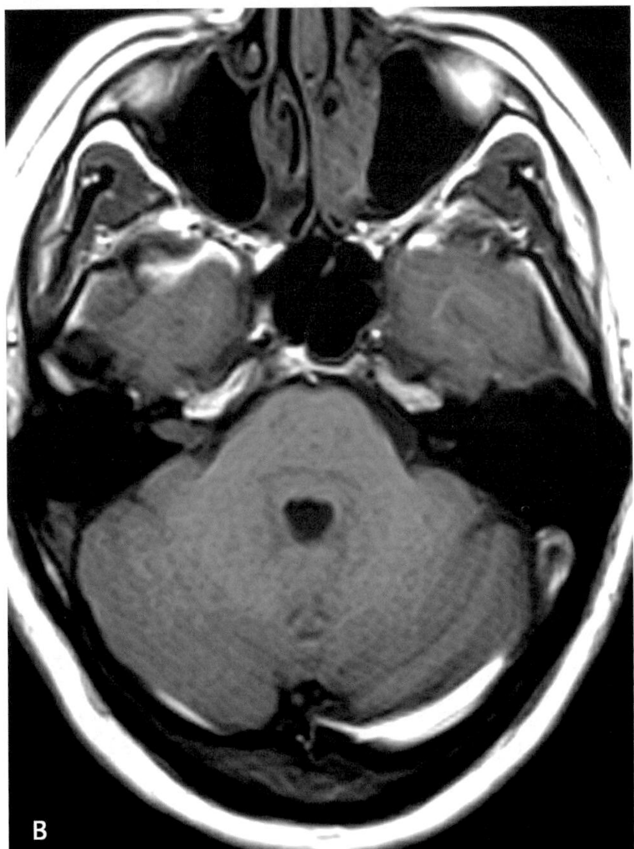

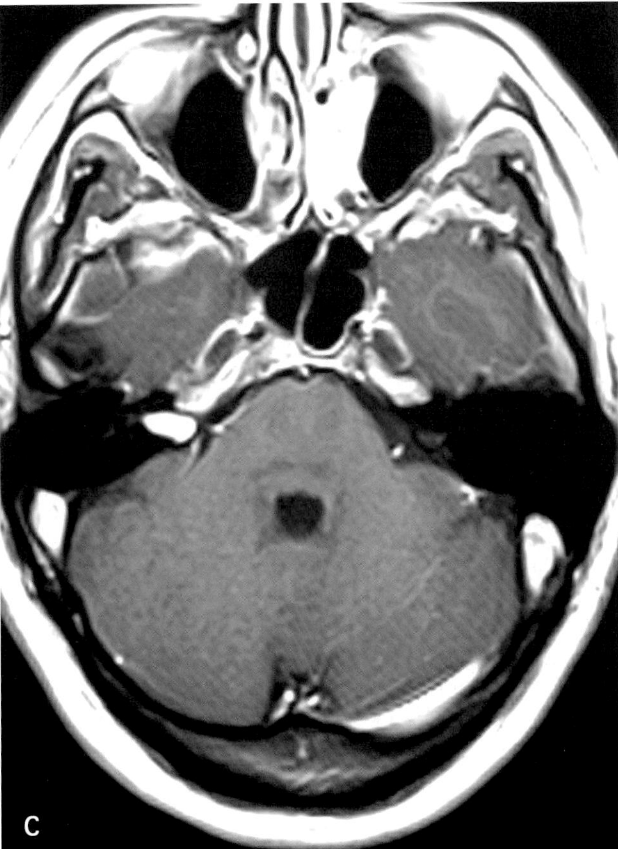

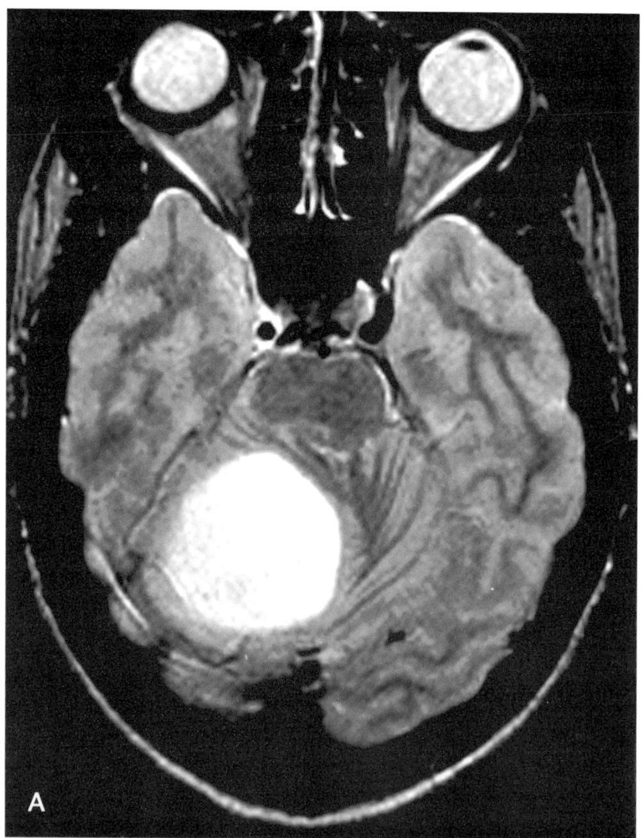

Figure 13. Hemangioblastoma. On (A) the intermediate T2-weighted scan, a high signal intensity abnormality is identified within the posterior fossa, which causes mass effect with compression of the fourth ventricle. The lesion is slightly higher in signal intensity than cerebrospinal fluid on this scan and (B) the pre-contrast T1-weighted scan, suggesting a neoplastic origin. (C) Post-contrast, there is enhancement of a small mural nodule, with a large prominent vein also identified adjacent to the mass. The most common presentation for an hemangioblastoma on imaging is that of a cystic mass with a peripheral mural nodule. Tumor vessels may also be apparent. Less commonly, these lesions present as solid masses. *(From Runge VM, Brack MA, Garneau RA, Kirsch JE. Magnetic resonance imaging of the brain. Philadelphia, JB Lippincott, 1994).*

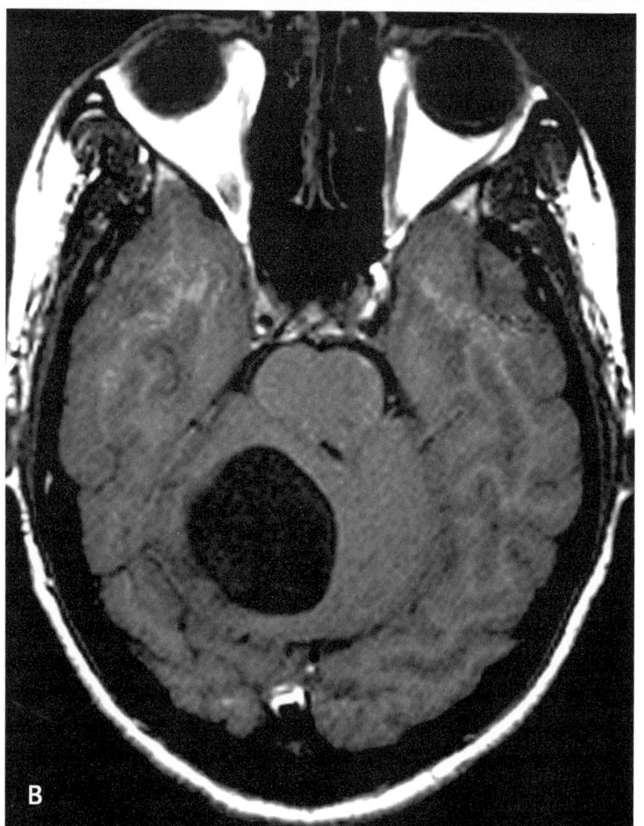

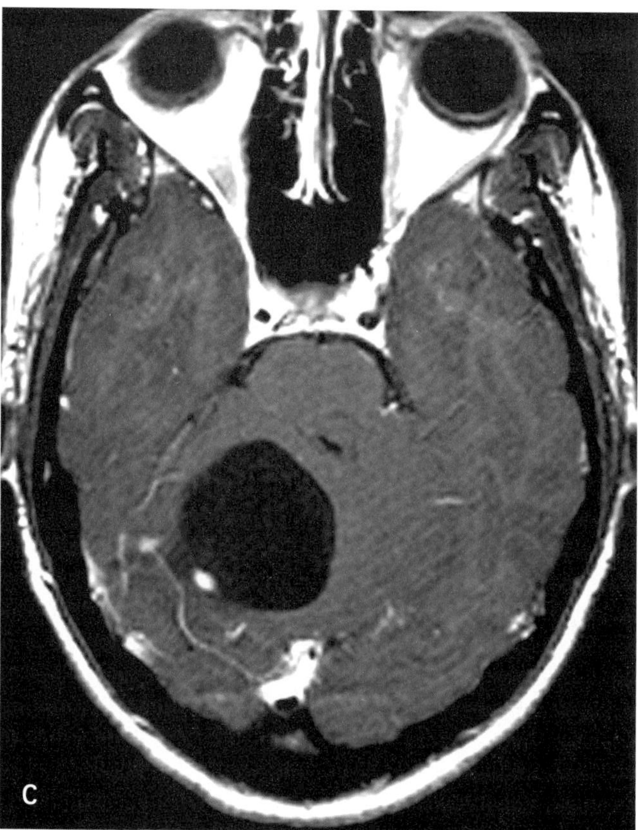

important (figure 14). Because there is no beam hardening artifact, a meningioma along a dural surface is more easily demonstrated with MR than with CT (figure 15). The extraaxial location with displacement of adjacent brain tissue is also better demonstrated by the multiplanar capability of MR.

Edema is a variable finding in patients with meningioma. Some lesions show no associated edema, while other meningiomas may incite impressive vasogenic edema. The extraaxial location, the relationship to the dura, and the presence on contrast enhanced studies of a "dural tail" (adjacent enhancing thickened dura) should strongly suggest the diagnosis.[44,45] The relationship of a convexity meningioma to the superior sagittal sinus is extremely important to establish prior to any surgical intervention, and MR angiography may be of value in this regard.

With contrast enhanced studies, meningiomas typically show intense homogeneous enhancement. On occasion, areas of cystic change or necrosis can be identified. However, the major benefit of contrast media is both to detect the lesion and define its extent. On unenhanced studies even moderate sized isointense lesions can be difficult to detect (figure 16). En plaque lesions are particularly difficult to identify without contrast enhancement (figure 17).

Craniopharyngioma

Although craniopharyngiomas account for less than 5% of all brain tumors, they account for about half of all suprasellar tumors of childhood.[46] There is a bimodal peak in incidence for this tumor. The first peak occurs in the first and second decades of life, while the second peak occurs in the early sixth decade. These lesions are slow growing, with symptoms often related to impingement on adjacent structures. Because of the relationship of this tumor to the optic chiasm, bitemporal hemianopsia often is a presenting symptom. Endocrinological abnormalities such as growth failure and diabetes insipidus can also be seen in patients with craniopharyngioma.[47] These tumors are markedly heterogeneous in consistency and can include cystic, solid, and fatty components. The MR appearance of craniopharyngiomas reflects their heterogeneous composition (figure 18). MR contrast enhancement does not play a major role in tumor detection, although enhancement can best define the extent of the lesion and its relationship to normal adjacent structures. MR is significantly better than CT in defining the relationship between the tumor and the optic chiasm and associated structures. Enhancement is relatively homogeneous within the solid portions of the tumor and can be rim-like within the cyst walls. The calcifications that are so clearly delineated on CT studies may not be visible at all on MR imaging, although gradient echo imaging can increase the sensitivity to this calcification.

Pituitary Macroadenomas/Microadenomas

Pituitary adenomas are either functioning or non-functioning in terms of hormonal secretions. Lesions which oversecrete hormones tend to become manifest when quite small. Lesions less than 10 mm in size are termed microadenomas. Non-functioning adenomas become manifest secondary to mass effect or pituitary failure. These lesions are invariably macroadenomas. Pituitary macroadenomas can be isointense with normal brain on both T1 and T2-weighted pulse sequences. However, variations from this appearance are common.[48] Pituitary macroadenomas demonstrate moderate enhancement post-contrast, which improves lesion depiction and definition of lesion borders (figure 19). These tumors usually are easily detected because of their size, the distortion of adjacent anatomical relationships, and their enhancement characteristics. Macroadenomas can hemorrhage, while functioning adenomas can exhibit bright signal after bromocriptine therapy. This signal is most likely secondary to hemorrhage or hemorrhagic infarction, although its precise etiology is uncertain.

Thin slice, high resolution imaging is quite helpful for evaluating the pituitary, particularly when searching for microadenomas. The coronal and sagittal planes are both valuable. However, the coronal plane best demonstrates the relationship of the pituitary adenoma to the optic chiasm, the third ventricle, and the cavernous sinuses. Even with careful attention to technique, microadenomas may be difficult to detect. Subtle alterations in the contour of the gland and deviation of the stalk may be helpful in detecting pituitary microadenomas. Contrast enhancement can also play a major role in small lesion detection (figure 20).[49] It has been suggested that half-dose MR contrast is advantageous in detecting pituitary microadenomas,[50] since the pituitary lacks a blood-brain barrier and enhances intensely. Microadenomas appear as less intense lesions against a more intense background on post-contrast studies.

Colloid Cyst

Colloid cysts are relatively rare tumors comprising less than one percent of all intracranial neoplasms. Most often they are located in the anterior aspect of the third ventricle. Colloid cysts usually present in the adult with headache secondary to obstruction of the foramen of Monro. The peak incidence of these lesions occurs between the ages of twenty to forty years. These tumors can be quite variable in size on presentation, ranging from a few millimeters to a few centimeters in diameter. Because the contents of colloid cysts vary, they have a variety of appearances. Lesions may be isointense on T1-weighted images and hyperintense on T2-weighted images or they may show diminished signal on T2-weighted images, with or without a surrounding high signal rim.

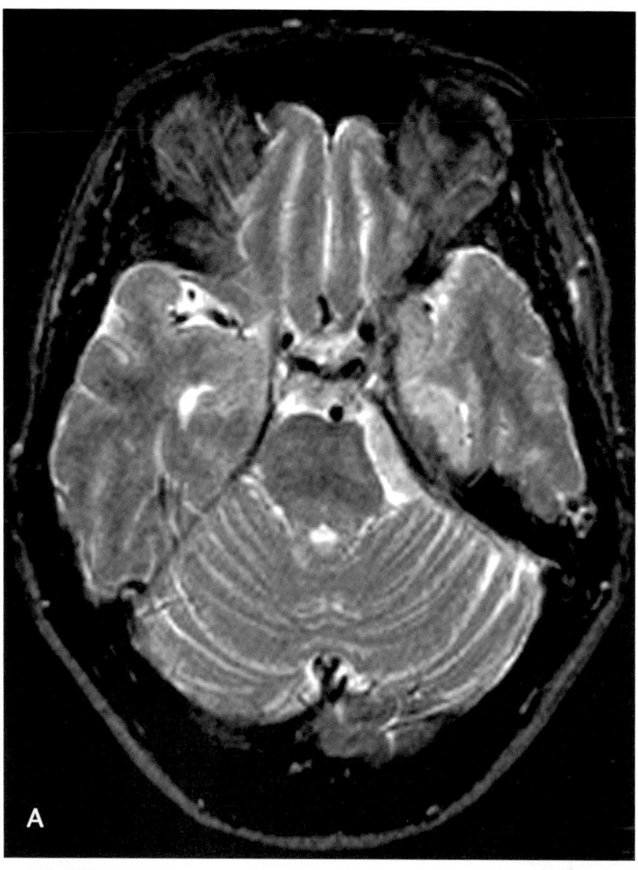

Figure 14. Sphenoid wing meningioma. A soft tissue mass that is isointense to brain is noted just to the left of the pons on pre-contrast (A) T2 and (B) T1-weighted scans. There is mild mass effect. (C) Post-contrast, the posterior fossa component of the mass is more easily identified, due to intense enhancement. A larger enhancing component within the middle cranial fossa is now also apparent. With extraaxial lesions in particular, unenhanced scans may fail to diagnose the abnormality, or as in the current case markedly underestimate its full extent. *(From Runge VM, Brack MA, Garneau RA, Kirsch JE. Magnetic resonance imaging of the brain. Philadelphia, JB Lippincott, 1994).*

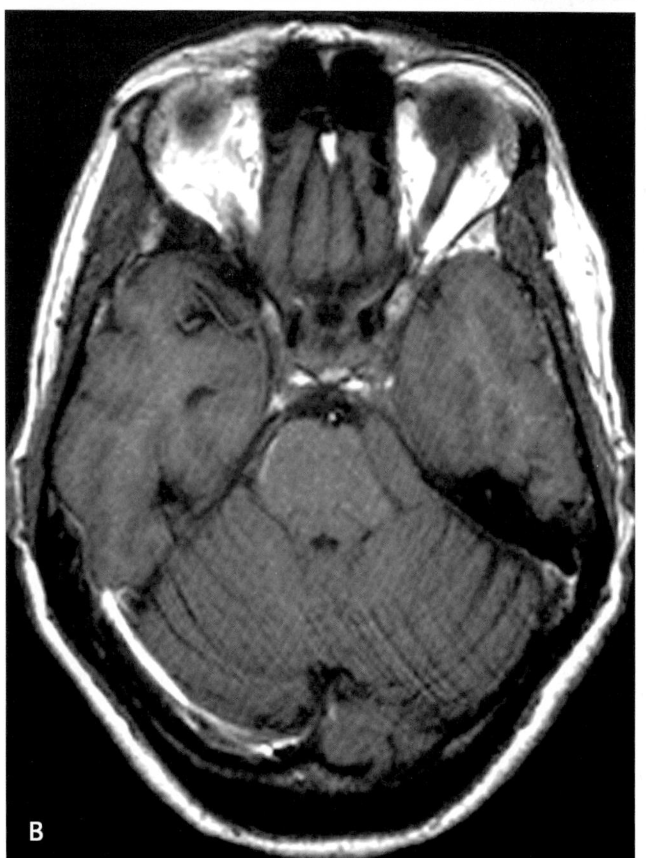

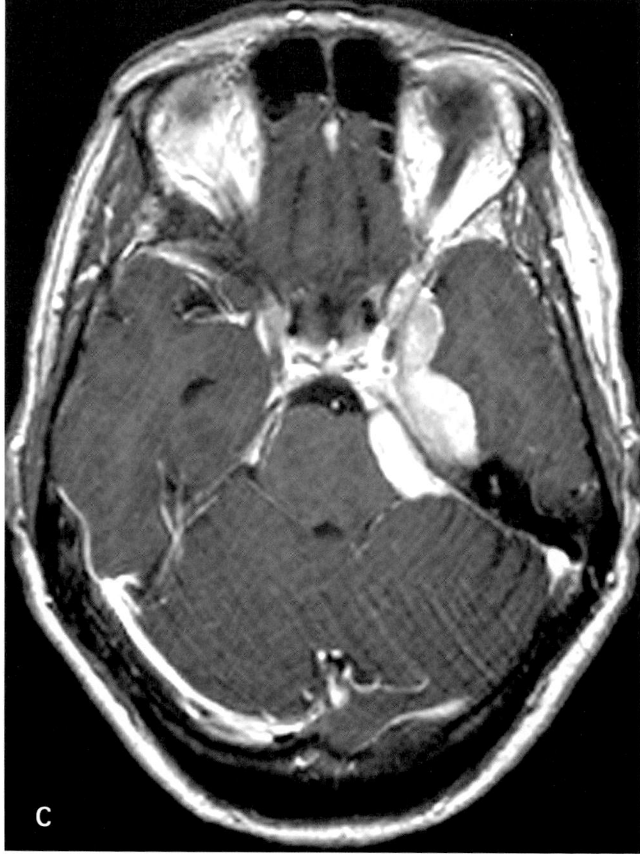

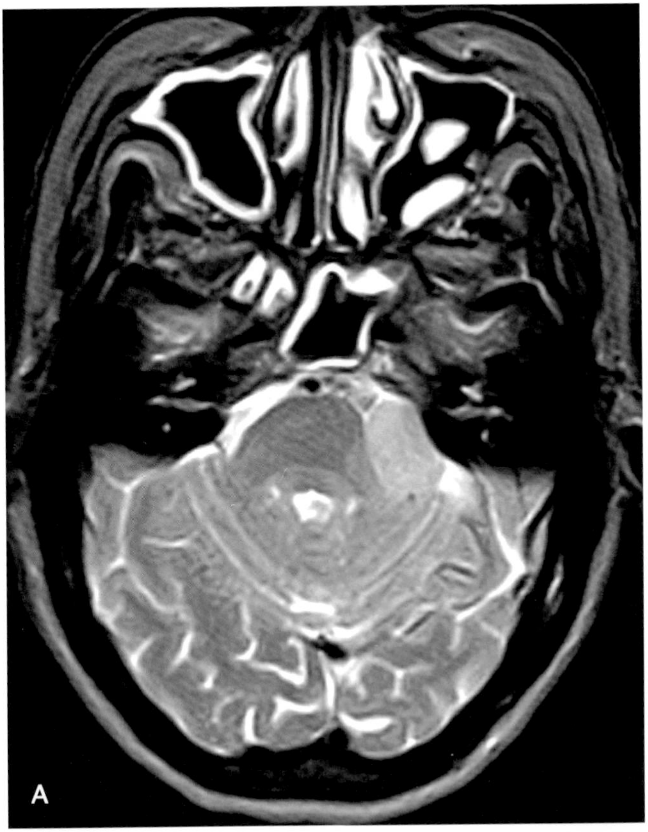

Figure 15. Cerebellopontine angle meningioma. On (A) the precontrast T2-weighted scan, a mass with intermediate signal intensity is noted in the left cerebellopontine angle. There is mild mass effect upon the pons. Comparison of (B) pre- and (C) post-contrast T1-weighted scans reveals intense homogeneous enhancement of the mass. The lesion is dural based, without extension into the internal auditory canal.

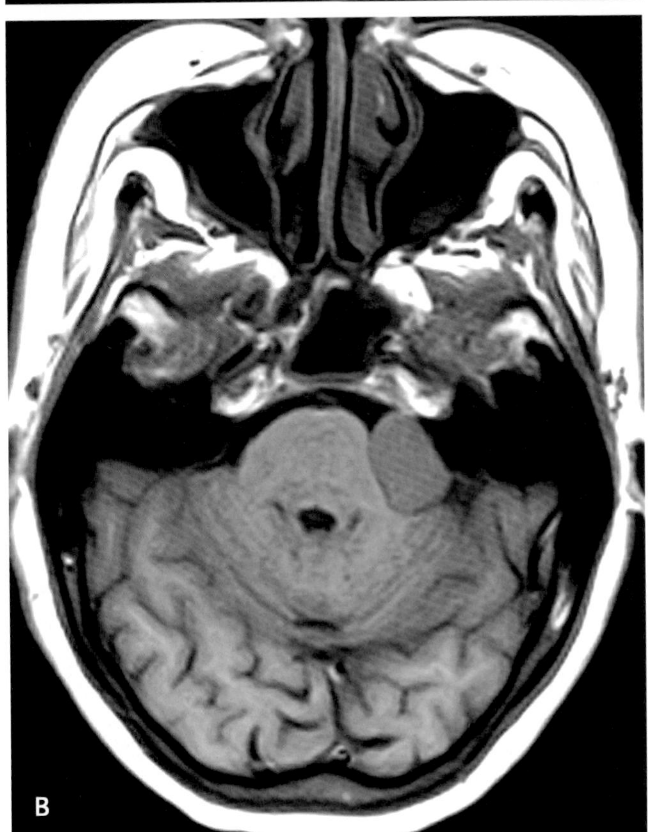

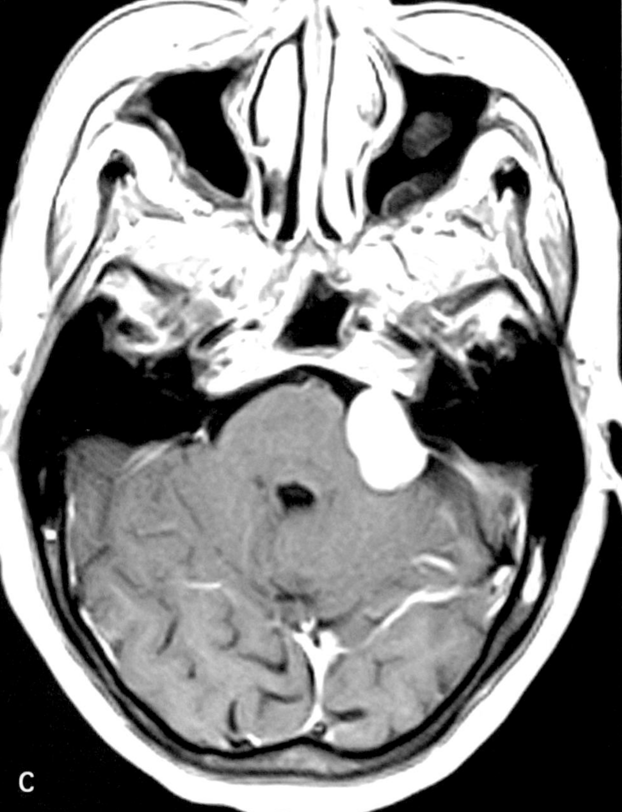

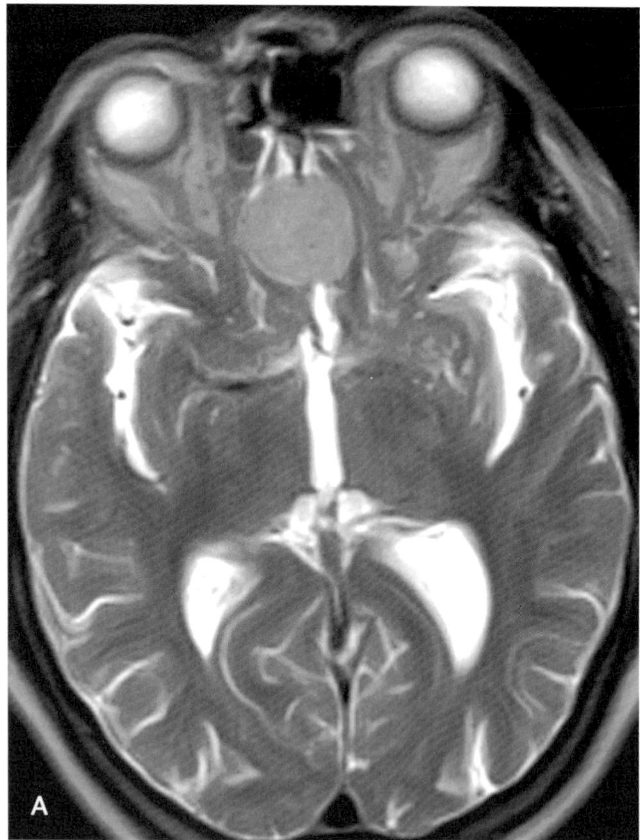

Figure 16. Olfactory groove meningioma. (A) The pre-contrast T2-weighted scan reveals a subtle midline lesion at the base of the low frontal lobe, with apparent displacement of surrounding brain. The mass is poorly visualized on (B) the pre-contrast T1-weighted scan. The lesion is best visualized, due to intense homogeneous enhancement, on (C) the post-contrast scan. Well-recognized sites for meningiomas at the skull base include the sphenoid ridge, olfactory groove, tuberculum sella, and parasellar region.

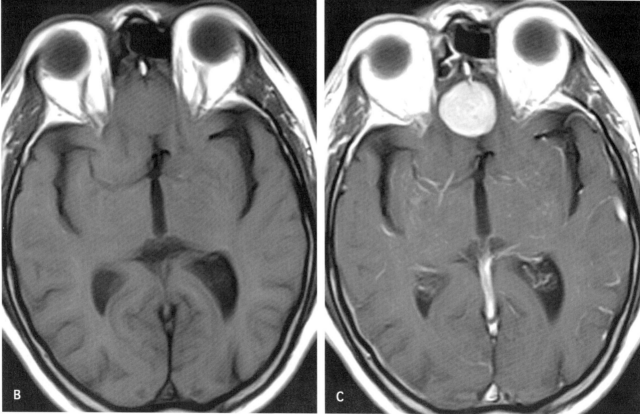

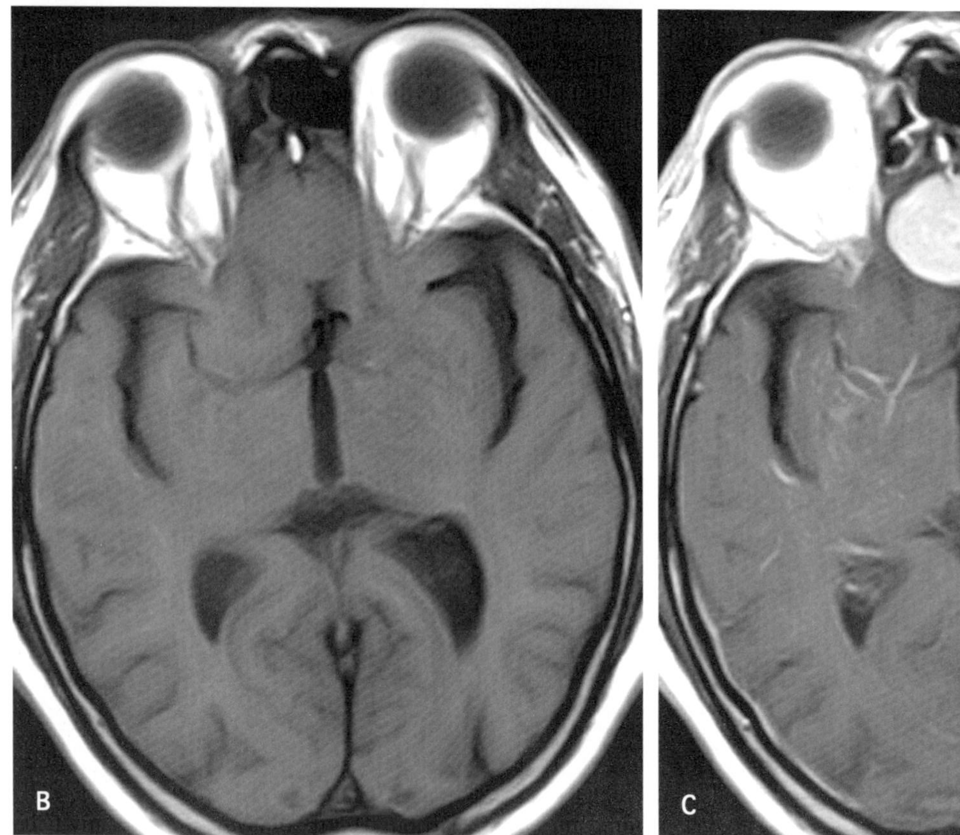

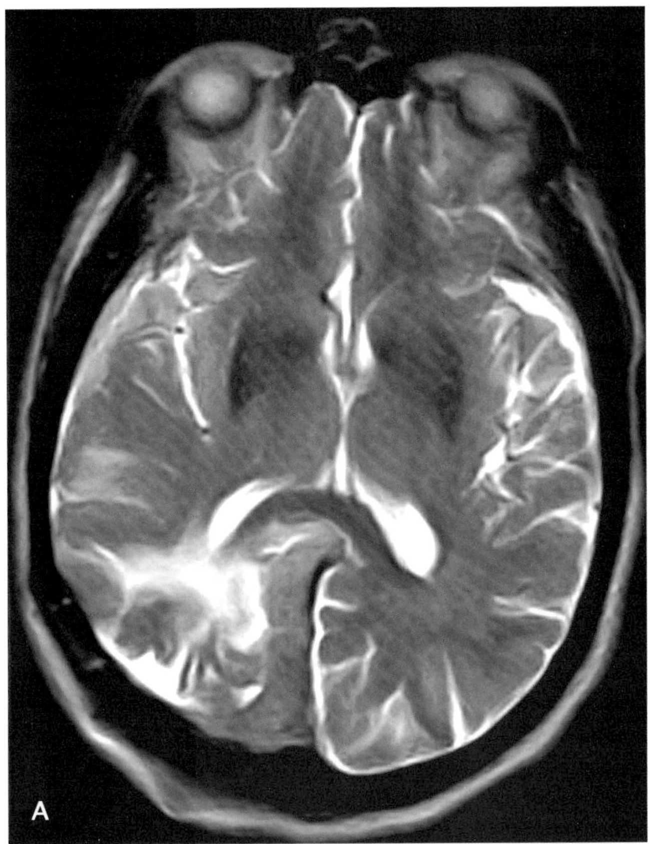

Figure 17. En plaque meningioma. (A) The pre-contrast T2-weighted scan reveals edema adjacent to the atria of the right lateral ventricle. (B) The pre-contrast T1-weighted scan is noncontributory. (C) Post-contrast, an extensive homogeneous enhancing mass is identified, extending along the posterior falx and right cerebral convexity. The mass follows the planes of the leptomeninges.

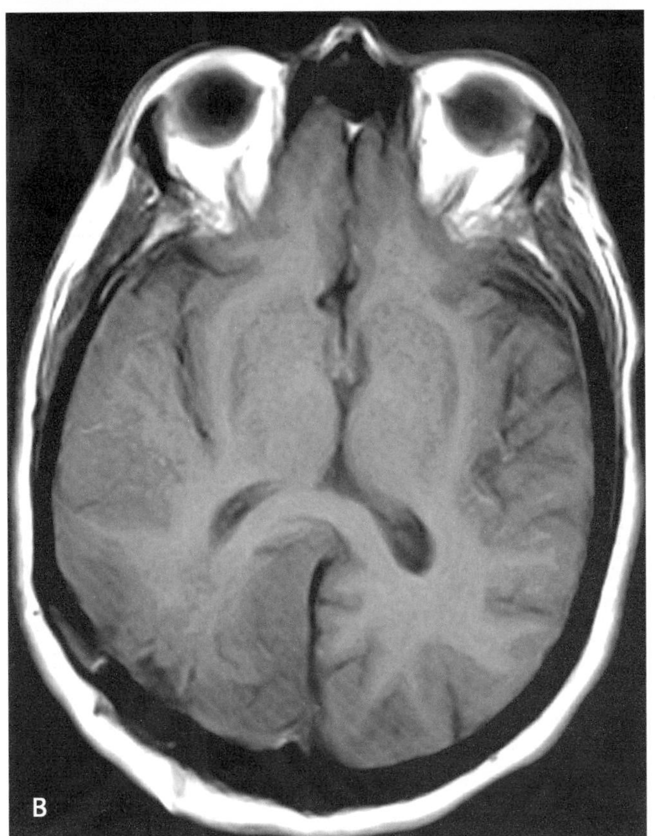

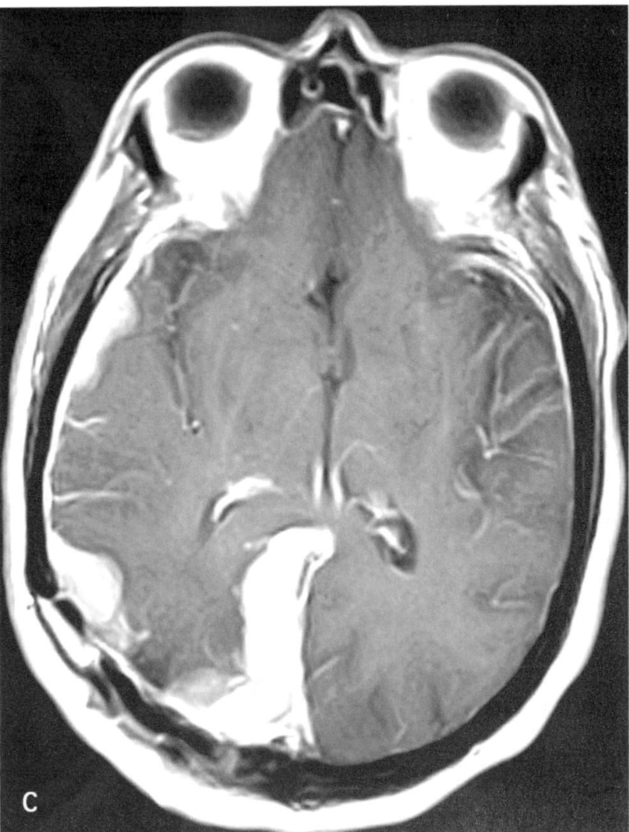

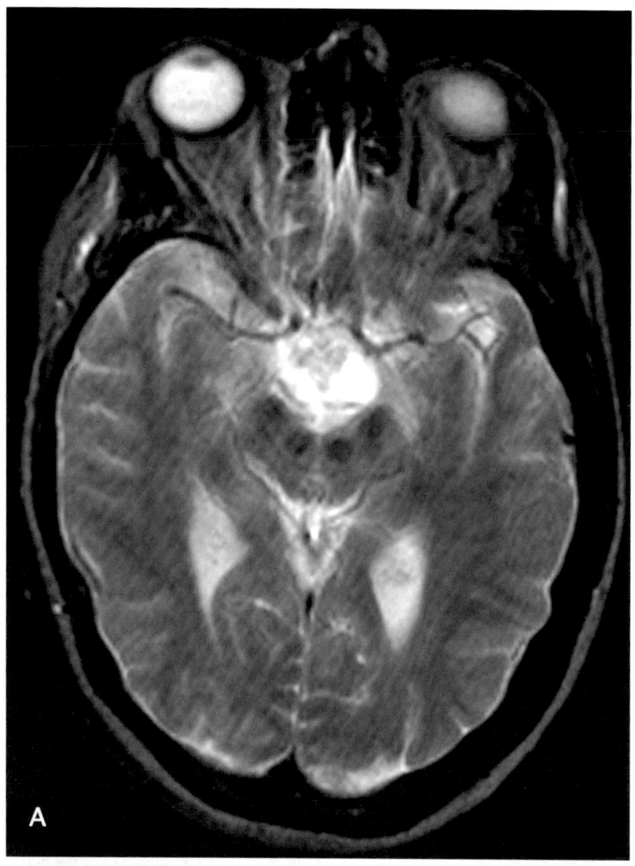

Figure 18. Craniopharyngioma. On (A) the pre-contrast T2-weighted scan, a predominantly high signal intensity suprasellar lesion is noted. Comparison of (B) pre- and (C) post-contrast T1-weighted scans reveals a solid enhancing nidus anteriorly, with a cystic component demonstrating rim enhancement posteriorly. Craniopharyngiomas are complex heterogeneous masses, with both cystic and solid components. Contrast administration aids in differential diagnosis and definition of lesion extent. *(From Runge VM, Brack MA, Garneau RA, Kirsch JE. Magnetic resonance imaging of the brain. Philadelphia, JB Lippincott, 1994).*

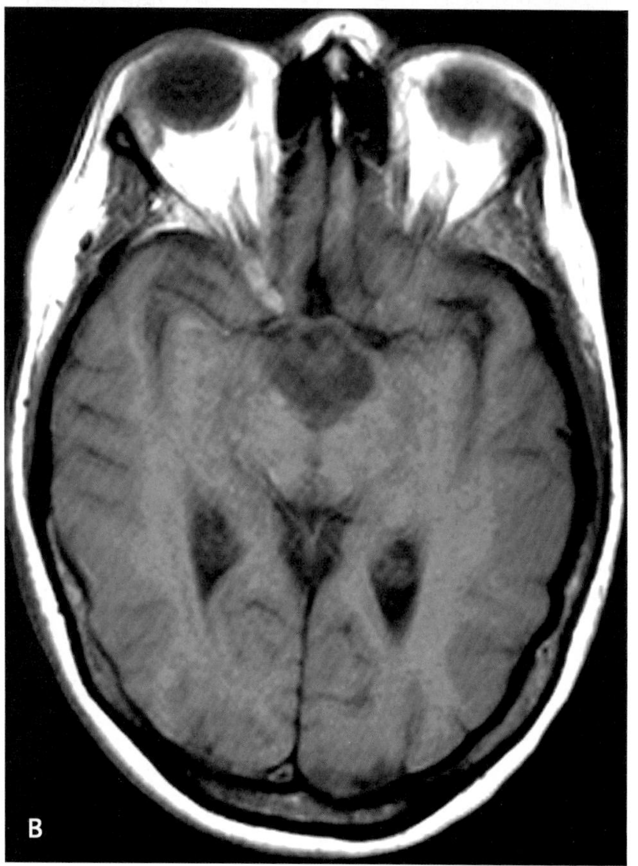

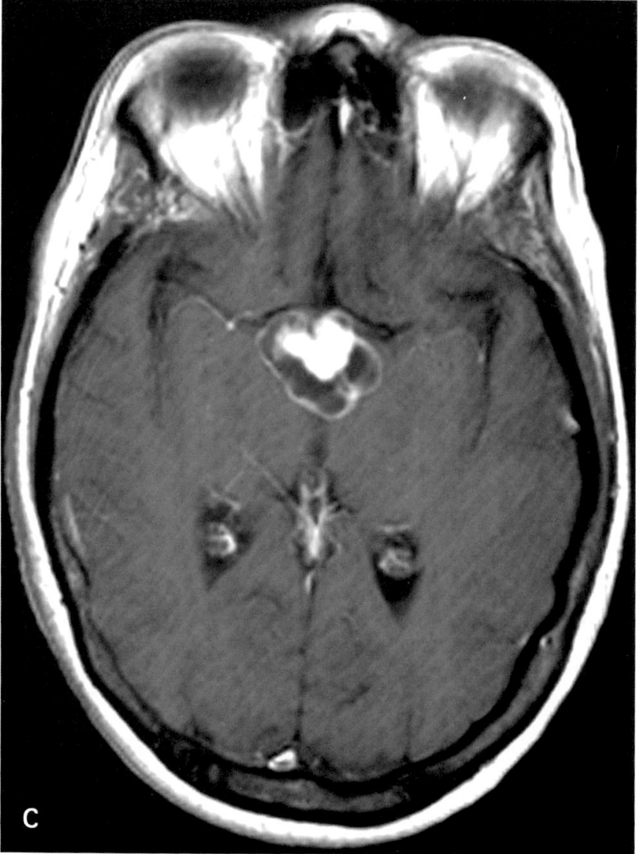

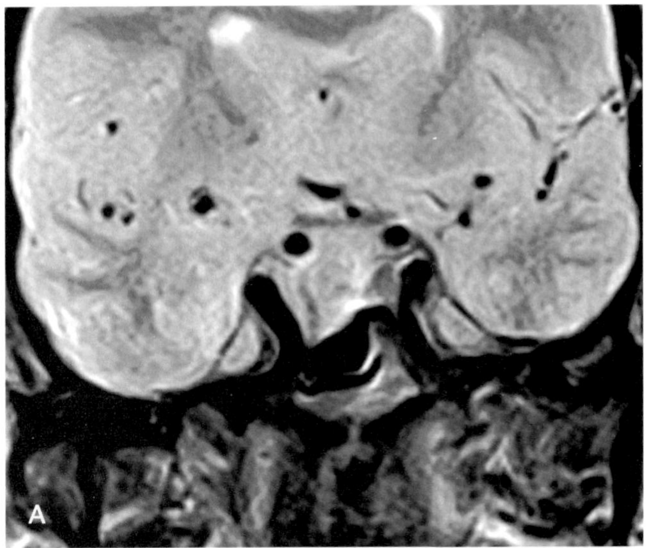

Figure 19. Pituitary macroadenoma. (A) T2 and (B) T1-weighted pre-contrast coronal scans reveal sella enlargement, with deviation of the pituitary infundibulum and erosion of the sellar floor. (C) Post-contrast, there is moderate enhancement of the lesion, which occupies the right side of the sella and can now be differentiated from the normal pituitary gland on the left (arrow).

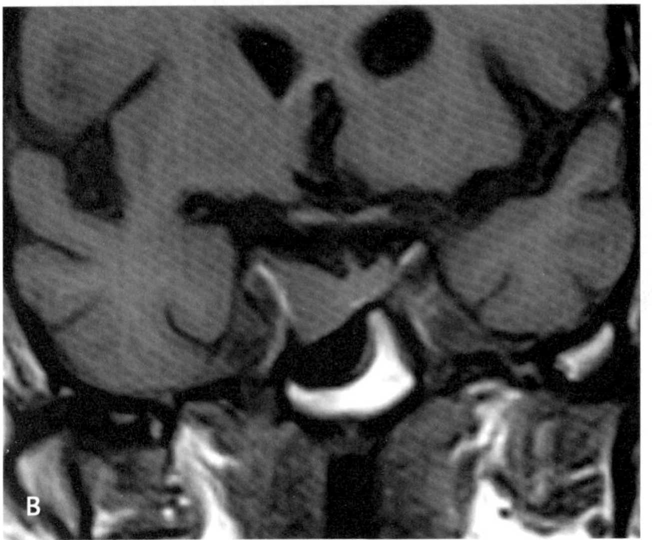

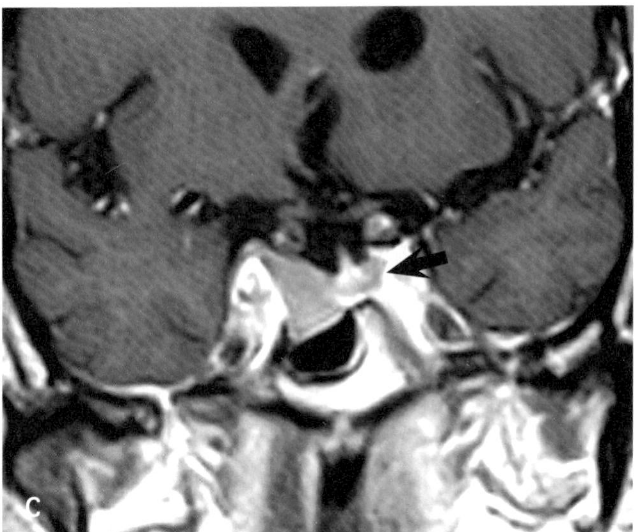

Arachnoid Cyst

Arachnoid cysts can be developmental or post-traumatic in origin. Developmental lesions are often seen in the temporal and sub-temporal region of the brain, although they may be parasagittal or even over the convexity. These lesions present as CSF signal on all pulse sequences. They do not exhibit contrast enhancement. Arachnoid cysts of developmental origin typically do not exhibit mass effect on adjacent normal structures, while those that are post-traumatic in etiology can exhibit substantial distortion of adjacent anatomy. The location and appearance of arachnoid cysts are usually sufficient to allow appropriate diagnosis and differentiation from other masses. On rare occasion the differentiation of arachnoid cysts from a low grade cystic glioma can be difficult. Comparison of the lesion appearance with CSF on multiple different sequences can be of help, as can the judicious use of MR contrast.

Pineal Cyst

Pineal cysts are commonly seen on MR studies. Typically, the lesions are round and well marginated. Their signal intensity may be different from that of CSF, reflecting a higher protein concentration. Contrast enhanced MR can be helpful in the identification of pineal cysts and their differentiation from other lesions. Pineal cysts do not enhance after gadolinium administration, although there may be homogeneous enhancement of the surrounding normal pineal tissue (figure 21).

Pineal cysts are most often asymptomatic, yet if they become large, they can cause symptoms secondary to the

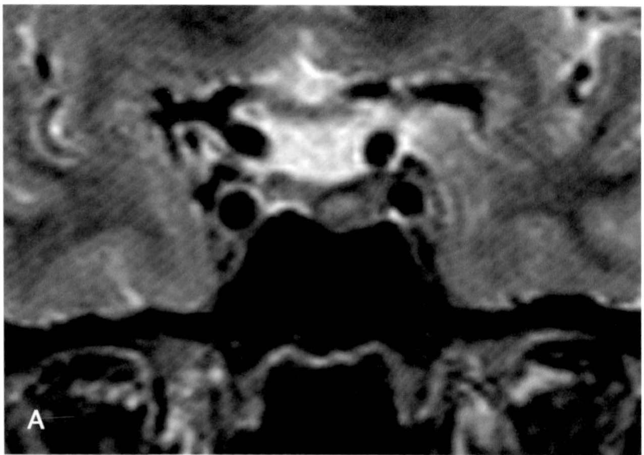

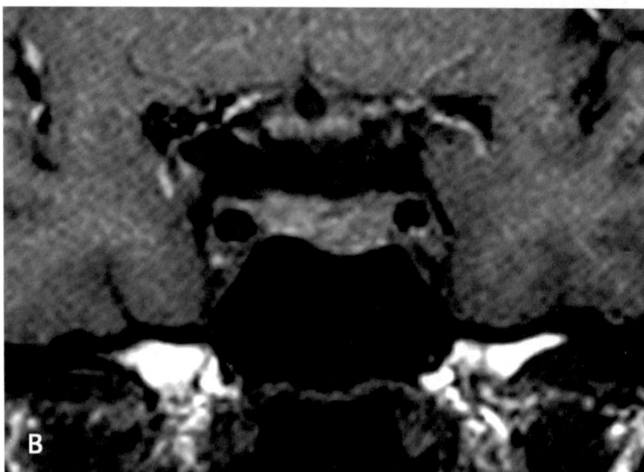

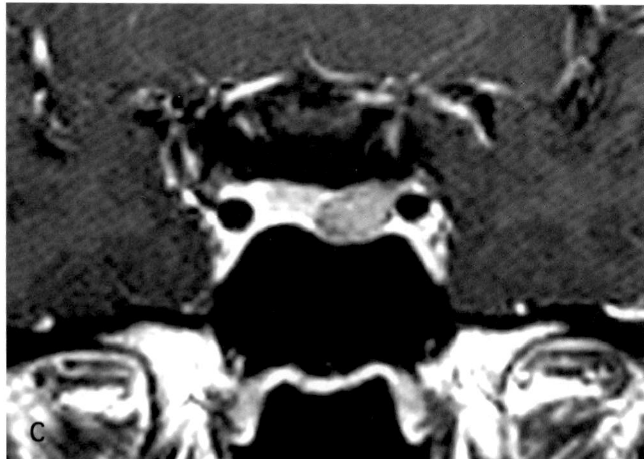

Figure 20. Pituitary microadenoma (prolactinoma). On (A) the thin section T2-weighted coronal scan, asymmetry of the sella floor is evident. A definite mass lesion cannot be identified on either this scan or (B) the thin section T1-weighted coronal scan. (C) Post-contrast, the normal pituitary demonstrates intense enhancement, revealing a large left-sided pituitary microadenoma, with less relative enhancement. Contrast administration improves lesion recognition, with identification in one study of a microadenoma only post-contrast in three of eleven patients. *(From Runge VM, Brack MA, Garneau RA, Kirsch JE. Magnetic resonance imaging of the brain. Philadelphia, JB Lippincott, 1994).*

development of hydrocephalus. However, this is quite unusual. Lesions showing irregular margins and internal enhancement represent other tumors of the pineal region.

Germ Cell Tumors

About half of all germ cell tumors are germinomas. These tumors typically present between the ages of five and twenty-five years. They can be seen in either the pineal region or in the suprasellar cistern or pituitary fossa. Germinomas can infiltrate and can also spread through the CSF. MR imaging typically will show a well-circumscribed homogeneous lesion. With gadolinium administration, these tumors show marked contrast enhancement (figure 22). They probably do not calcify. However, they tend to engulf pineal calcifications and thus may appear inhomogeneous after contrast administration. Contrast is also helpful in depicting CSF spread of these tumors. Germinomas are extremely radiosensitive, and respond to chemotherapy as well.

Teratoma is a less common germ cell tumor that contains all three germ cell layers — ectoderm, mesoderm, and endoderm. These tumors typically present on MR as heterogeneous lesions secondary to the presence of cystic and fatty components. Chemical shift artifact may be demonstrated. Calcification, which can be more readily visualized on computed tomography, may not be visualized on MR imaging.

Miscellaneous Pineal Tumors

Other tumors of the pineal region include pineoblastomas, pineocytomas, and rare germ cell tumors such as choriocarcinomas and embryonal tumors. Pineoblastomas have a male predominance, while pineocytomas are somewhat more common in females. Pineoblastomas are highly malignant, seed through the CSF, and carry a uniformly poor prognosis. They have been classified as a primitive neuroectodermal tumor (PNET). These lesions are seen on both CT and MR as irregular, invasive tumors. Contrast enhancement is typical, and can be helpful in the assessment of the extent of the tumor and its relationship to normal structures.

Pineocytomas are more benign lesions. They are well circumscribed, although hemorrhage and cystic degenera-

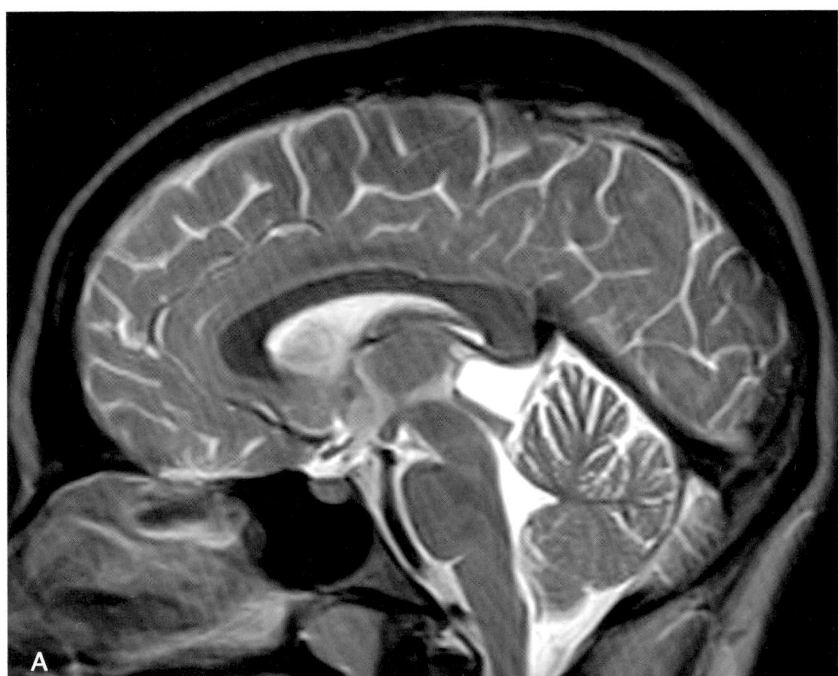

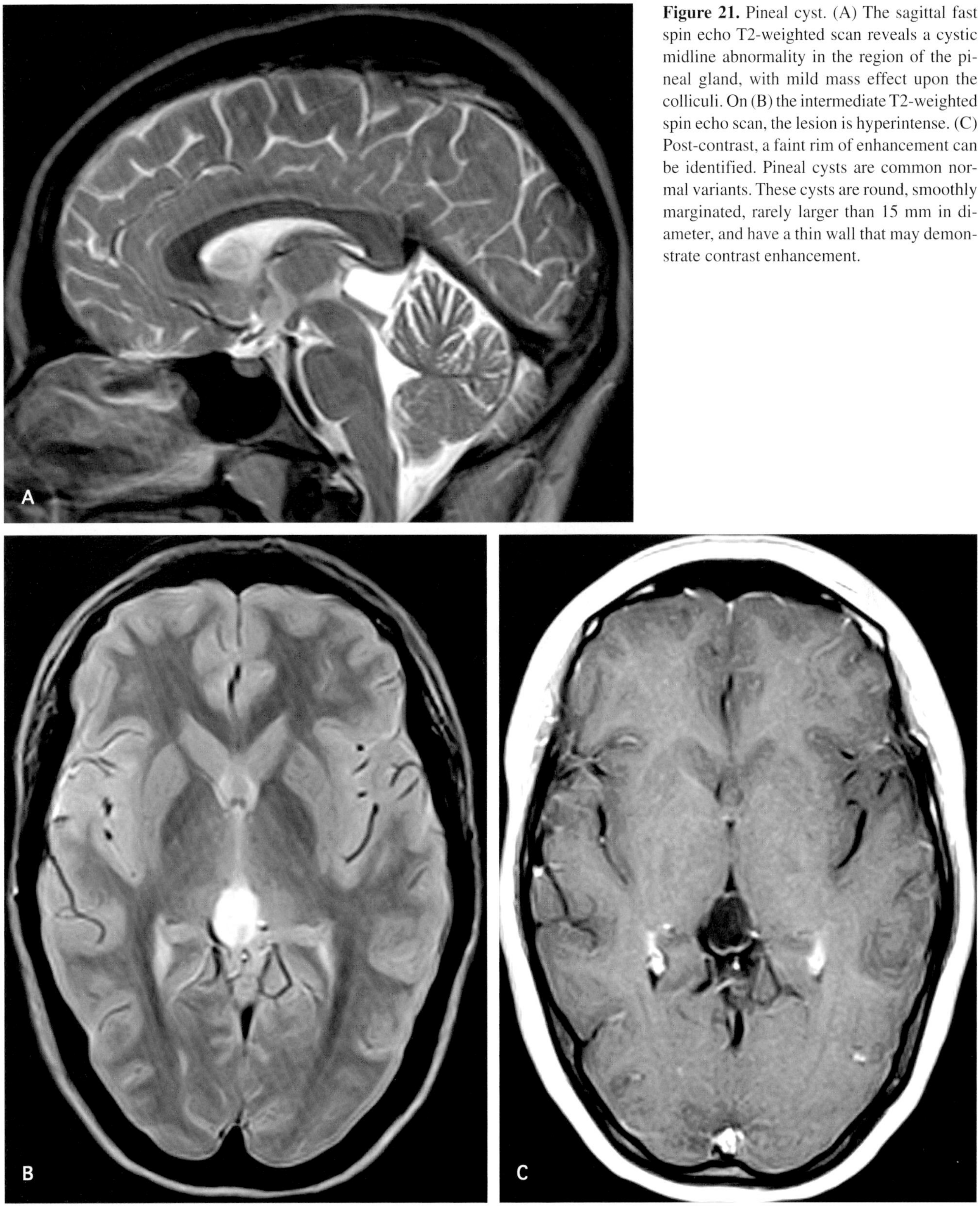

Figure 21. Pineal cyst. (A) The sagittal fast spin echo T2-weighted scan reveals a cystic midline abnormality in the region of the pineal gland, with mild mass effect upon the colliculi. On (B) the intermediate T2-weighted spin echo scan, the lesion is hyperintense. (C) Post-contrast, a faint rim of enhancement can be identified. Pineal cysts are common normal variants. These cysts are round, smoothly marginated, rarely larger than 15 mm in diameter, and have a thin wall that may demonstrate contrast enhancement.

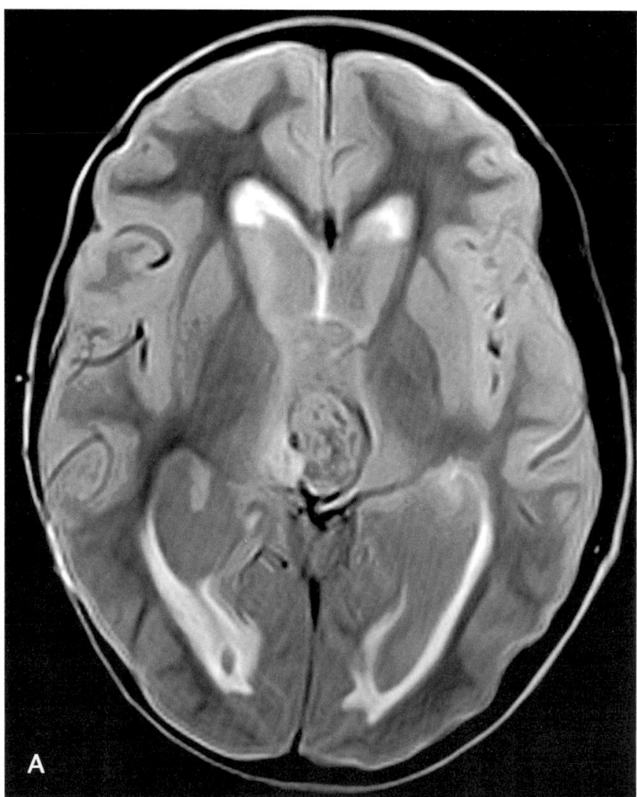

Figure 22. Mixed germ cell tumor. The most evident finding on (A) the intermediate T2-weighted scan is the abnormal high signal intensity surrounding the ventricles, consistent with transependymal flow (due to acute obstructive hydrocephalus). With the addition of (B) the pre-contrast T1-weighted scan, a mass just posterior to the third ventricle that demonstrates mild internal inhomogeneity is easily recognized. (C) Post-contrast, there is intense lesion enhancement. Although contrast enhancement improves lesion identification, imaging characteristics for pineal region tumors on MR are nonspecific in regard to lesion type. *(From Runge VM, Brack MA, Garneau RA, Kirsch JE. Magnetic resonance imaging of the brain. Philadelphia, JB Lippincott, 1994).*

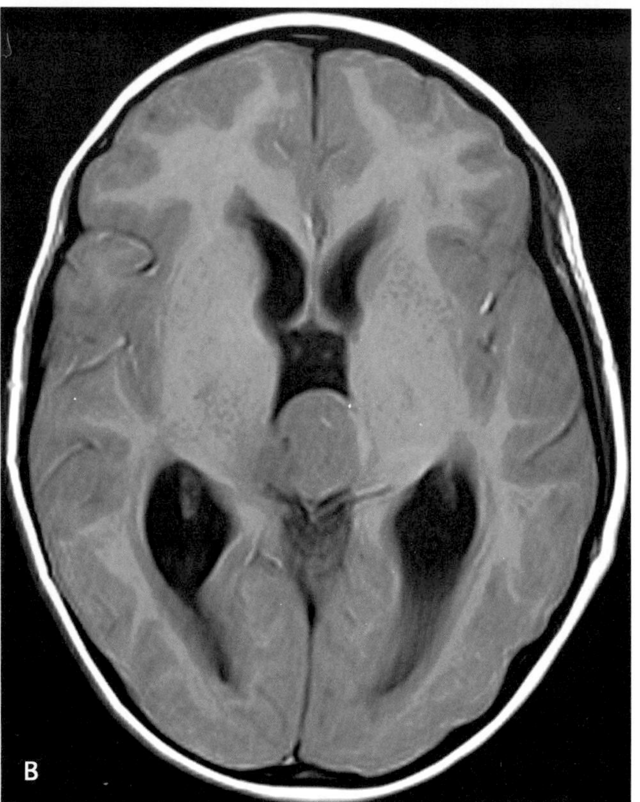

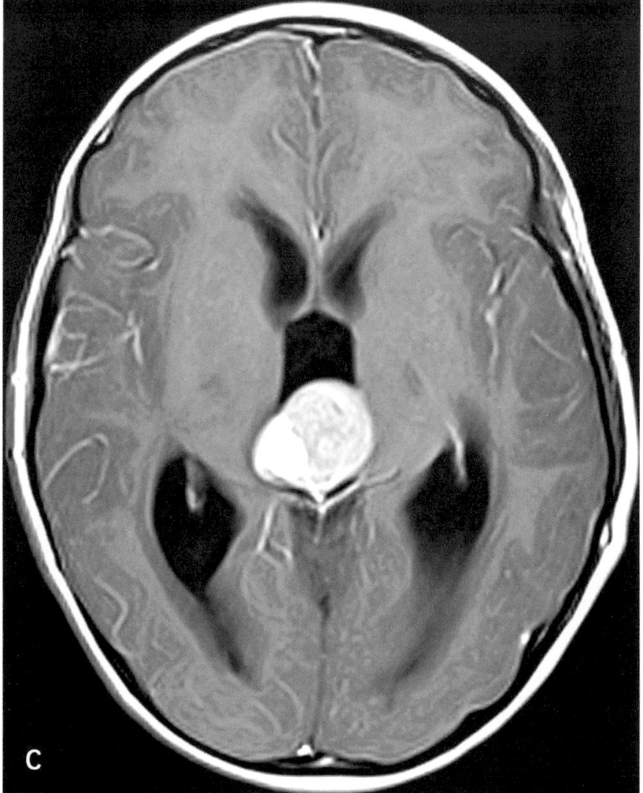

tion may be present. The use of contrast both defines the lesion and confirms its homogeneous appearance.

All other pineal tumors are quite rare. A distinguishing feature of choriocarcinomas is their tendency to hemorrhage. However, the differential diagnosis of these unusual tumors is difficult, even after contrast administration.

Epidermoid/Dermoid

Epidermoids are relatively rare tumors, accounting for about 1% of all intracranial neoplasms.[51] Although they result from epidermal inclusions occurring during early embryogenesis, they usually do not become manifest until age 20 to 50. Most epidermoids are located in the basal cisterns, with the cerebellopontine angle the most frequent site of occurrence. These tumors can occur in the fourth ventricle and obstruct the outflow of CSF.

On occasion an epidermoid tumor can be mistaken for an arachnoid cyst since both show low signal on T1-weighted sequences and increased signal on T2-weighted sequences. Proton density weighted imaging can be quite helpful since epidermoids will be hyperintense to both brain and CSF, while arachnoid cysts are isointense to CSF on all pulse sequences.

Dermoids are far more rare then epidermoid tumors. They are typically seen in children, and tend to have a midline location. About half of all patients with dermoid tumors have associated congenital abnormalities.[52]

The MR appearance of dermoid tumors reflects their fatty composition. Lesions have markedly increased signal on T1-weighted images and slightly decreased intensity on T2-weighted images. Some of these tumors contain fluid, and on occasion they can rupture with fat-like droplets seen scattered over the convexity (figure 23).

Metastatic Disease

Metastatic lesions account for about twenty to thirty percent of brain tumors in adults. The highest incidence of brain metastases occurs in patients in the fourth to seventh decades of life.[53] Approximately eighty percent of metastases are located in the supratentorial compartment, typically at the gray-white interface. This, most likely, is a feature reflective of their hematogenous spread, as it can be seen with other intracranial embolic phenomena.

Lesions which most commonly spread to brain include primary carcinoma of the lung, breast, and gastrointestinal tract. Melanomas also commonly spread to the brain, and there are a significant number of metastases from unknown primary cancers. Patients with breast, pelvic, and abdominal primary tumors often present with single lesions, while those with melanoma, lung cancer, and unknown primary tumors more often present with multiple lesions.[54,55] There are, of course, sufficient exceptions to this observation to make it unreliable for diagnostic purposes. For example, patients with primary carcinoma of the breast often demonstrate multiple lesions, particularly when studied with contrast enhanced MR.

Most metastases show decreased signal on T1-weighted sequences and increased signal on T2-weighted sequences. However, some lesions can be relatively isointense on T1-weighted images. Most metastatic lesions incite some vasogenic edema and some metastases are associated with impressive edema (figure 24). However, this is a variable finding. The amount of edema does not appear to correlate with lesion size or tumor type. While a substantial number of metastatic lesions can be seen without gadolinium contrast enhancement, MR contrast markedly increases the sensitivity of detection of intracerebral metastases. Because of their non-cerebral origin, metastases do not have a blood-brain barrier. Therefore they usually enhance intensely after gadolinium administration. In some patients, lesions can be seen only on enhanced studies (figure 25). Triple-dose (0.3 mmol/kg) not only improves lesion detection, but in selective patient populations also results in significant cost savings realized through the elimination of unnecessary surgery (figure 26).

It is common practice to utilize MR contrast in the evaluation of all patients with suspected metastatic disease. However, cost constraints may make this approach less feasible in the future. The following circumstances mandate MR contrast use.

1. Metastatic disease is suspected clinically, but the unenhanced MR scan is negative.
2. One lesion is found on the unenhanced study that is considered amenable to surgical removal.
3. The number of lesions detected is few, suggesting the possibility of either surgical removal or gamma knife therapy.
4. The patient is on an experimental therapeutic protocol, and the detection and follow-up of all lesions is required.

For intraaxial metastatic disease, the typical appearance is a single or multiple rounded lesions located at the gray-white junction. Edema is frequently present, a finding that is best seen on T2-weighted sequences. Contrast enhancement is almost always demonstrated, except with some small lesions. In these patients, triple-dose (0.3 mmol/kg) contrast imaging can visualize lesions not seen with unenhanced studies or even with conventional contrast doses (0.1 mmol/kg). Mass effect may be seen secondary to either lesion size or associated vasogenic edema. However with small lesions that incite no vasogenic edema, mass effect may not be apparent. Such lesions are best demonstrated on contrast enhanced MR studies, and often are not seen on unenhanced images.

Although most metastatic disease presents as increased signal on T2-weighted images, on occasion decreased sig-

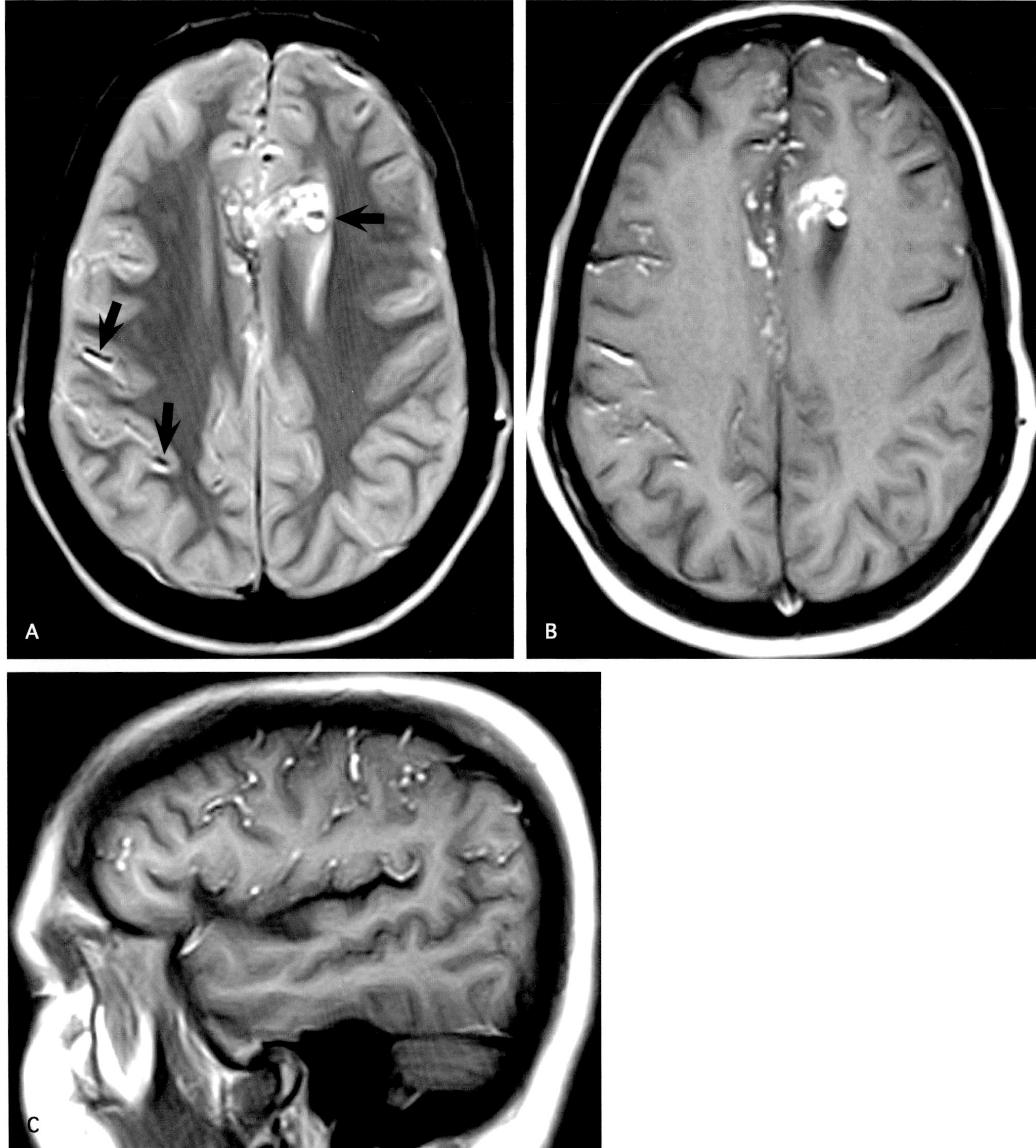

Figure 23. Ruptured dermoid. (A) The intermediate T2-weighted scan reveals scattered areas of abnormal hyperintensity (arrows), with many exhibiting a low signal intensity border along the frequency encoding direction (chemical shift artifact). (B) Axial and (C) sagittal pre-contrast T1-weighted scans confirm the presence of scattered abnormalities, which are also hyperintense on T1. The more peripheral globules are noted to lie within cortical sulci. By recognition of chemical shift, high signal intensity due to fat (as in this case) can be differentiated from methemoglobin. The case also illustrates the importance of obtaining pre-contrast T1-weighted scans, to identify fat or blood that might otherwise be mistaken for abnormal contrast enhancement.

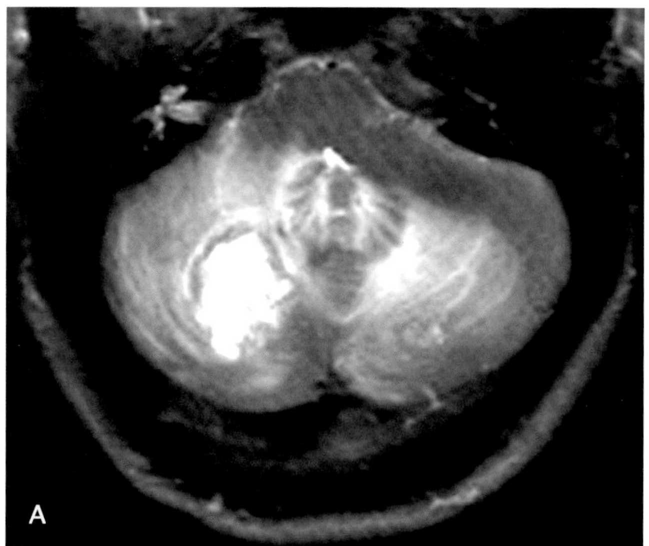

Figure 24. Brain metastases. A cystic and/or necrotic mass is noted in the right cerebellum on (A) the pre-contrast T2-weighted scan. Vasogenic edema, with abnormal high signal intensity, is seen bilaterally. Comparison of (B) pre- and (C) post-contrast T1-weighted scans reveals three enhancing lesions. These include a large necrotic right-sided metastasis, a one cm diameter solid left-sided metastasis, and a smaller pin point metastasis just anterior and lateral to this lesion (arrow). The case illustrates the value of contrast enhancement in aiding identification of metastatic lesions. Although the left cerebellar hemisphere appears abnormal pre-contrast, focal lesions cannot be identified.

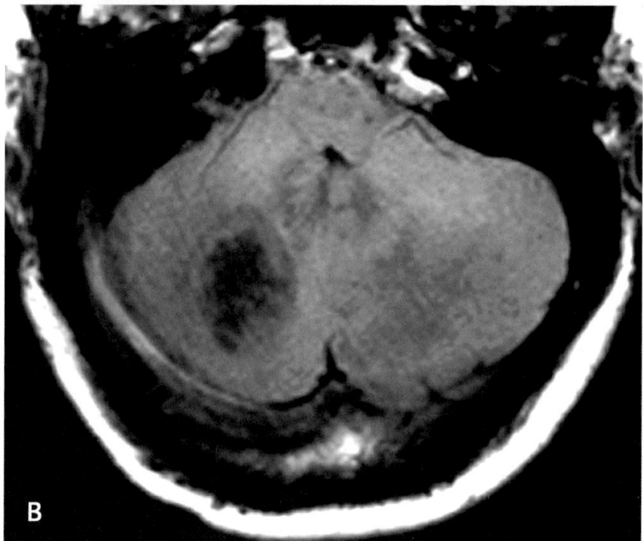

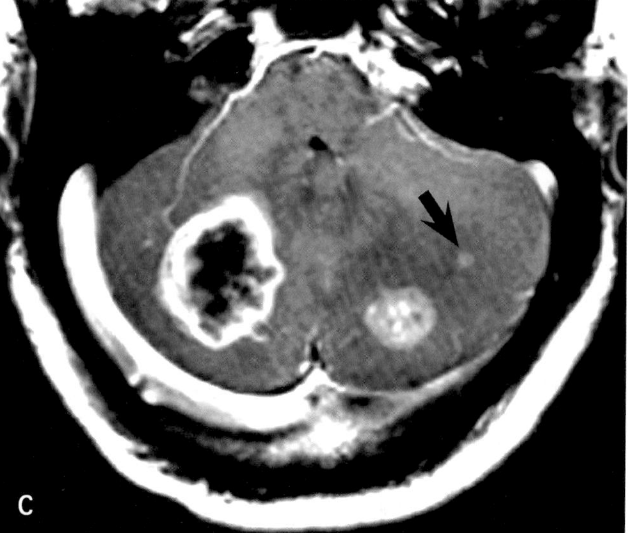

nal on T2-weighted sequences can be seen. This should suggest the possibility of calcification, hemorrhage, paramagnetic effects, or mucin. Hemorrhage can be seen with renal cell carcinoma, choriocarcinoma, carcinomas of the breast and thyroid, oat cell carcinoma, and melanoma (figure 27). Melanoma can also present with decreased signal on T2-weighted sequences because of the paramagnetic effect of melanin. Finally, mucinous adenocarcinoma of the bowel can present with decreased signal on T2-weighted images.

The differentiation of metastatic disease from other intracranial pathology is usually not a problem. Because metastases do not have a blood-brain barrier, they tend to enhance uniformly and intensely. Metastases also tend to present as multiple, small, rounded lesions all located at the gray-white junction.

In the elderly patient with chronic small vessel disease, contrast enhancement is particularly important. Small lesions (or those without substantial surrounding edema) are often overlooked or mistaken for ischemic disease without contrast administration (figure 28).

Differentiating metastases from abscesses can, on occasion, be difficult, and history is quite important. Both lesions are embolic in etiology and thus can have a similar distribution. The enhancement characteristics are usually different. Metastases enhance uniformly, while abscesses usually exhibit rim-like enhancement. When necrosis occurs in metastases, the rim seen is usually thicker and more irregular than that seen with an inflammatory process.

Extraaxial metastases typically involve the leptomeninges, dura, and/or the calvarium. Dural and calvarial lesions will be discussed later in this chapter. Leptomeningeal metastases most commonly come from lung, breast, or primary CNS neoplasms. Leukemia and lymphoma can also present with leptomeningeal involvement, as can melanoma.

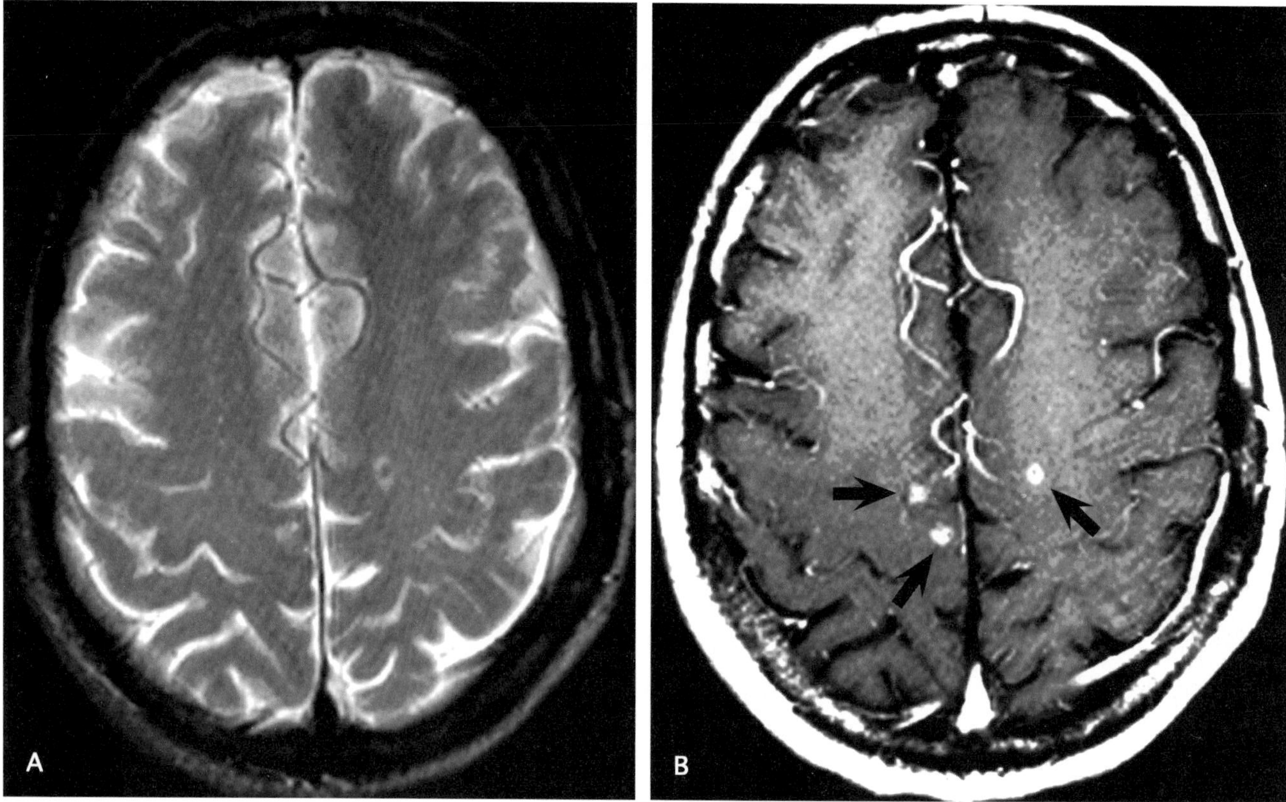

Figure 25. Brain metastases, visualized only following IV contrast administration. (A) The pre-contrast T2-weighted scan is normal. Only on (B) the post-contrast T1-weighted scan can three punctate enhancing lesions be identified (arrows), all at the gray-white matter junction along the falx. Small brain metastases may not elicit sufficient surrounding vasogenic edema to be recognized on pre-contrast MR scans. Identification of blood-brain barrier disruption, provided by IV contrast administration, permits diagnosis of such lesions. *(From Runge VM, Brack MA, Garneau RA, Kirsch JE. Magnetic resonance imaging of the brain. Philadelphia, JB Lippincott, 1994).*

Enhanced MR imaging is extremely valuable in the detection of leptomeningeal tumor involvement (figure 29). Nonenhanced MR and even enhanced CT can be relatively insensitive to these lesions.[56] All patients suspected of extraaxial metastases should be evaluated with contrast enhanced MR imaging.

Bony Lesions

Clivus Chordoma

Chordomas are tumors of notochordal tissue remnants. Although they more commonly involve the sacrum, they not infrequently arise from the clivus. The peak incidence of these tumors is between the third and fourth decades. Males are twice as likely to be affected as females.

The MR appearance of chordoma is that of a bulky midline lesion with marked destruction of bone. Chordomas can extend into the middle or posterior cranial fossae, as well as into the nasopharynx. These tumors may compress adjacent brain, but rarely invade it. Chordomas are highly vascular and enhance with contrast administration. MR contrast can help delineate tumor extent and the relationship of the tumor to normal adjacent structures. The sagittal view can be important to show the clival origin and the full extent of the lesion. CT scanning may be more sensitive in depicting tumoral calcification and bony destruction.

Calvarial/Dural Metastases

Involvement of the calvarium is invariably secondary to tumor emboli in the diploic space. This is a common occurrence in children, where hematogenous spread to the bone and dura is often seen (particularly with neuroblastoma and Ewing's sarcoma). Intraaxial metastases in children are quite rare.[57] The dura usually serves as an effective barrier to limit the spread of neoplasms between the calvarium and the cortical surface of the brain. Therefore, metastatic disease rarely spreads from the calvarium to the cortex or from the parenchyma to the calvarium.

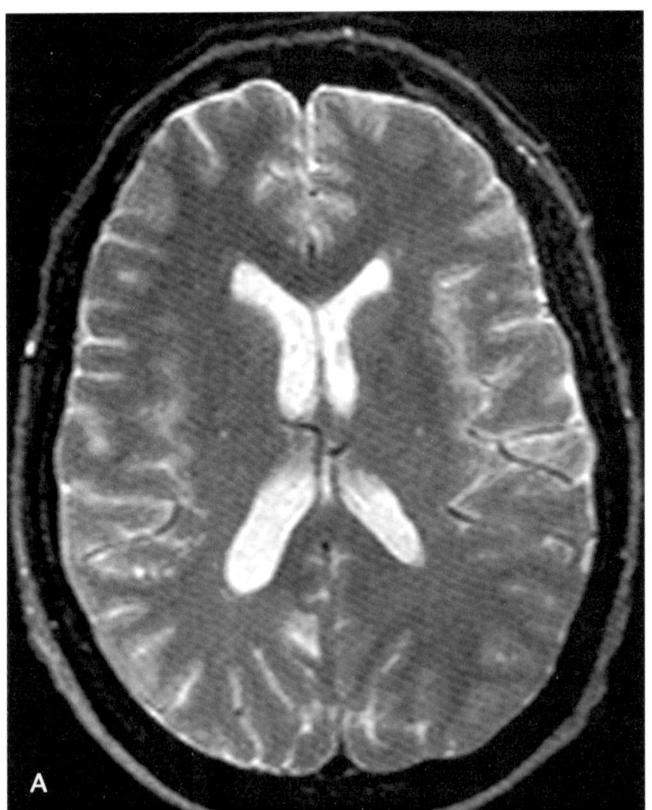

Figure 26. Brain metastasis, visualized only following high dose IV contrast administration (0.3 mmol/kg gadoteridol). The (A) pre-contrast T2-weighted and (B) post-contrast T1-weighted scans, the latter using standard dosage (0.1 mmol/kg), are normal. A repeat (C) post-contrast T1-weighted scan, using a dose of 0.3 mmol/kg, reveals a small right sided metastasis (arrow). This lesion was confirmed on follow-up exam some months later, with interim growth despite whole brain radiation. In a recent multi-institutional study, 32% more metastatic lesions were identified on MR following high dose as compared with standard dose (0.3 versus 0.1 mmol/kg) contrast administration. *(Reprinted with permission from Runge VM, Wells JW, Nelson KL, Linville PM. MR imaging detection of cerebral metastases with a single injection of high dose gadoteridol. J Magn Reson Imaging 1994;4:669-673).*

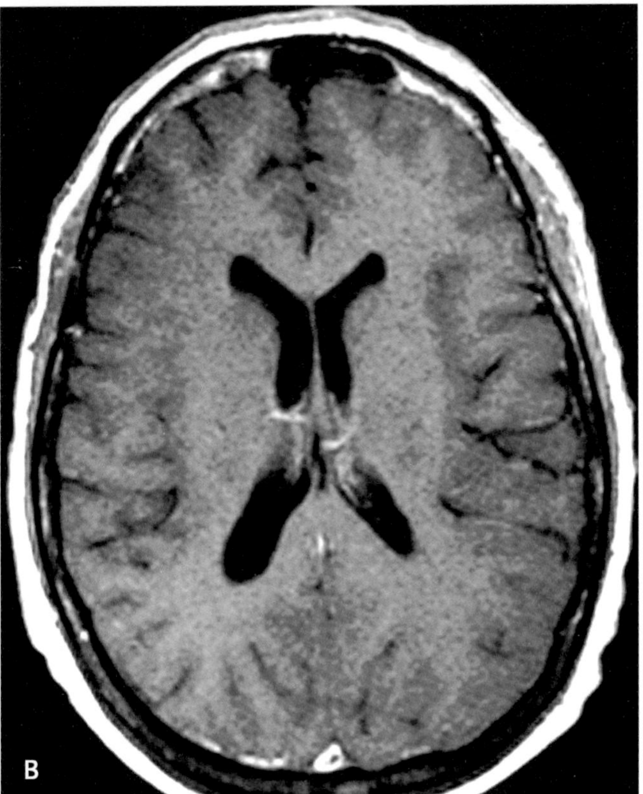

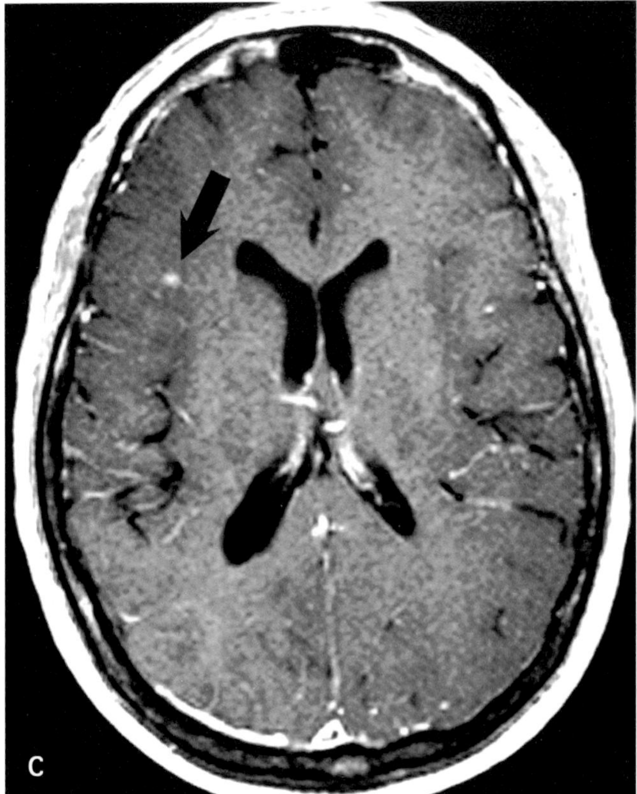

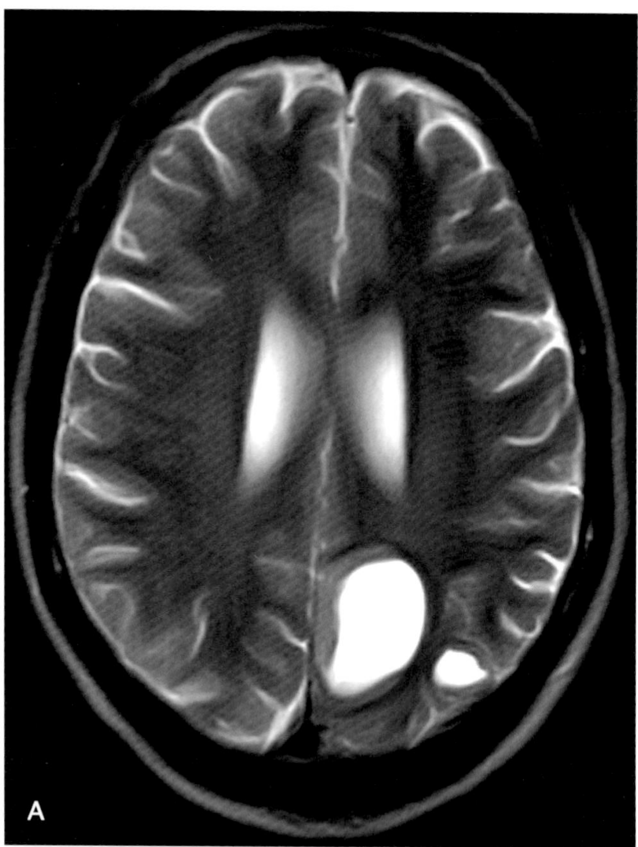

Figure 27. Hemorrhagic brain metastases. (A) The pre-contrast T2-weighted scan reveals two hyperintense lesions. On (B) the pre-contrast T1-weighted scan, the larger of the abnormalities remains hyperintense, while the smaller is difficult to identify. The imaging characteristics are compatible with the presence of two intra-parenchymal hematomas, with slightly different composition. (C) Post-contrast, there is enhancement of abnormal soft tissue along the medial border of the larger lesion, with a thick circumferential rim of enhancement surrounding the smaller lesion. Both abnormalities were confirmed to represent metastatic disease. In the presence of acute and subacute hemorrhage, careful inspection of post-contrast scans is mandated to rule out an underlying abnormality, such as metastatic disease in this instance.

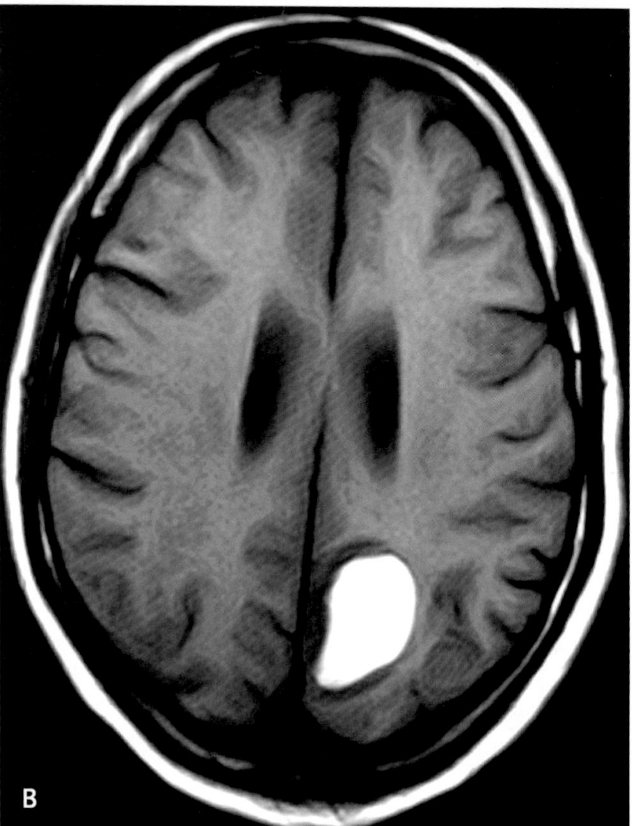

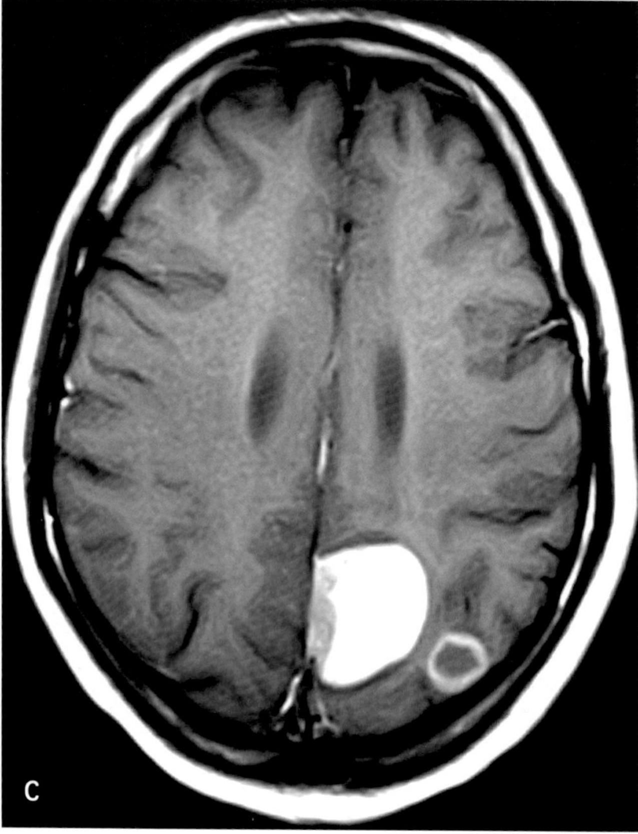

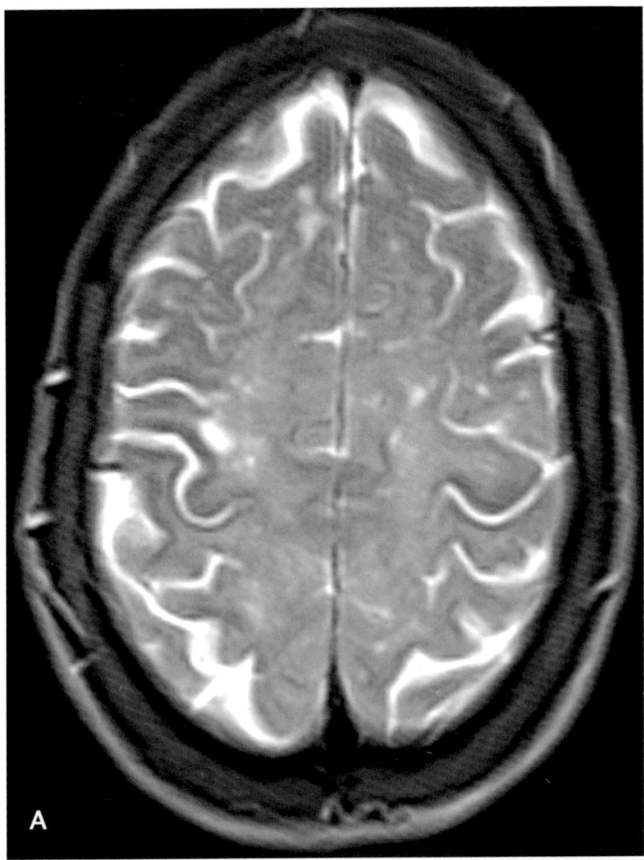

Figure 28. Brain metastases, differentiation from small vessel ischemia. (A) The pre-contrast T2-weighted scan in this elderly patient reveals multiple abnormal, nonspecific high signal intensity foci. (B) The pre-contrast T1-weighted scan is non-contributory. (C) Post-contrast, abnormal enhancement is noted within a single lesion located on the right at the gray-white matter junction. This was subsequently confirmed to be a metastasis. In the older population, chronic ischemic white matter changes can be common and difficult to differentiate from small metastatic lesions without IV contrast administration.

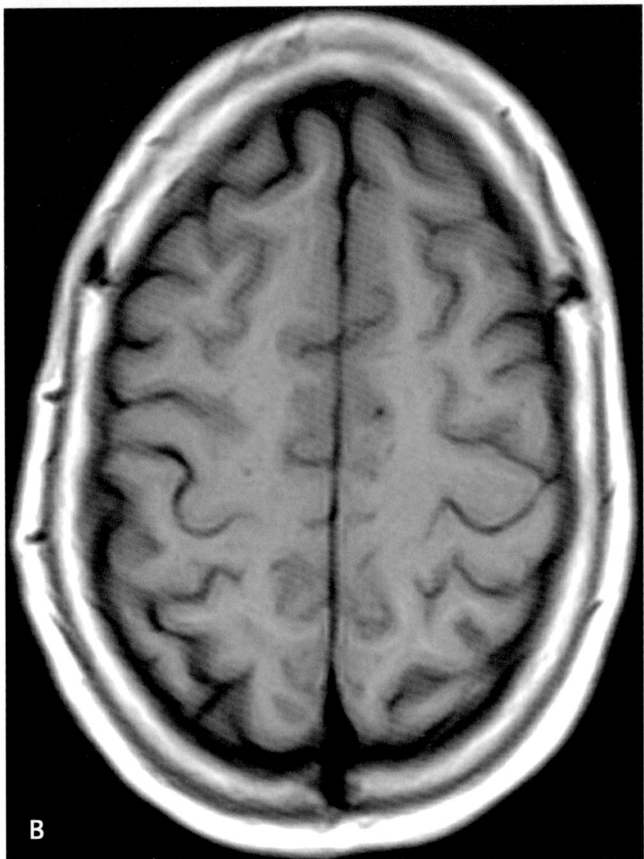

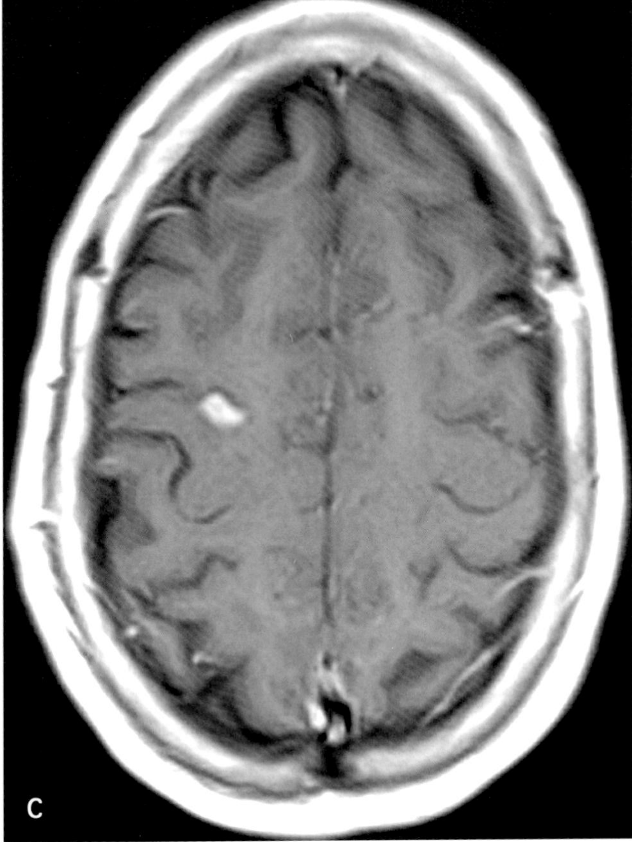

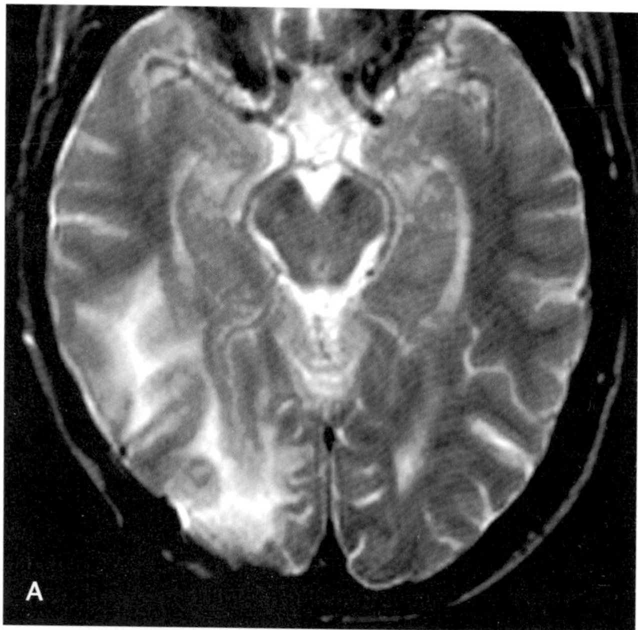

Figure 29. Meningeal carcinomatosis. The patient is one year following surgical resection and whole brain radiation for a right occipital metastasis from breast carcinoma. Abnormal high signal intensity, without a specific focal lesion, is noted in the right parietal and occipital lobes on (A) the pre-contrast T2-weighted scan. No additional information is provided by (B) the pre-contrast T1-weighted scan. (C) Following contrast administration, recurrent tumor is identified, marked by intense enhancement, along the surface of the brain in the right parietal and occipital regions. *(From Runge VM, Brack MA, Garneau RA, Kirsch JE. Magnetic resonance imaging of the brain. Philadelphia, JB Lippincott, 1994).*

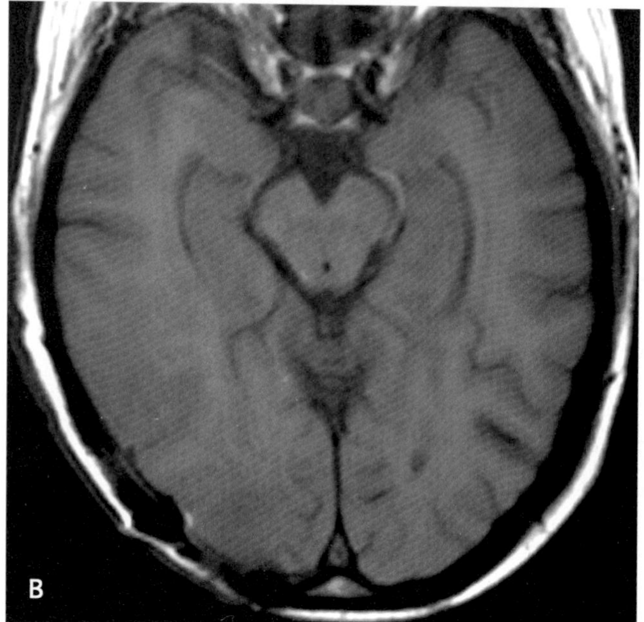

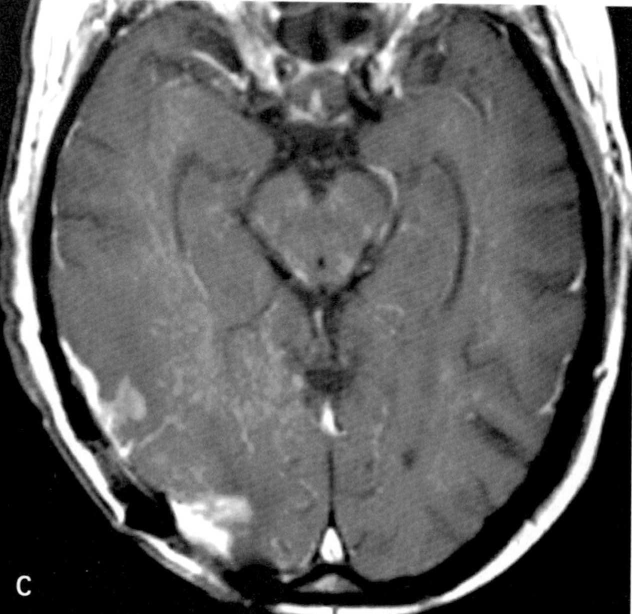

Tumor involvement of the diploic space is most commonly visualized on magnetic resonance imaging due to focal marrow replacement. Lesions demonstrate decreased signal on unenhanced T1-weighted sequences as compared to the higher signal of adjacent normal fat. Pre-contrast images are very important, since MR contrast enhancement may make lesions of the diploic space become isointense with the adjacent fat.[58] If lesions extend to the dura, contrast may facilitate the detection of these metastases by demonstrating abnormal dural enhancement. A careful comparison of the unenhanced study with gadolinium enhanced MR imaging (figure 30) can enable the diagnosis of metastases to the calvarium (and at times the adjacent dura) that might otherwise escape detection.

Not all calvarial lesions represent metastatic disease of course. Correct scan interpretation requires correlative clinical information and construction of an appropriate differential diagnosis (figure 31).

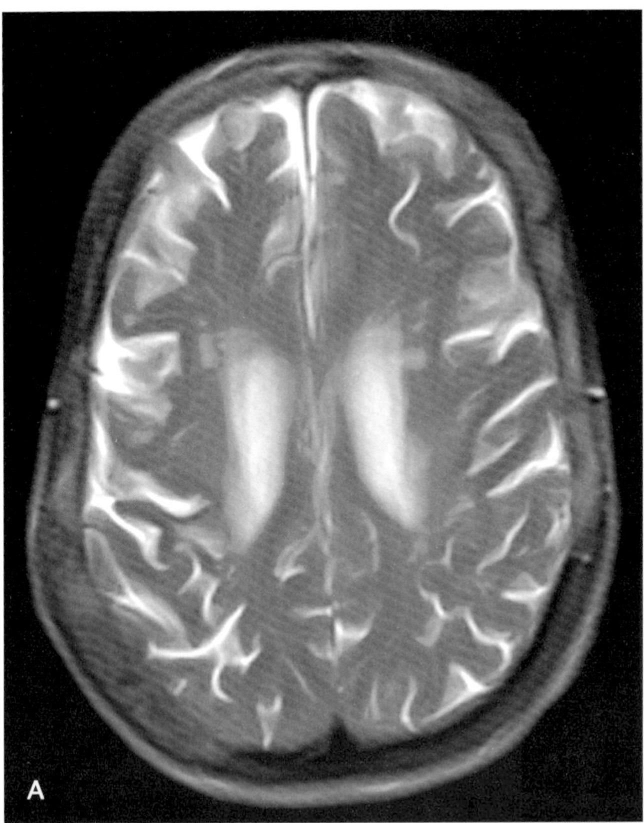

Figure 30. Calvarial metastases. On (A) the pre-contrast T2-weighted scan, there is widening of the diploic space in the right parietal and left frontal regions. On (B) the pre-contrast T1-weighted scan, the marrow space in the left frontal region appears enlarged, and the soft tissue within is of lower signal intensity than normal marrow fat. (C) Post-contrast, there is intense enhancement of soft tissue within the diploic space in the right parietal and left frontal regions, consistent with bony metastatic disease. Contrast administration, as in this case, may improve recognition of metastatic involvement of the diploic space due to intense enhancement of neoplastic tissue. Comparison with pre-contrast scans is mandatory.

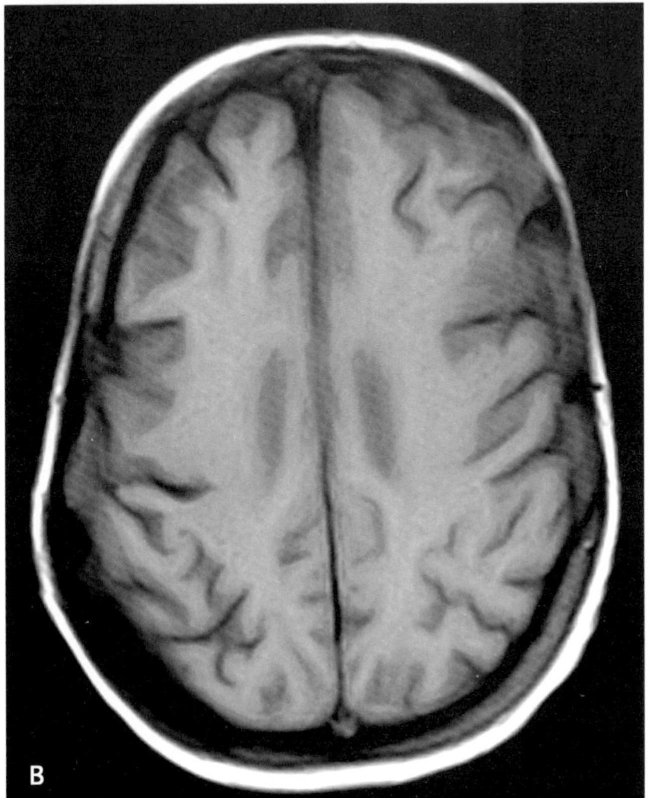

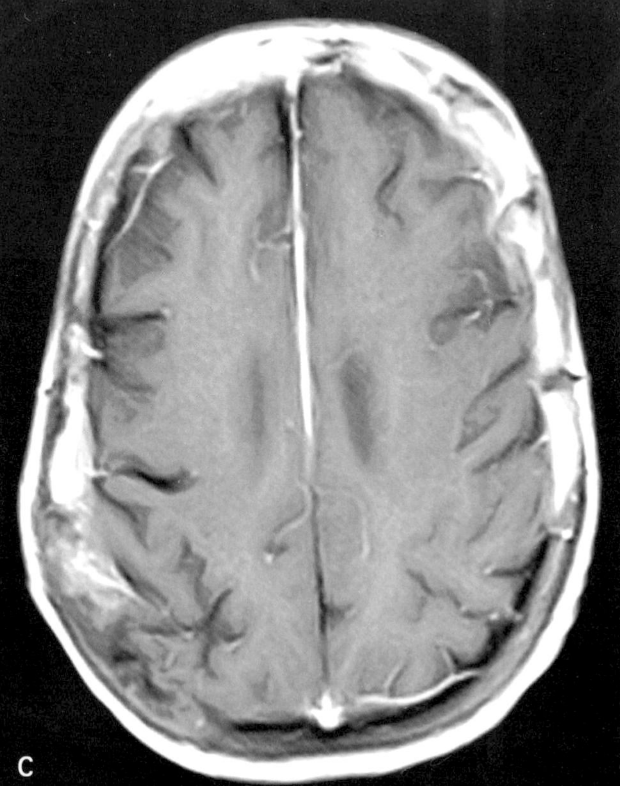

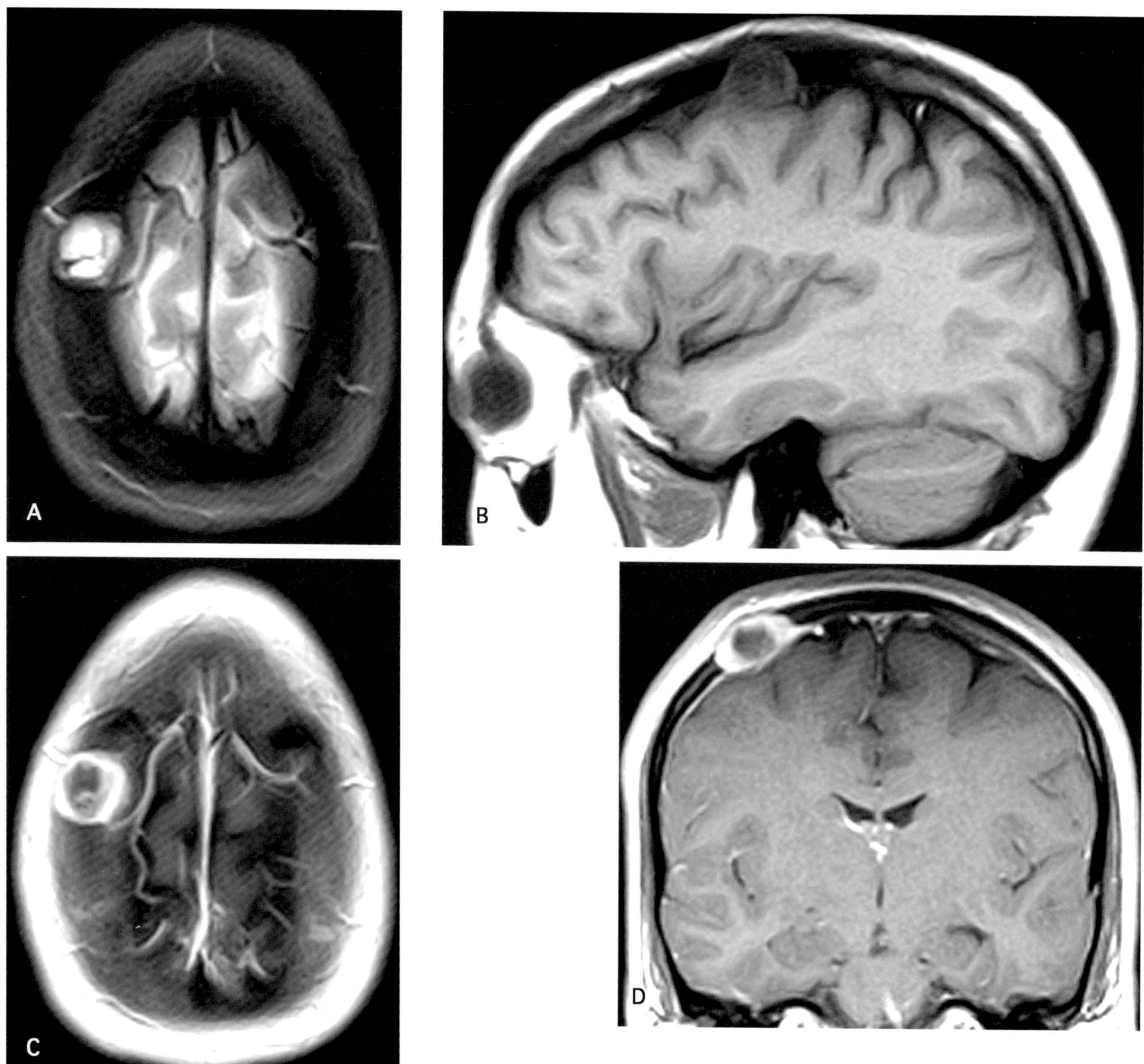

Figure 31. Eosinophilic granuloma. An expansile diploic space lesion is identified on (A) axial T2 and (B) sagittal T1-weighted images. On (C) axial and (D) coronal post-contrast scans, there is a thick peripheral rim of abnormal contrast enhancement. The sagittal and coronal scans demonstrate focal expansion of the diploic space. Differential diagnosis plays an important role in scan interpretation in this instance, with imaging findings (a solitary lesion) and clinical information (a young man with headaches and a "bump" on his head) favoring a diagnosis of eosinophilic granuloma. This was proven on excision.

Neurophakomatoses

Neurofibromatosis Type 1 (von Recklinghausen's Disease)

Neurofibromatosis Type 1 (NF 1) affects one in five thousand births. NF 1 represents an abnormality of chromosome 17. The average age of presentation is three to seven years. The disorder is characterized by cafe-au-lait spots, mesenchymal deformities, and visual pathway gliomas.[59,60,61] These visual pathway gliomas are typically low grade neoplasms that may extend from the optic nerve through the optic chiasm and along the optic tracks. These neoplasms rarely enhance with contrast administration. Optic nerve gliomas and optic sheath meningiomas can have a similar appearance.

However, with gliomas the optic nerve appears enlarged and ectatic, while the major finding with meningioma is that of a straightened, more rigid appearing optic nerve. About twenty percent of these visual pathway gliomas tend to be more aggressive. Thus, it has been recommended that children with this diagnosis be followed with MR imaging one year after the initial diagnosis to assess for tumor aggressiveness.[62] Other brain and spinal tumors can be seen in patients with NF 1, although an increased incidence of spinal tumors is much more commonly associated with patients who have Neurofibromatosis Type 2. Finally, with NF 1 there may be abnormal areas of increased signal intensity seen on T2-weighted images in the diencephalon and upper brainstem. These lesions are non-neoplastic and have been referred to as hamartomas. They may represent areas of late myelination or dysmyelination.

Neurofibromatosis Type 2

Neurofibromatosis Type 2 (NF 2) is a much less common disorder than NF 1, affecting approximately one in fifty thousand births. This condition relates to an abnormality of chromosome 22. Classically, these patients are noted to have bilateral acoustic schwannomas, although they also have a higher incidence of other brain and spinal cord tumors (figure 32). Thus, these patients can present with intracranial gliomas, meningiomas, and cranial nerve schwannomas, as well as ependymomas, meningiomas, and neurofibromas of the spinal cord. The occurrence of meningioma in a child or young adult should raise the question of NF 2. Because of the common association with CNS tumors, it is recommended that patients with NF 2 be examined by MR imaging on an annual basis to assess for both intracranial and spinal tumors. Contrast enhanced imaging can be most helpful in the detection of these lesions.

Tuberous Sclerosis

Tuberous sclerosis is an autosomal dominant condition seen with a frequency of one in twenty thousand births. Affected children present with mental retardation, seizures, and sebaceous adenomas of the nasolabial region.[63]

Subependymal and cortical hamartomas are the hallmarks of tuberous sclerosis. These hamartomas (tubers) are most commonly located between the caudate nuclei and the bodies of the lateral ventricles. They range in size from a few millimeters to over one centimeter. In younger patients, they may be mistaken for areas of heterotopic gray matter. As patients become older, this differentiation is more easily made (particularly by CT) because of the tendency of the tubers to calcify.

Subependymal hamartomas may degenerate into giant cell astrocytomas. While these are usually low grade lesions, they may develop into more aggressive tumors. MR contrast may be helpful in diagnosing giant cell astrocytomas since these lesions tend to enhance while tubers usually show little or no contrast enhancement. Giant cell astrocytomas can cause obstructive hydrocephalus, because of their common location near the foramen of Monro (figure 33). Because the lesions usually have a relatively benign course, often affected patients may be shunted without removal of the tumor, although tumor removal may now be the treatment of choice.[64]

The Post-Therapy Patient

Changes secondary to surgery or radiation therapy can cause findings on imaging studies that are identical to residual or recurrent tumor. Contrast enhanced studies are helpful in the evaluation of the post-treatment brain tumor patient (figure 34). However, both surgical and radiation induced change can enhance in a manner similar to that of neoplasm.[65,66]

It is best to image a post-operative patient within the first four days post-surgery. This minimizes the problems with differentiating residual tumor from the surgical reparative process (this process will not be evident on MR imaging within the first four post-operative days). However, blood from the surgical procedure may make interpretation of the early post-operative scan difficult, and it is very important to obtain both pre- and post-contrast images to facilitate correct diagnoses. Within a week or two post-surgery, there can be extensive enhancement along the margin of the resection. Without a baseline study it can be extremely difficult to distinguish this benign surgically induced change from residual tumor.[67,68]

Radiation injury is usually a delayed phenomenon that most often takes many months to become manifest. This delayed necrosis is a serious complication of radiotherapy. Brain tissue is replaced by a tumefactive mass, which demonstrates enhancement post-contrast (figure 35), and can resemble an aggressive glioma. Edema and cavitation can occur.[69,70] Differentiation of tumor from radiation necrosis can be impossible on both CT and MR imaging. Positron emission tomography can effectively differentiate these entities since gliomas are associated with increased metabolic activity while radiation necrosis has decreased metabolism.[71] However, access to PET scanners is limited, reimbursement from third party payers is variable, and thus this modality is not optimally utilized.

Conclusion

MR plays an important role in both the diagnosis and management of patients with brain tumors. It can define the lo-

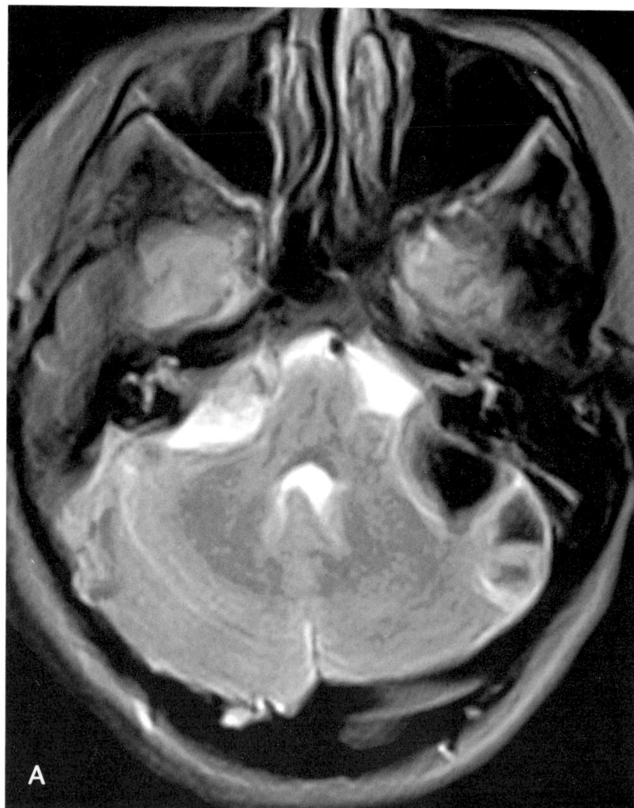

Figure 32. Neurofibromatosis type 2. (A) The pre-contrast T2-weighted scan reveals abnormal hypointensity within the posterior fossa on the left along the petrous apex (due to dense calcification). The question of a right cerebellopontine angle (CPA) soft tissue mass is also raised. Bilateral soft tissue masses, at the CPA, are questioned on the basis of (B) the pre-contrast T1-weighted scan. (C) Post-contrast, at least four lesions are identified, which include bilateral acoustic neuromas and two dural based meningiomas.

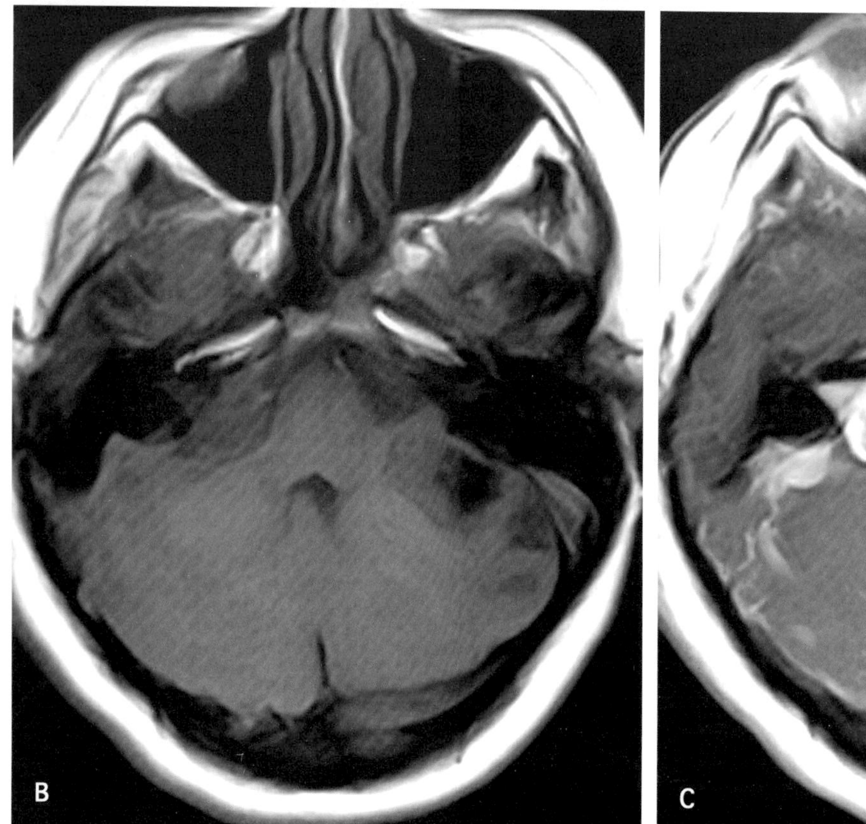

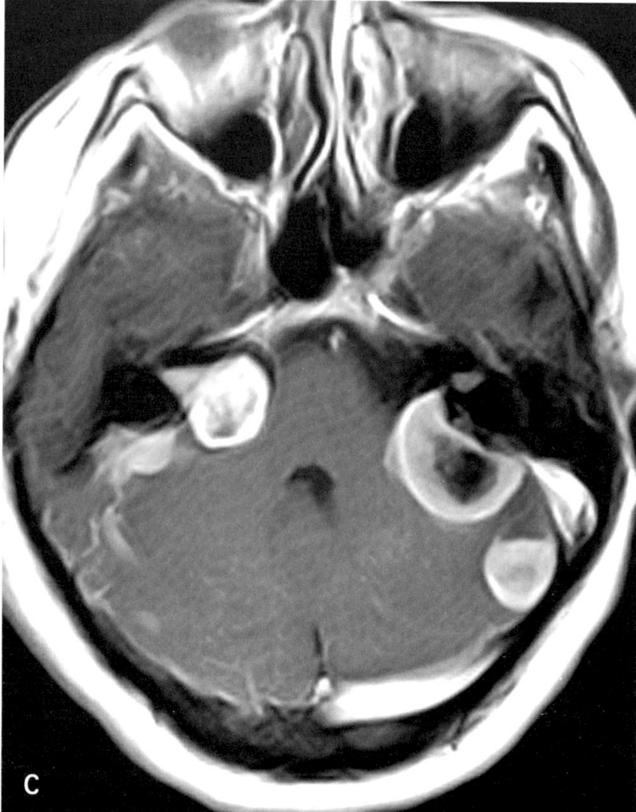

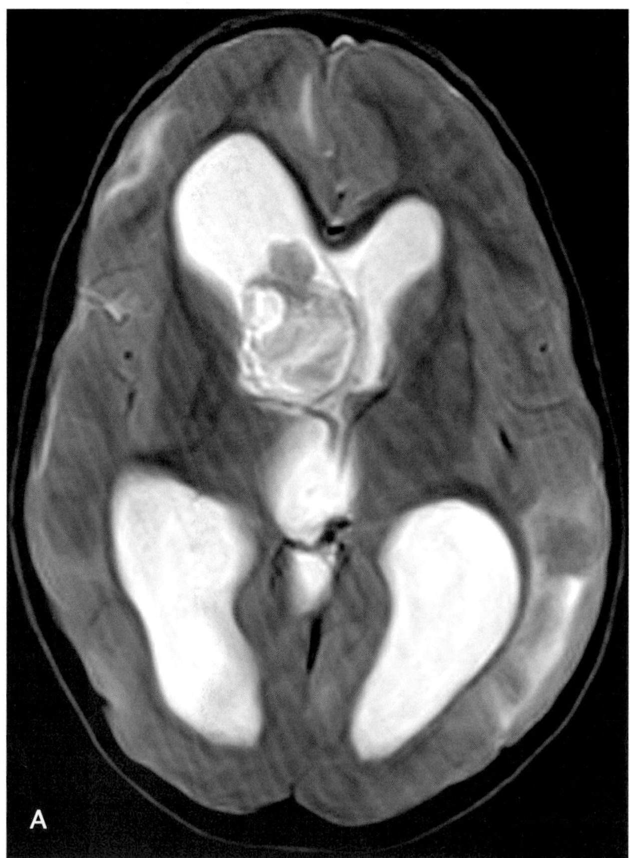

Figure 33. Subependymal giant cell astrocytoma. On (A) the T2-weighted scan, an intraventricular mass is noted at the level of the foramen of Monro. There is ventricular enlargement. The mass is isointense with brain on (B) the pre-contrast T1-weighted scan. (C) Post-contrast, there is intense lesion enhancement. Recognition of abnormal parenchymal hyperintensity on the T2-weighted exam (most prominent in the left parietal region) aids in diagnosis, suggesting tuberous sclerosis with a giant cell astrocytoma causing obstruction of the lateral ventricles.

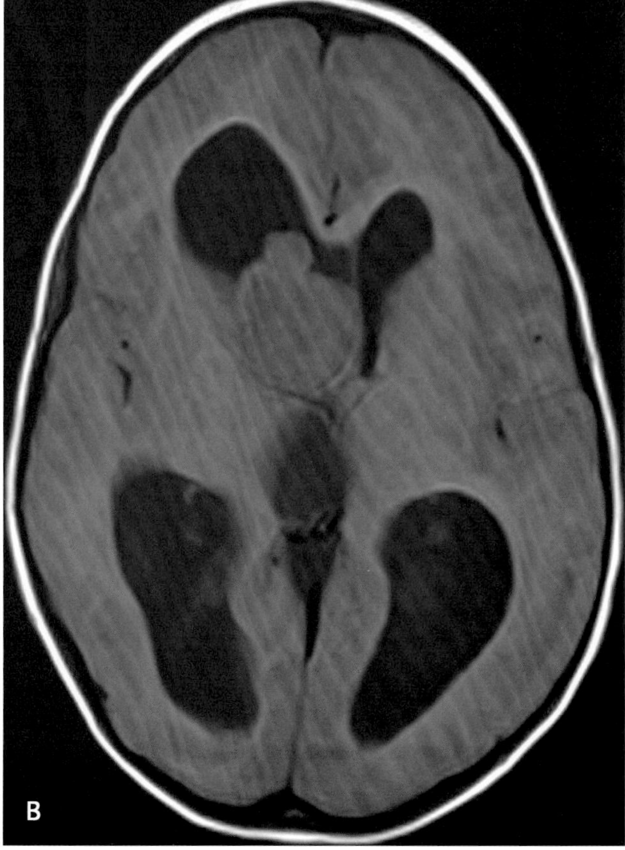

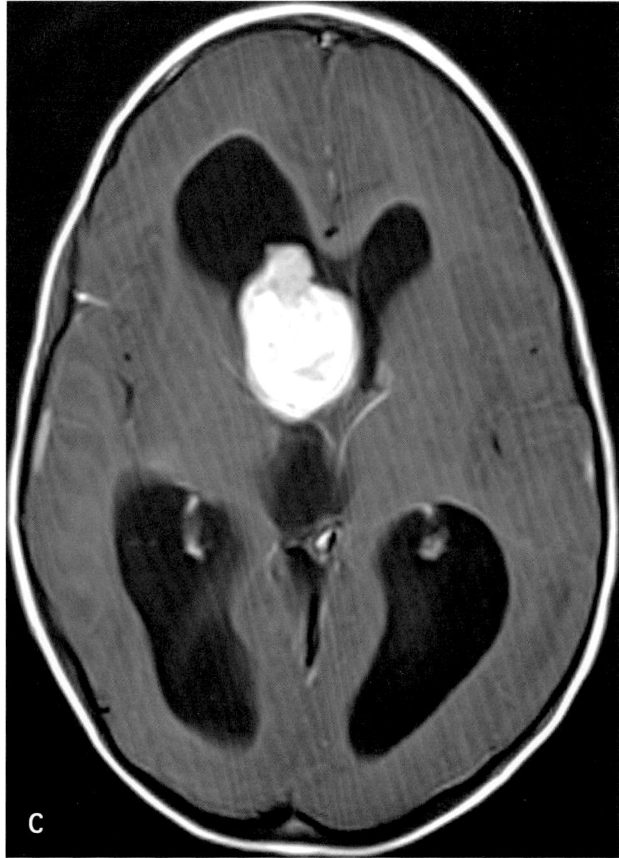

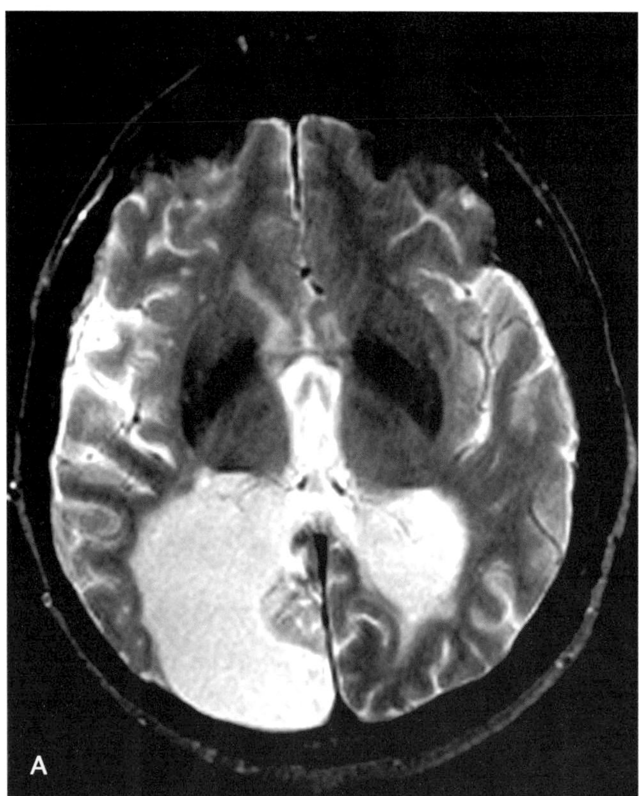

Figure 34. Recurrent astrocytoma. A large post-surgical defect, communicating with the atria of the right lateral ventricle, is noted on pre-contrast (A) T2 and (B) T1-weighted scans. The exam was performed to rule out tumor recurrence in this elderly patient with resection of a glioma four years earlier. Medial to the post-surgical defect is soft tissue with signal intensity similar to that of normal brain. The question of tumor recurrence is raised by the slight hyperintensity of this soft tissue on the pre-contrast T1-weighted scan. (C) Following contrast administration, there is intense enhancement, making possible definitive diagnosis of recurrent tumor. *(From Runge VM, Brack MA, Garneau RA, Kirsch JE. Magnetic resonance imaging of the brain. Philadelphia, JB Lippincott, 1994).*

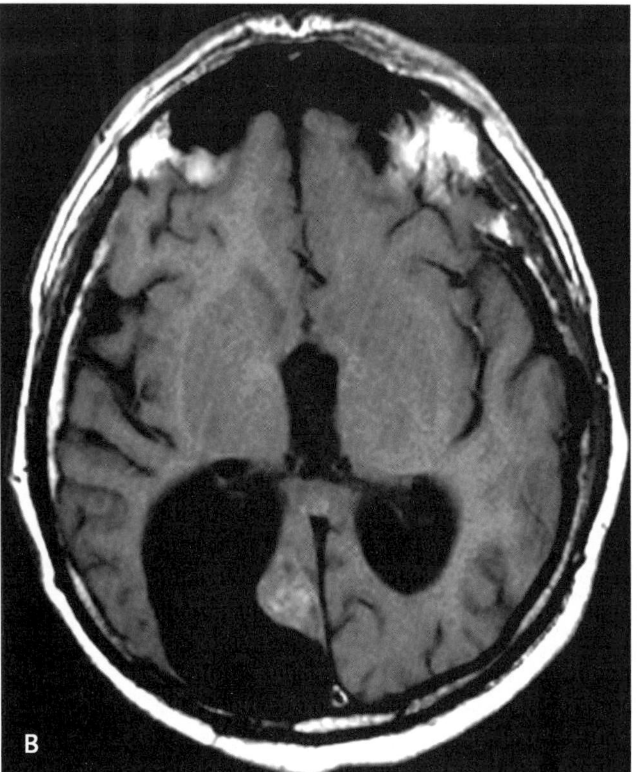

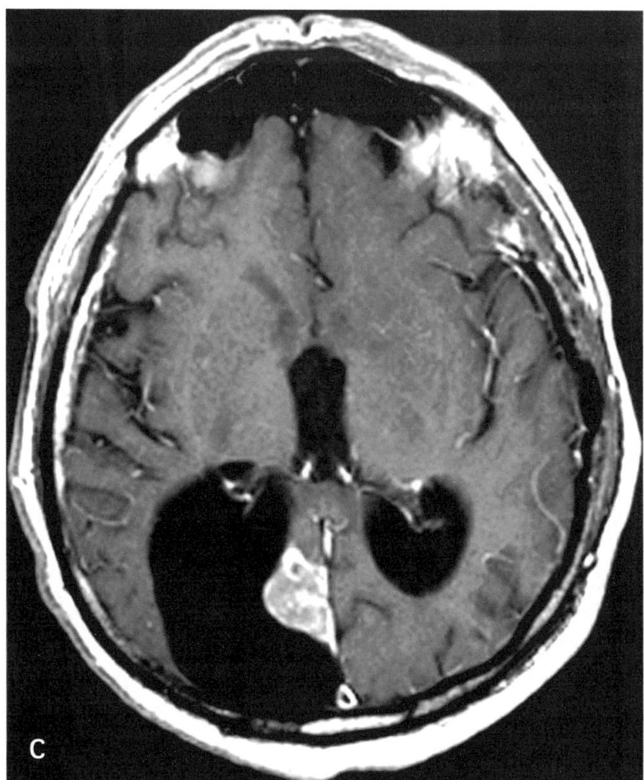

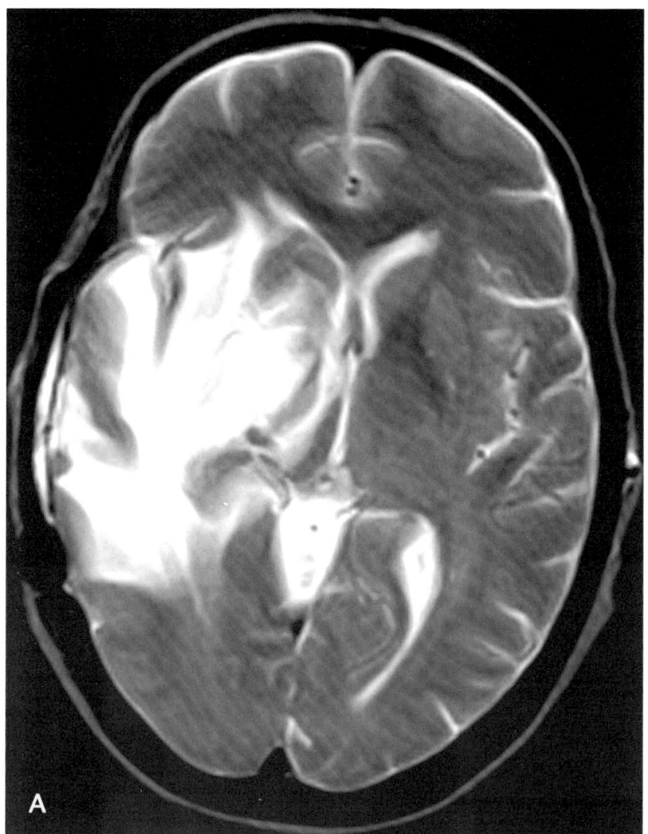

Figure 35. Radiation necrosis. Extensive edema, with moderate mass effect, is identified on (A) the T2-weighted scan. Comparison of (B) pre- and (C) post-contrast T1-weighted scans reveals abnormal contrast enhancement centrally. On histologic exam, this represented a combination of tumor recurrence (astrocytoma) and radiation necrosis. The appearance is typical for radiation necrosis, with a central enhancing mass and surrounding vasogenic edema. Recurrent tumor cannot be differentiated by conventional imaging alone, either CT or MR, from radiation necrosis.

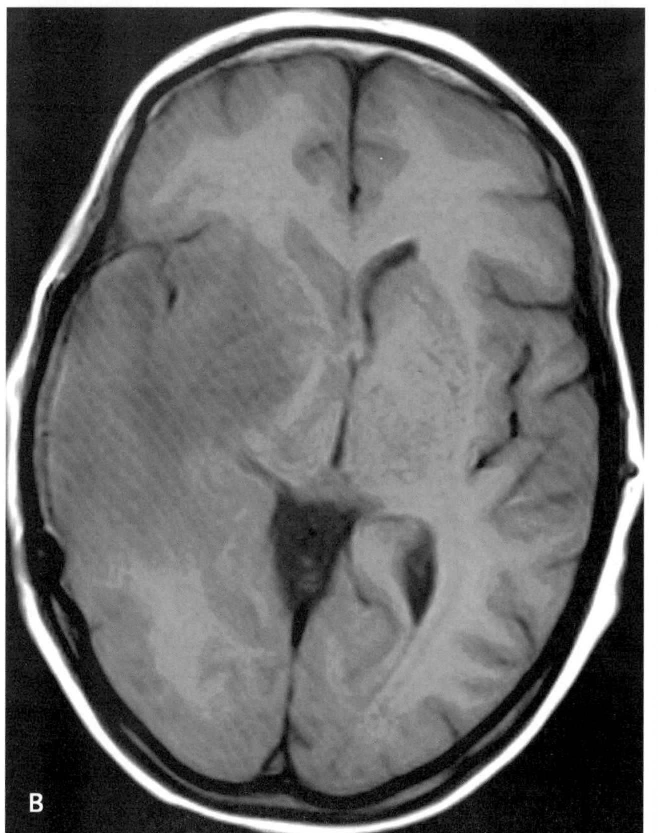

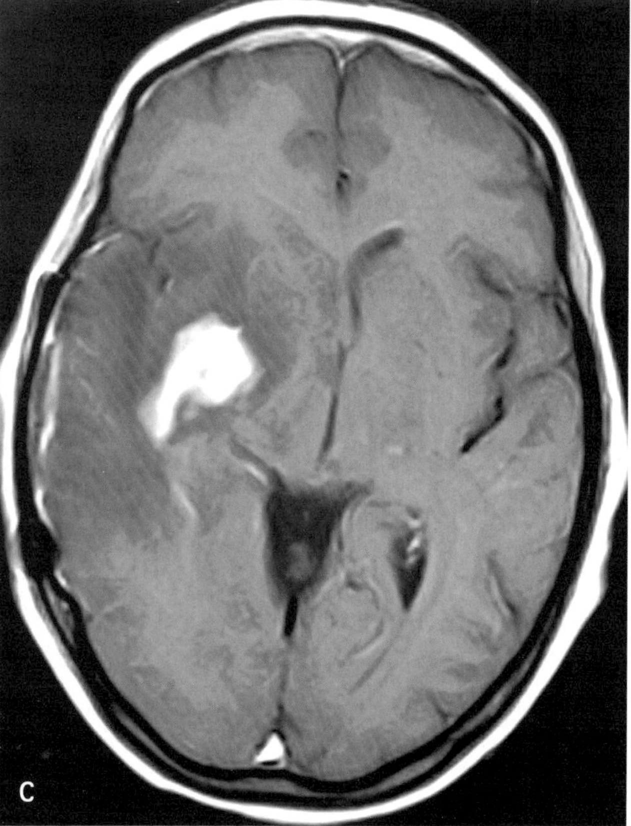

cation and the extent of neoplastic involvement, as well as establish the relationship of the tumor to normal adjacent structures. Contrast agents provide increased diagnostic sensitivity and specificity. Imaging with MR contrast can also establish whether a tumor is well circumscribed or infiltrative. Biopsy sites can be defined more appropriately, and the surgical decision-making can be facilitated by the anatomical information available. For example, the patency of the sagittal sinus or the location of the motor strip in relationship to the tumor can be better established by contrast enhanced MR. Newer developments such as MR angiography (MRA) and functional MR imaging may add significantly to the efficacy of conventional MR.

MR, and in particular contrast enhanced MR, have important cost containment consequences. Unnecessary surgery can be avoided when multiple lesions are demonstrated in patients with metastatic disease. Appropriate therapy can be more readily instituted when both the extent of tumor involvement and its relationship to normal structures are adequately demonstrated. Contrast enhanced MR imaging often is the only way to demonstrate leptomeningeal tumor involvement. In an era of cost containment and limited resources, optimum patient care demands accurate and timely diagnostic information. MR imaging, and contrast enhanced MR in selected patient populations, provides the sensitivity, lesion delineation, and characterization that is essential for time-efficient diagnosis and cost-effective patient management.

References

1. Runge VM, Gelblum DY. The role of gadolinium diethylenetriaminepentacetic acid in the evaluation of the central nervous system. Magn Reson Q 1990;2:85-107.

2. Muroff LR. MR contrast agents for the CNS. In: Bradley WG, Muroff LR, eds. MR of non-neoplastic disease in the brain. Tampa: Gilham Press, 1994:1-7.

3. Tweedle MF. Physico-chemical properties of gadoteridol and other magnetic resonance contrast agents. Invest Rad 1992;27:S2-6.

4. Wedeking P, Kumar K, Tweedle MF. Dissociation of gadolinium chelates in mice: relationship to chemical characteristics. Magn Reson Imaging 1992;10:641-648.

5. Muroff LR. Normal enhancement patterns and the role of contrast in non-neoplastic disease in the brain. In: Bradley WG, Muroff LR, eds. MR of non-neoplastic disease in the brain. Tampa: Gilham Press, 1994:73-82.

6. Burke JW, Podrasky AE, Bradley WG. Meninges: benign postoperative enhancement on MR images. Radiology 1990;1174:99-102.

7. Yuh WTC, Tali ET, Nguyen H, et al. Application of delayed imaging and dose increment in the evaluation of CNS metastatic disease. Proceedings of the Thirtieth Annual Meeting of the American Society of Neuroradiology 1992.

8. Levin VA, Gutin PH, Leibel S. Neoplasms of the central nervous system. In: DeVita VT, Hellman S, Rosenberg SA, eds. Cancer: principles of practice and oncology. Philadelphia: J.B. Lippincott Company, 1993:1679-1737.

9. Atlas SW. Adult supratentorial tumors. Semin Roentgenol 1990;25:130-154.

10. Muroff LR. Supratentorial brain tumors in adults. In: Bradley WG, Muroff LR, eds. MR of brain tumors and tumor mimics. Tampa: Gilham Press, 1994:28-39.

11. Muller W, Afra D, Schroder R. Supratentorial recurrances of gliomas. Morphological studies in relation to time intervals with astrocytomas. Acta Neurochir 1977;37:75-91.

12. Earnest F, Kelly PJ, Scheithauer BW, et al. Cerebral astrocytomas: histopathologic correlation of MR and CT contrast enhancement with stereotactic biopsy. Radiology 1988;166:823-827.

13. Runge VM, Kirsch JE, Burke VJ, et al. High-dose gadoteridol in MR imaging in intracranial neoplasms. J Magn Reson Imaging 1992;2:9-18.

14. Yuh WTC, Fisher DJ, Engelken JD, et al. MR evaluation of CNS tumors, dose comparison study with Gd-DTPA and gadoteridol. Radiology 1991;180:485-491.

15. Yuh WTC, Engelken JD, Muhonen MG, et al. Experience with high-dose gadolinium MR imaging in the evaluation of brain metastases. AJNR 1992;13:335-345.

16. Kernahan JW, Sayre GP. Tumors of the central nervous system. In: Atlas of tumor pathology. Washington, DC: Armed Forces Institute of Pathology, 1952: section 10; fascicle 35.

17. Zulch KJ. Principles of the new World Health Organization (WHO) classification of brain tumors. Neuroradiol 1980;19:59-66.

18. Lee YY, Tassel PV, Brunner JJ, et al. Juvenile pilocytic astrocytomas: CT and MR characteristics. AJNR 1989;10:363-370.

19. Grossman RI, Yousem DM. Neoplasms of the brain. In: Grossman RI, Yousem DM, eds. Neuroradiology — the requisites. St. Louis: Mosby-Yearbook Inc., 1994:67-104.

20. Vignaud J, Bocquet M, Aubin ML, et al. NMR imaging of intraaxial tumors of the posterior fossa. J Neuroradiol 1984;11:249-261.

21. Mork SJ, Lindegaard KF, Halvorsen TB, et al. Oligodendroglioma: incidence and biological behavior in a defined population. J Neurosurg 1985;63:881-889.

22. Lee YY, Tassel PV. Intracranial oligodendrogliomas: imaging findings in 35 untreated cases. AJNR 1989;10:119-127.

23. Atlas SW, Grossman RI, Hackney DB, et al. Calcified intracranial lesions: detection with gradient echo-acquisition rapid MR imaging. AJNR 1988;9:253-259.

24. Castillo M, Davis P, Takel Y, et al. Intracranial ganglioglioma: MR, CT, and clinical findings in 18 patients. AJNR 1990;11:109-114.

25. Cohen BH, Bury E, Packer RJ, et al. Gadolinium-DTPA-enhanced magnetic resonance imaging in childhood brain tumors. Neurology 1989;39:1178-1183.

26. Kucharczyk W, Brant-Zawadzki M, Sobel D, et al. Central nervous system tumors in children: detection by magnetic resonance imaging. Radiology 1985;155:131-136.

27. Spoto GP, Press GA, Hesselink JR, Solomon M. Intracranial ependymoma and subependymoma: MR manifestations. AJNR 1990;11:83-91.

28. Hasso AN, Fahmy JL, Hinshaw DB. Tumors of the posterior fossa. In: Stark DD, Bradley WG, eds. Magnetic resonance imaging. St Louis: Mosby, 1988:425-450.

29. Bradley WG. Pediatric brain tumors. In: Bradley WG, Muroff LR, eds. MR of brain tumors and tumor mimics. Tampa: Gilham Press, 1994:90-101.

30. Figueroa RE, El Gammal T, Brook BS, et al. MR findings in

primitive neuroectodermal tumors. J Comput Assist Tomogr 1989;13:773-778.
31. Koci TM, Chiang F, Mehringer CM, et al. Adult cerebellar medulloblastoma: imaging features with emphasis on MR findings. AJNR 1993;14:929-939.
32. Lee YY, Bruner JM, Tassel PV, Libshitz HI. Primary central nervous system lymphoma, CT and pathologic correlation. AJR 1986;147:747-752.
33. Poon T, Matoso I, Tchertkoff V, et al. CT features of primary cerebral lymphoma in AIDS and non-AIDS patients. J Comput Assist Tomogr 1989;13:6-9.
34. Schwaighofer BW, Hesselink JR, Press GA, et al. Primary intracranial CNS lymphoma: MR manifestations. AJNR 1989;10:725-729.
35. Hasso AN, Kortman KE, Bradley WG. Supratentorial neoplasms. In: Stark DD, Bradley WG, eds. Magnetic resonance imaging. St. Louis: Mosby-Yearbook Inc., 1992:770-818.
36. Dina TS. Primary central nervous system lymphoma vs toxoplasmosis in AIDS. Radiology 1991;179:823-828.
37. Jackson A, Panizza BJ, Hughes D, Reid H. Primary choroid plexus papilloma of the cerebellopontine angle: magnetic resonance imaging, computed tomographic, and angiographic appearances. Br J Radiol 1992;65:754-757.
38. Stack, JP, Ramsden RT, Antoun NM, et al. Magnetic resonance imaging of acoustic neuromas: the role of gadolinium DTPA. Br J Radiol 1988;61:800-805.
39. Cass SP, Kartush JM, Wilner HI, Graham MD. Comparison of computerized tomography and magnetic resonance imaging for postoperative assessment of residual acoustic tumor. Otolaryngol Head Neck Surg 1991;104:182-190.
40. Huson SM, Harper PS, Hourihan MD, et al. Cerebellar hemangioblastoma and von Hippel-Lindau disease. Brain 1986;109:1297-1310.
41. Hubschmann OR, Vijayanathan T, Countee RW. Von Hippel-Lindau disease with multiple manifestations: diagnosis and management. Neurosurgery 1981;8:92-95.
42. Rosenbaum AE, Rosenbloom SB. Meningiomas revisited. Semin Roentgenol 1984;19:8-26.
43. Haughton VM, Rimm AA, Czervionke LF, et al. Sensitivity of Gd-DTPA-enhanced MR imaging of benign extraaxial tumors. Radiology 1988;166:829-833.
44. Elster AD, Challa VR, Gilbert TH, et al. Meningiomas: MR and histopathologic features. Radiology 1989;170:857-862.
45. Goldberg HI. Extraaxial brain tumors. In: Atlas SW, ed. Magnetic resonance imaging of the brain and spine. New York: Raven Press, 1991:327-378.
46. Freeman MP, Kessler RM, Allen JH, Price AC. Craniopharyngioma: CT and MR imaging in 9 cases. J Comput Assist Tomogr 1987;11:810-814.
47. Zimmerman RA. Imaging of intrasellar, suprasellar, and parasellar tumors. Semin Roentgenol 1990;25:174-197.
48. Newton DR, Dillon WP, Norman D, et al. Gd-DTPA-enhanced MR imaging of pituitary adenomas. AJNR 1989;10:949-954.
49. Doppman JL, Frank JA, Dwyer AJ, et al. Gadolinium DTPA enhanced MR imaging of ACTH-secreting microadenomas of the pituitary gland. J Comput Assist Tomogr 1988;12:728-735.
50. Davis PC, Gokhale KA, Joseph GJ, et al. Pituitary adenoma: correlation of half-dose gadolinium enhanced MR imaging with surgical findings in 26 patients. Radiology 1991;180:779-784.
51. Atlas SW. Intraaxial brain tumors. In: Atlas SW, ed. Magnetic resonance imaging of the brain and spine. New York: Raven Press, 1991:223-326.
52. Wilson CB. Epidermoid cysts of the posterior fossa. J Neurosurg 1985;62:214-219.
53. Vieth RG, Odom GL. Intracranial metastases and their neurosurgical treatment. J Neurosurg 1965;23:375-383.
54. Healy ME, Hesselink JR, Press GA, Middleton GS. Increased detection of intracranial metastases with intravenous Gd-DTPA. Radiology 1987;165:619-624.
55. Sze G, Milano E, Johnson C, Heier L. Detection of brain metastases: Comparison of contrast enhanced MR with unenhanced MR and enhanced CT. AJNR 1990;11:785-791.
56. Davis PC, Friedman NC, Fry SN, et al. Leptomeningeal metastases: MR imaging. Radiology 1987;163:449-454.
57. Zimmerman RA. Pediatric supratentorial tumors. Semin Roentgenol 1990;25:225-248.
58. West, MS, Russell, EJ, Breit R, et al. Calvarial and skull base metastases: Comparison of non-enhanced and Gd-DTPA-enhanced MR images. Radiology 1990;174:85-91.
59. Byrd SE. Central nervous system manifestations of inherited syndromes. In: Atlas SW, ed. Magnetic resonance imaging of the brain and spine. New York: Raven Press, 1991:539-566.
60. Braffman BH, Bilaniuk LT, Zimmerman RA. The central nervous system manifestations of the phakomatoses on MR. Radiol Clin North Am 1988;26:773-800.
61. Braffman BH, Bilaniuk LT, Zimmerman RA. MR of central nervous system neoplasia of the phakomatoses. Semin Roentgenol 1990;25:198-217.
62. Elster AD. Neurofibromatosis. AJNR 1992;13:1071-1077.
63. Morris JH. The nervous system. In: Cotran RS, Kumar V, Robbins SL, eds. Robbins pathologic basis of disease. Philadelphia: WB Saunders, 1989:1385-1449.
64. Nagib MG, Haines SJ, Erickson DL, et al. Tuberous sclerosis: a review for the neurosurgeon. Neurosurgery 1984;14:93-98.
65. Sherman JL. Evaluation of the post-operative brain. In: Bradley WG, Muroff LR, eds. MR of brain tumors and tumor mimics. Tampa: Gilham Press, 1994:14-27.
66. Hudgins PA, Davis PC, Hoffman JC. Gadopentetate dimeglumine enhanced MR imaging in children following surgery for brain tumor: spectrum of meningeal findings. AJNR 1991;12:301-307.
67. Forsting M, Albert F, Kunze S, et al. Extirpation of glioblastoma: MR and CT followup of residual tumor and regrowth patterns. AJNR 1993;14:77-87.
68. Forsting M, Albert F, Sartor K. Baseline CT and MR after brain resection: prognostic value [abstract]. American Society of Neuroradiology Annual Meeting, June 1991:29.
69. Volk PE, Dillon WP. Radiation injury of the brain. AJNR 1991;12:45-52.
70. Tsuruda JS, Kortman, KE, Bradley WG, et al. Radiation effects on cerebral white matter: MR evaluation. AJNR 1987;8:431-437.
71. Schwartz RB, Carvalho PA, Alexander E, et al. Radiation necrosis versus recurrent glomia: Dual-isotope SPECT. AJNR 1991;12:1187-1192.

Chapter 3

Brain: Non-Neoplastic Disease

Val M. Runge, M.D.

Introduction

Intravenous contrast use in magnetic resonance (MR) was first clinically evaluated in neoplastic disease of the brain. Subsequent trials included non-neoplastic disease, with widespread applications quickly noted. Today, contrast use in MR is as important in non-neoplastic disease of the brain as in neoplastic disease. This chapter describes the utility of contrast administration and the patterns of abnormal enhancement in infection, vascular disorders (arteriovenous malformations and infarction), diseases of white matter, and trauma. Contrast enhancement assumes a prominent position in the routine clinical evaluation by MR of non-neoplastic disease, with advances in instrumentation driving additional new applications including the assessment of brain perfusion.

Infection

Toxoplasmosis is an important pathogen in patients with compromise of the immune system. It is also the most common intracranial infection in the acquired immunodeficiency syndrome (AIDS). Ineffective cell-mediated immunity permits reactivation of latent infection, and results in a more fulminant acquired infection. 25% to 75% of the US population have been exposed to toxoplasmosis, with chronic seropositive antibody titers. Lesions are commonly located in the basal ganglia and at the gray-white matter junction in the cerebral hemispheres.[1] Post-contrast, nodular or ring enhancement is noted on MR (figure 1). Surrounding edema, best seen on T2 weighted images, is common. Contrast administration plays an important role in differential diagnosis and assessment of disease activity. In the immunocompromised patient, with multiple ring enhancing brain lesions, lymphoma should also be considered in differential diagnosis.[2] Contrast administration in human immunodeficiency virus (HIV) positive patients is particularly useful in disease characterization, detection of meningeal pathology, and patient management.[3,4]

In both the immunocompromised and immunocompetent populations, it is important to consider other organisms in differential diagnosis. With *mycobacterium tuberculosis*, involvement both of the leptomeninges and the brain parenchyma, the latter as granulomas, can occur. Important fungal infections to consider include cryptococcosis (figure 2), coccidioidomycosis, and histoplasmosis. Parasitic infections, in addition to toxoplasmosis, include amebiasis and cysticercosis (figure 3).

Herpes simplex virus type 1 (HSV-1) is the most common cause of viral encephalitis in the US. HSV-1 causes cold sores in the mouth, with nearly every adult exposed. Brain involvement results from reactivation of latent infection in the trigeminal ganglion. The virus then spreads along branches of the trigeminal nerve (cranial nerve V) as it innervates the meninges of the anterior and middle cranial fossae. Thus HSV-1 most commonly affects the temporal and inferior frontal lobes. Early diagnosis, best made by MR,[5] and treatment[6] are critical to prevent substantial morbidity and mortality. Abnormal high signal intensity on T2 weighted scans in the cortex and white matter of involved areas is seen as early as the second day following onset. Unilateral involvement is common initially, with bilateral involvement not unusual. Post-contrast scans can show meningeal inflammation (figure 4),[7] and less commonly parenchymal enhancement.

The use of a gadolinium chelate for improved lesion detection in the brain, and indeed the superiority of enhanced MR over enhanced computed tomography (CT), was first demonstrated in a brain abscess model.[8] In this study, it was also shown that early parenchymal infection is best detected on MR following contrast administration. New lesions may go unrecognized on pre-contrast T1 and T2 images alone.

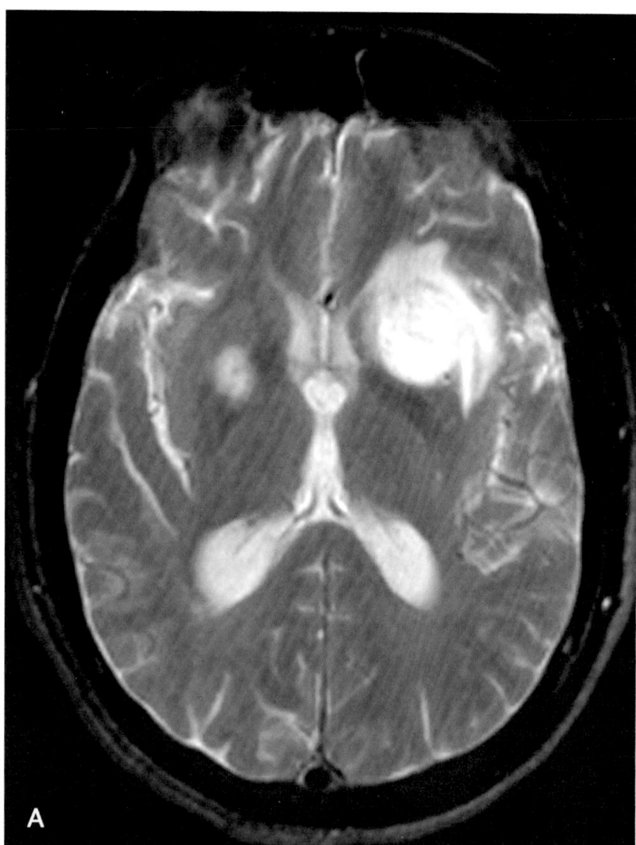

Figure 1. Toxoplasmosis. Bilateral high signal intensity abnormalities are noted in the basal ganglia on (A) the T2 weighted scan. Comparison of (B) pre- and (C) post-contrast T1 weighted scans reveals faint rim enhancement, indicative of active disease. Cerebral edema, depicted as high signal intensity on T2 and low signal intensity on T1, is noted surrounding the larger lesion, specifically extending beyond the thin rim of enhancement defined on the post-contrast scan. In this instance, contrast enhancement provides information regarding differential diagnosis. The presence of multiple nodular or ring-enhancing basal ganglia (or gray-white matter junction) lesions in the immunocompromised patient suggests the diagnosis of toxoplasmosis, which is the most common intracranial opportunistic infection in AIDS. Other considerations include metastatic disease and lymphoma. *(From Runge VM, Brack MA, Garneau RA, Kirsch JE. Magnetic resonance imaging of the brain. Philadelphia, JB Lippincott, 1994.)*

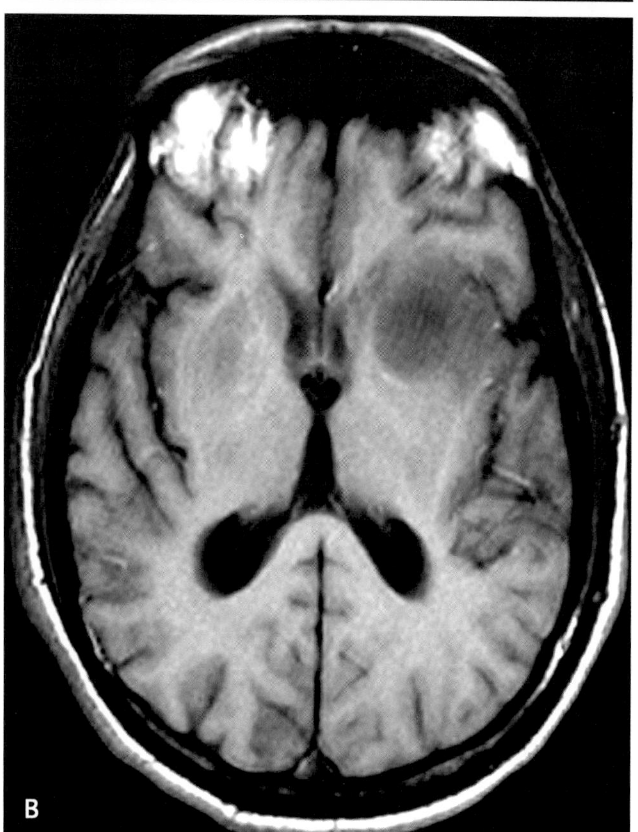

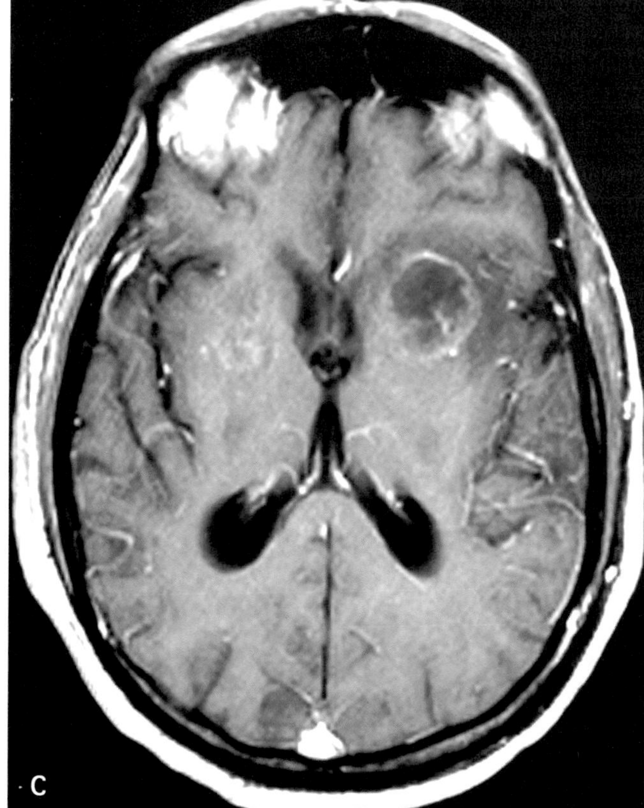

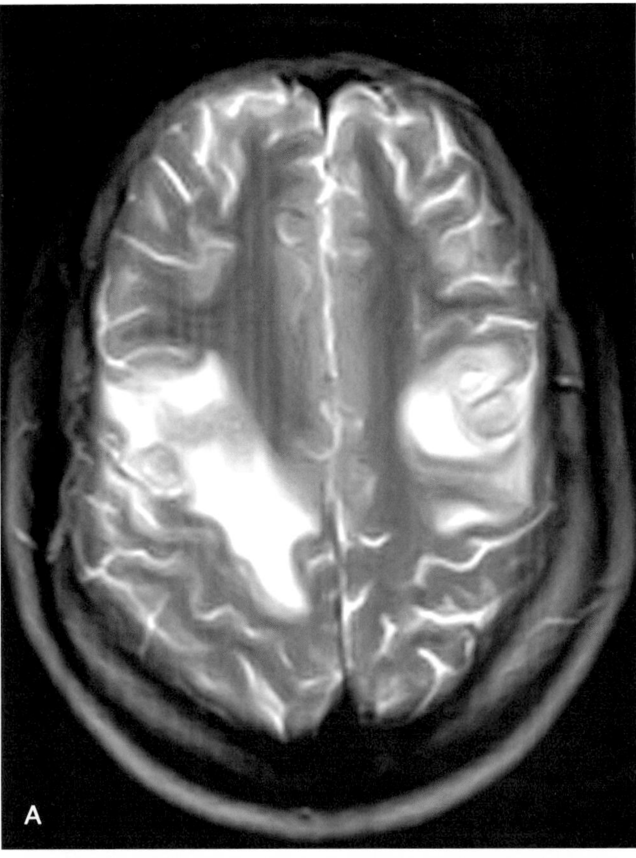

Figure 2. Cryptococcosis. Two areas of abnormal high signal intensity are noted on (A) the T2 weighted scan, consistent with cerebral edema. Comparison of (B) pre- and (C) post-contrast T1 weighted scans reveals three ring enhancing lesions, two of which (on the patient's left) are adjacent to one another. *Cryptococcus* is a ubiquitous fungus, which grows in tissue as yeast cells and spreads hematogenously. This organism usually causes leptomeningitis, which may be either acute or chronic. Parenchymal lesions, as featured in this case, are less common.

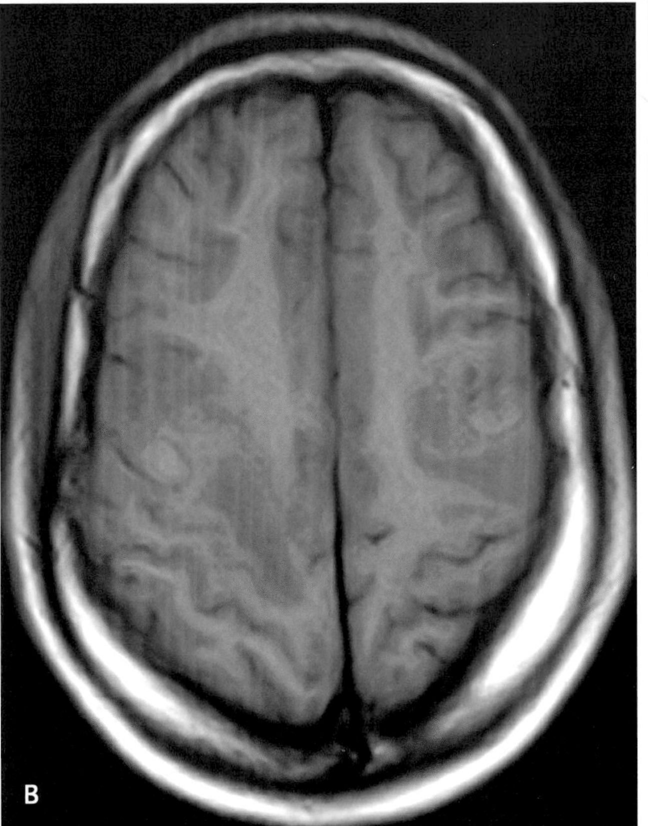

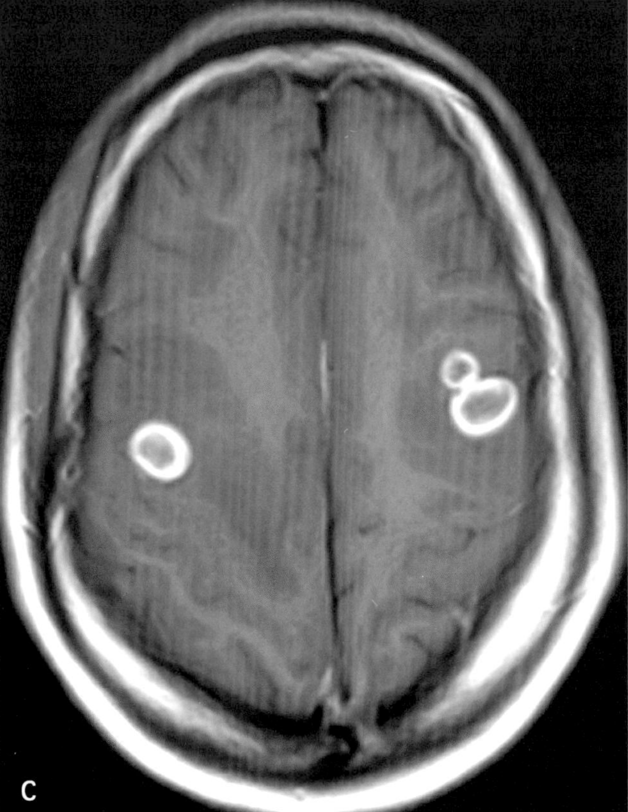

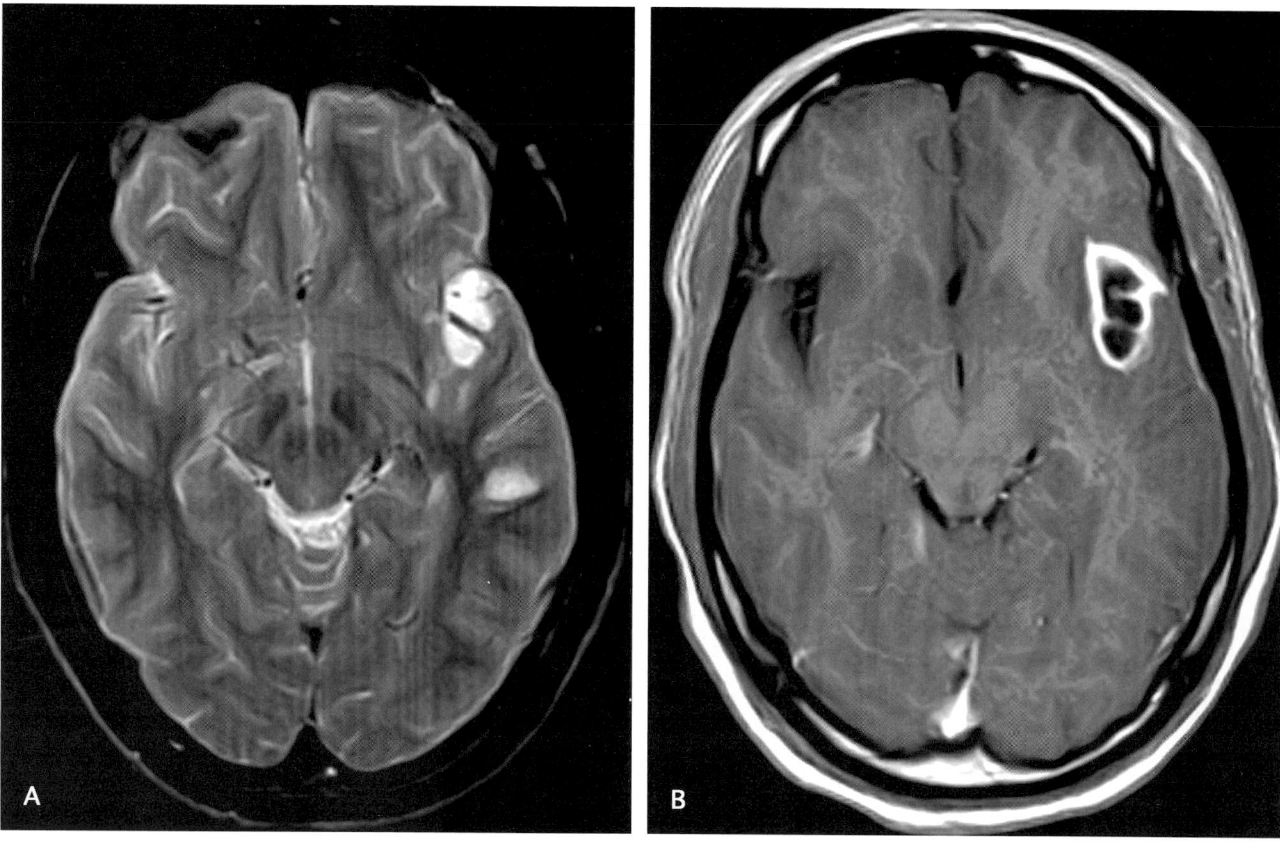

Figure 3. Neurocysticercosis. On (A) the pre-contrast T2 weighted scan, an ovoid area of abnormal high signal intensity is noted in the region of the sylvian fissure. (B) On the T1 weighted scan following contrast administration, there is ring enhancement of the lesion, with a suggestion of septations. In neurocysticercosis (infection by the larval stage of the pork tapeworm), the patient may present with either seizures, because of parenchymal cysts, or obstructive hydrocephalus, because of intraventricular cysts. On MR, the cysts have fluid signal intensity, with ring enhancement post-contrast of the cyst wall.

In both the cerebritis and capsule stages of abscess formation in the brain, contrast enhancement is seen on the basis of blood-brain barrier (BBB) disruption. In early disease, associated edema may be minimal and difficult to recognize, with contrast enhancement improving lesion detection. At this stage, high dose contrast administration may also prove useful for improved lesion visualization, because of partial BBB disruption. In the late cerebritis and capsular stages of abscess formation, ring enhancement is typical. This identifies the lesion rim, as separate from surrounding edema (figure 5). Contrast enhancement also provides an assessment of lesion activity, and thus is recommended in the follow-up of parenchymal brain infection.

Animal experimentation[9] and clinical trials[10] have also demonstrated the superiority of contrast enhanced scans for the detection and delineation of meningeal involvement by infection. Gadolinium chelate enhanced MR is more effective than both unenhanced MR and enhanced CT for demonstrating meningitis and its complications (figure 6). Pre-contrast scans are needed for evaluation of complications, which can include edema, infarction, and hemorrhage.

It is important to appreciate that meningeal disease as demonstrated on contrast enhanced MR is not specific for infection. Prominent meningeal enhancement can be observed following surgery or trauma, due to neoplastic disease,[11] or with infection.[12] When meningeal disease is nodular, neoplasia can be suggested as the etiology.[13] Otherwise, on the basis of MR images alone, a specific diagnosis is often difficult to establish. Dural enhancement can be chronic in nature and seen many years following surgery. This enhancement is more intense and persists longer on MR than noted on CT. Post-operative meningeal enhancement may be focal or diffuse.[14] This reaction is felt to represent either a local inflammatory response or a chemical arachnoiditis. In one clinical series, all patients imaged within one year of surgery had abnormal dural enhancement on post-contrast MR.[15] Enhancement of the pia mater is indicative of more recent disease involve-

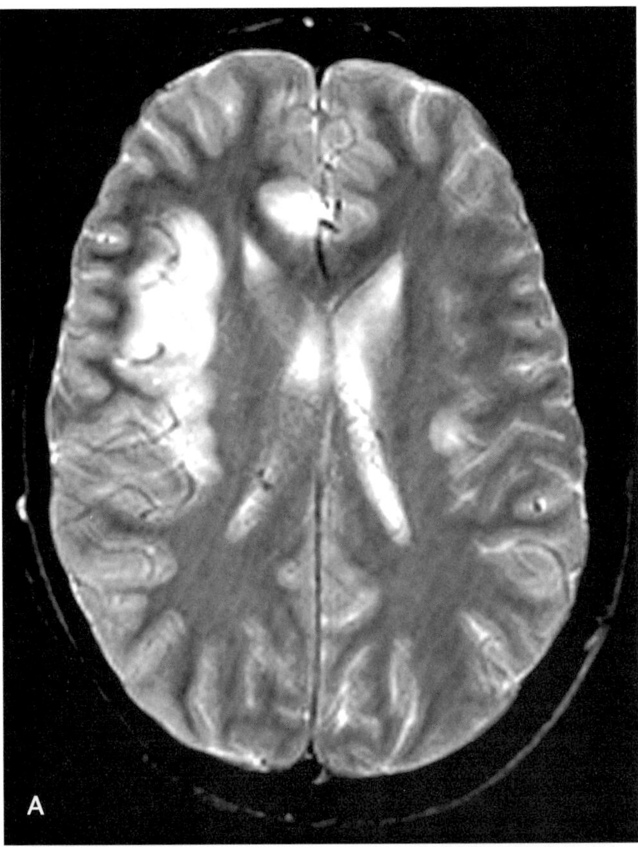

Figure 4. Herpes encephalitis (type 1). (A) The T2 weighted scan reveals abnormal high signal intensity in the insula bilaterally, and in the right frontal lobe. Comparison of (B) pre- and (C) post-contrast T1 weighted scans reveals abnormal meningeal enhancement within the sylvian fissure on the right. Herpes encephalitis in the adult most often affects the temporal and inferior frontal lobes. Meningeal enhancement is seen in the acute phase of the disease. *(From Runge VM, Brack MA, Garneau RA, Kirsch JE. Magnetic resonance imaging of the brain. Philadelphia, JB Lippincott, 1994.)*

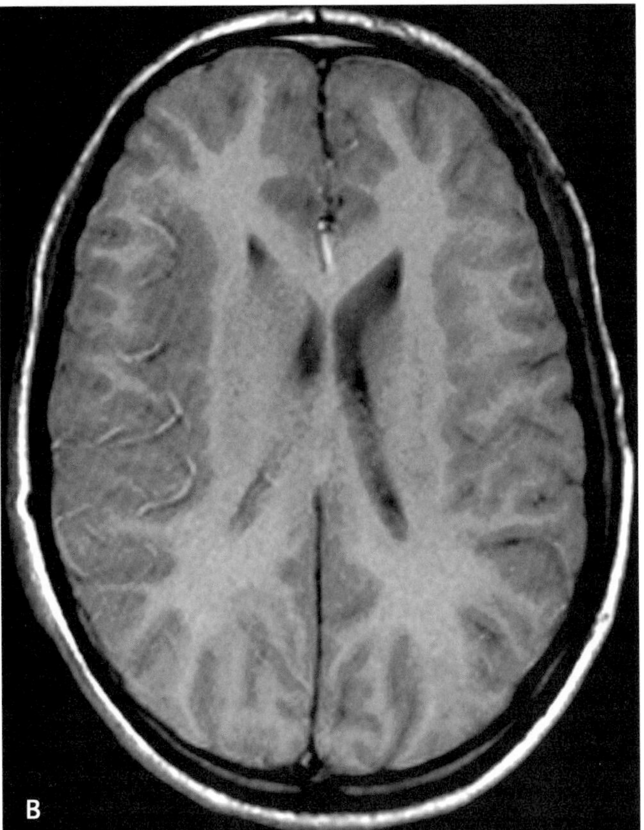

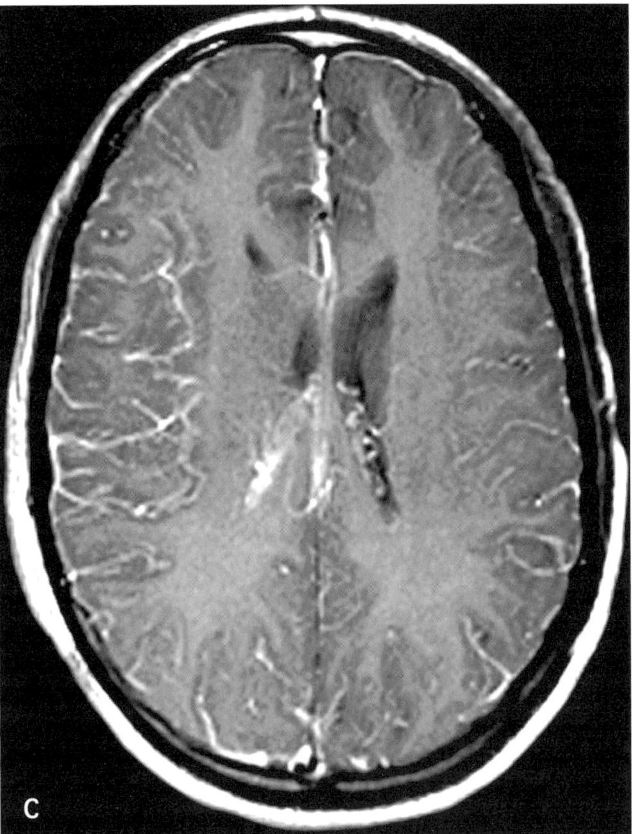

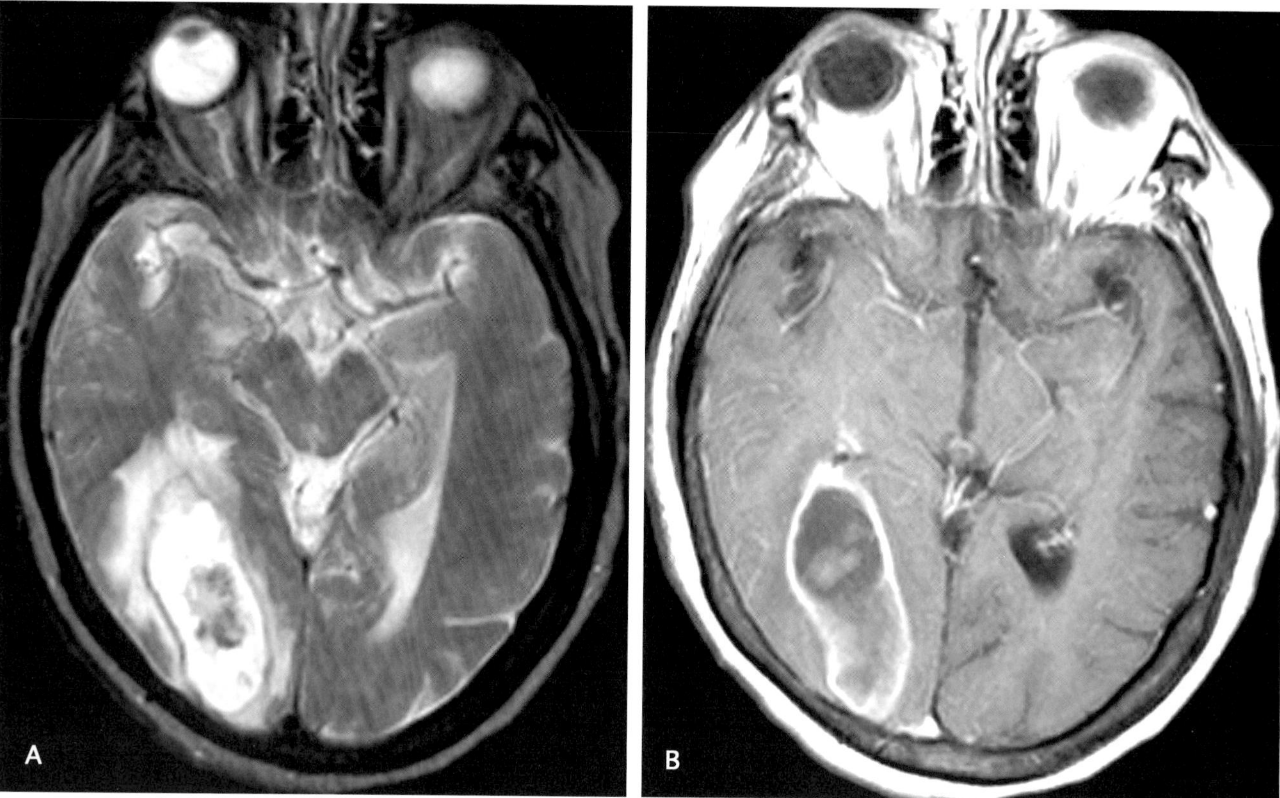

Figure 5. Brain abscess. A mixed low and high signal intensity abnormality, with a thin hypointense rim and surrounding high signal intensity edema, is noted on (A) the T2 weighted scan. On (B) the post-contrast T1 weighted scan, a thin uniform rim of abnormal enhancement is noted. Characteristic features of a brain abscess include location at the corticomedullary junction and the presence of a smooth, well defined, enhancing capsule. Necrotic contents are typically heterogeneous in signal intensity. *(From Runge VM, Brack MA, Garneau RA, Kirsch JE. Magnetic resonance imaging of the brain. Philadelphia, JB Lippincott, 1994.)*

ment and should not be seen as part of the normal postoperative appearance more than one year after surgery.

Whether due to surgery, infection, or neoplasm, the depiction of meningeal disease by contrast enhanced MR is superior to enhanced CT. Disease commonly is also revealed to be more extensive on MR. The improved efficacy of MR is in part because of the absence of beam hardening effects and excellent visualization of soft tissue immediately adjacent to dense bone, such as the cranial vault and the skull base. Improved depiction of ventriculitis and cerebritis on contrast enhanced MR, however, is due to the greater innate sensitivity of this modality.

Intracranial involvement with sarcoidosis occurs in about 15% of patients with this disease. The common presentation is that of a granulomatous leptomeningitis (figure 7). Progression to involve the adjacent brain via the perivascular spaces can occur. Less often, single or multiple parenchymal mass lesions may be observed.

Sinus infection can be difficult to identify on MR because of the prevalence of incidental non-clinical sinus inflammation. Prominent enhancement is observed routinely in viral and allergic sinus disease, with enhancement thus unable to provide differentiation between incidental disease and flagrant infection requiring medical or surgical therapy. Secondary changes in the brain because of sinus infection, in particular meningeal enhancement, when present do allow for differentiation.

Vascular disorders

Contrast administration can improve the detection of small arteriovenous lesions. In recent years, motion compensation techniques such as gradient moment nulling have become standard in clinical imaging. Implementation of these techniques has led to a reduction in the visualization of vessel abnormalities, which were originally well depicted on single slice MR as "flow voids." Signal from the vessels that would otherwise have been displaced, remains and leads to vessels that are isointense or hyperintense to brain tissue. Thus contrast between the brain and vessels has been reduced since MR's clinical introduction, decreasing the sensitivity of

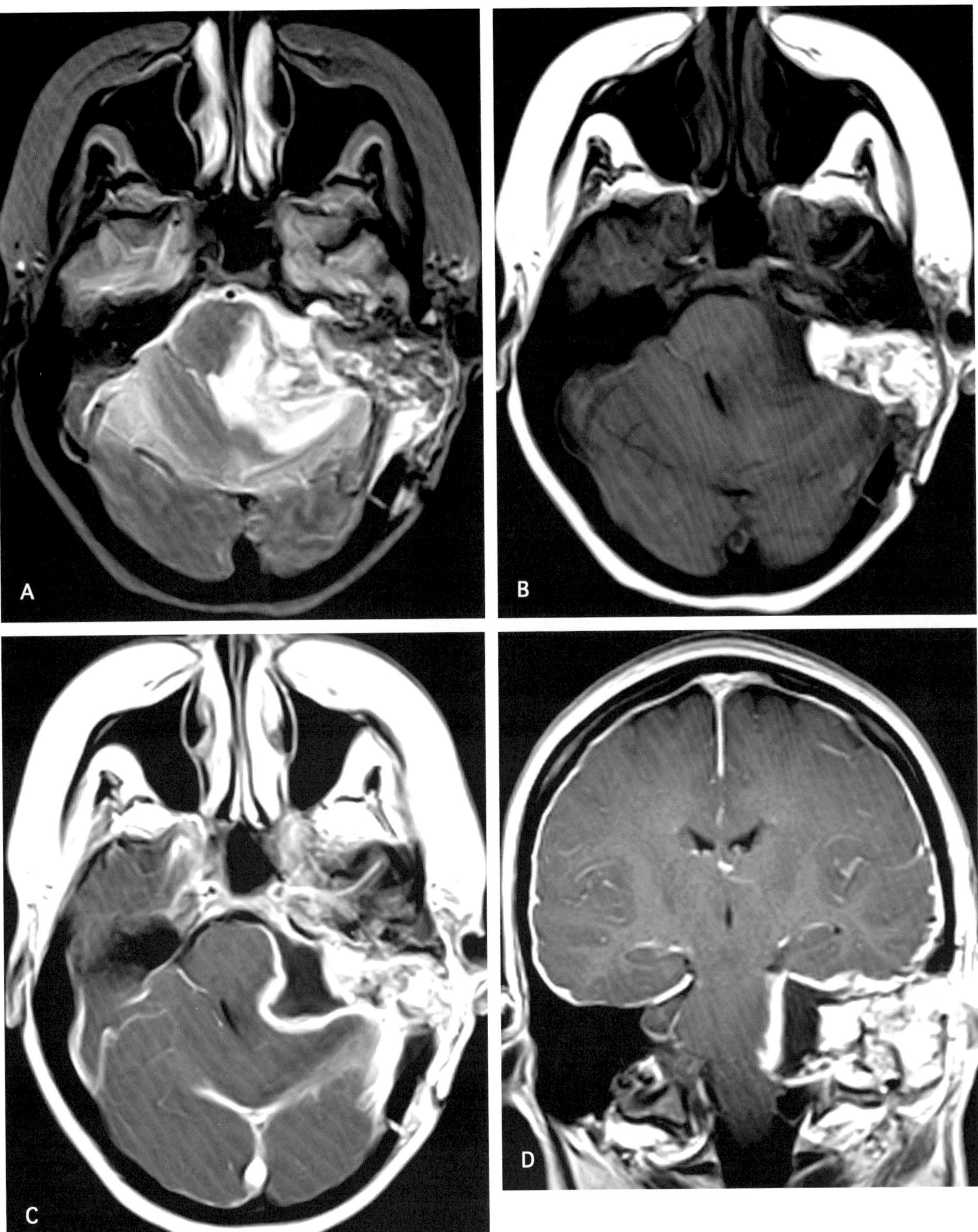

Figure 6. Bacterial meningitis (post-operative). On (A) the T2 weighted scan, edema in the pons, middle cerebellar peduncle, and cerebellar hemisphere is noted. Post-operative changes are present, including fat packing. The latter is best seen on (B) the pre-contrast T1 weighted scan. The patient is in the early post-operative period following resection of a large acoustic neuroma. There is mass effect on the brainstem and fourth ventricle. On the post-contrast (C) axial and (D) coronal T1 weighted scans, there is intense enhancement of the dura, in particular at the site of recent surgery. Mild cases of meningitis may show no abnormality on MR scans. Severe disease will display marked enhancement of the coverings of the brain.

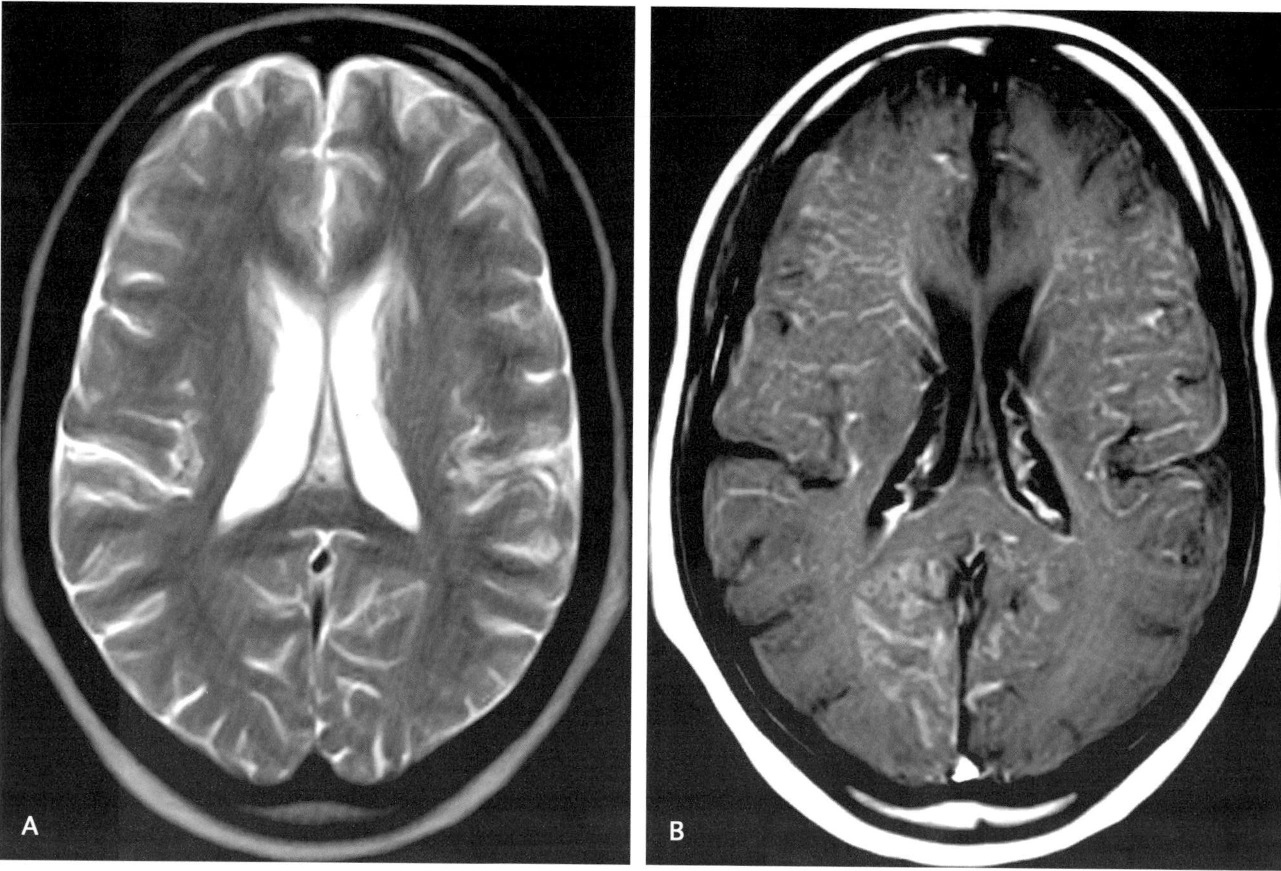

Figure 7. Neurosarcoidosis. (A) The T2 weighted scan is grossly normal. On (B) the post-contrast T1 weighted scan, there is diffuse enhancement of the leptomeninges. On imaging, two major patterns of brain involvement are seen with neurosarcoidosis. The first is a granulomatous leptomeningitis, and the second parenchymal involvement because of spread along Virchow-Robin spaces.

unenhanced studies to vascular abnormalities. To some extent this is compensated for today by the use of MR angiography. However, MR angiograms are typically employed for specific indications, and are not generally implemented on every patient exam.

Contrast administration causes a marked increase in vessel signal intensity, most prominent with slow flow in the venous system. In large arteriovenous malformations, contrast enhancement is often dramatic, primarily occurring in large draining veins (figure 8). In small arteriovenous malformations, enhancement of vascular structures can improve recognition of the lesion itself (figure 9).

MR angiography (MRA) can in certain instances be improved when obtained post-contrast.[16,17] This is particularly true for venous lesions when studied with 3D time-of-flight techniques.[18] Portrayal of small arteries, and specifically stenoses and slow flow, is also improved post-contrast on such images. Care should be exercised with maximum intensity projection (MIP) display of images, with selection of a small volume important to minimize vessel overlap. However, MRA is most commonly acquired today prior to the administration of intravenous contrast.

Slow flow in aneurysms is another situation that leads to marked lesion enhancement following gadolinium chelate administration on MR. With giant aneurysms, opacification post-contrast of the majority of the patent lumen can occur (figure 10). Imaging sequences with correction for pulsation artifacts, for example utilizing gradient moment nulling, maximize such enhancement. The blood jet into a large patent lumen may remain low signal intensity. With small berry aneurysms, detection is occasionally facilitated post-contrast, because of enhancement of slow flow (figure 11).

The depiction of venous lesions on conventional spin echo imaging is in particular improved post-contrast. Slow flow, combined with the use of gradient moment nulling and the reduction of blood T1 because of the presence of the contrast agent, leads to very high signal intensity venous structures on post-contrast scans. Venous angiomas commonly go unrecognized when scans without contrast are

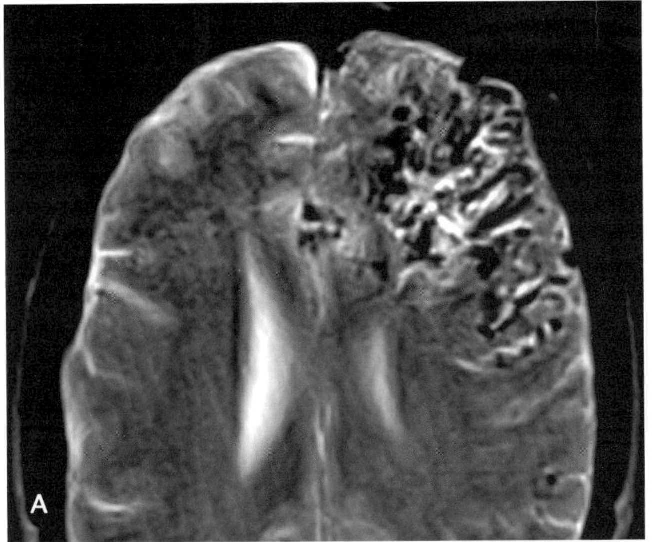

Figure 8. Arteriovenous malformation (AVM). On (A) the T2 weighted scan, a large lesion in noted in the left frontal lobe, with mixed high and low signal intensity suggestive of flow. Tubular-like signal voids are present on (B) the pre-contrast T1 weighted scan. (C) Post-contrast, a large enhancing nidus is identified. Also seen is enhancement of multiple large draining veins. AVMs are well depicted on conventional planar spin echo MR images, because of flow phenomena. On pre-contrast scans, multiple serpiginous structures can be identified, most with low signal intensity because of rapid flow. Following IV contrast administration, enhancement can be noted in areas of slower flow, in particular within draining veins.

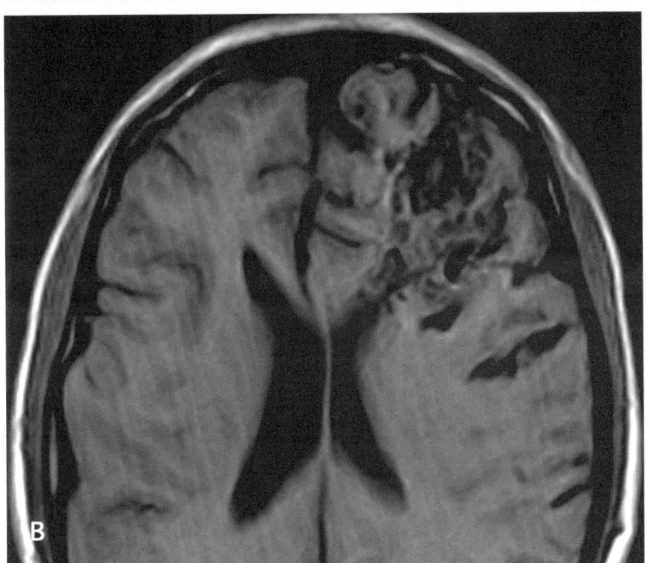

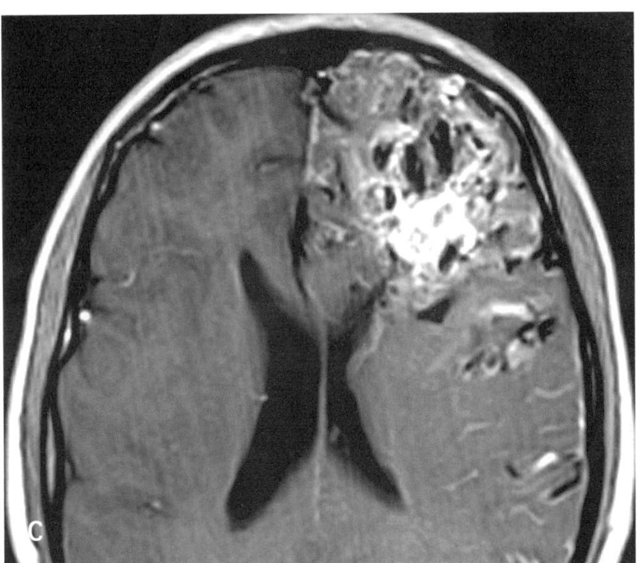

employed (figure 12).[19] In one study, 9 of 28 venous angiomas were detected only following gadolinium chelate administration. Depiction of the type of venous drainage, superficial or deep, is also improved post-contrast. In the case of cavernous angiomas, contrast administration leads to enhancement of the large vascular spaces within these lesions, improving differential diagnosis (figure 13).[20]

Three patterns of enhancement can be seen in cerebral infarction.[21] Intravascular enhancement is the earliest type of abnormal contrast enhancement identified, and is seen from day 0 to 7 following clinical presentation (figure 14). Prominent vessel enhancement occurs in the anatomic region of involvement, reflecting slow flow and vascular engorgement. Meningeal enhancement can be seen adjacent to the area of damaged tissue (figure 15). This pattern is the most uncommon, and is typically seen from day 1 to 3. Parenchymal enhancement, gyriform in nature, is usually not present prior to day 6. It is consistently seen in subacute infarction, from day 7 to 30, and may persist for up to 8 weeks (figures 16 and 17). This is one instance in which a slight delay in scan acquisition following contrast administration may be helpful for detection of abnormal enhancement. A gradual increase in the degree of enhancement is seen in subacute infarcts during the first hour post-contrast.[22] Recognition of these patterns of contrast enhancement improves differential diagnosis and permits lesion dating. In particular, gyriform enhancement in the subacute time period allows differentiation of a subacute infarct from chronic white matter ischemic changes. As on CT, on occasion a subacute infarct will not manifest sufficient vasogenic edema to be recognized on unenhanced scans, with contrast administration in this instance providing for lesion diagnosis (figure 18). High dose contrast administration with an agent such as Gd HP-DO3A provides for identification of subtle blood-

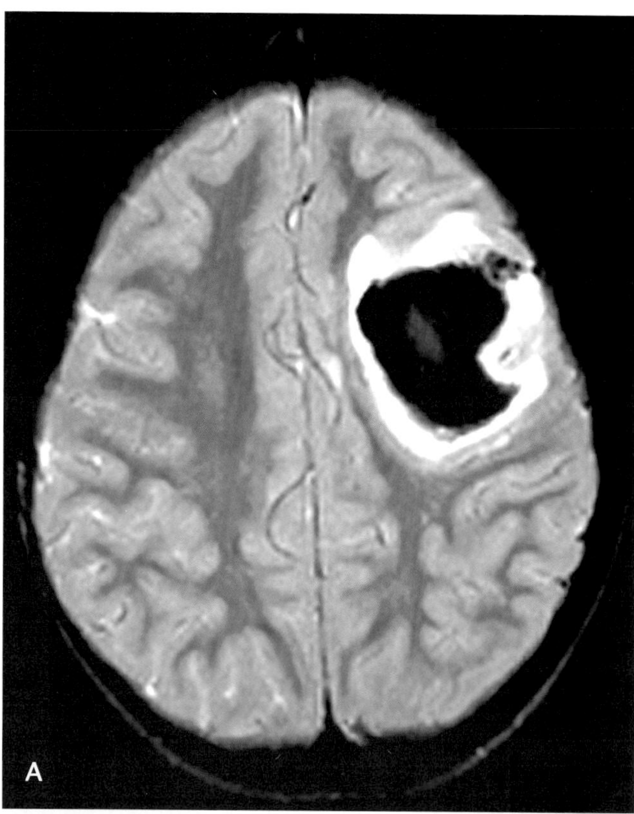

Figure 9. Arteriovenous malformation with subacute hemorrhage. On (A) the T2 weighted scan, a low signal intensity abnormality with surrounding high signal intensity edema is noted in the left frontal lobe. The signal characteristics of the mass are consistent with hemorrhage, specifically either deoxyhemoglobin or intracellular methemoglobin. Comparison of (B) pre- and (C) post-contrast T1 weighted scans reveals a small enhancing focus (arrow) just anterior and lateral to the bulk of the mass. This abnormality is well seen in retrospect, and is of low signal intensity, on the T2 weighted scan. The signal intensity characteristics (extreme low signal intensity pre-contrast on both T1 and T2, with enhancement post-contrast) and serpiginous nature are consistent with an arteriovenous malformation, which was confirmed angiographically. Contrast administration aids in this instance in both lesion identification and characterization. *(From Runge VM, Brack MA, Garneau RA, Kirsch JE. Magnetic resonance imaging of the brain. Philadelphia, JB Lippincott, 1994.)*

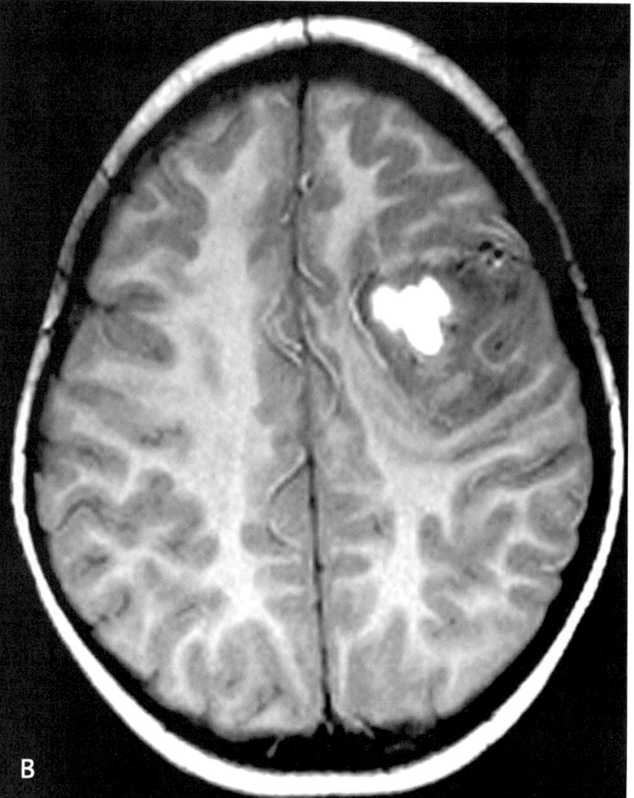

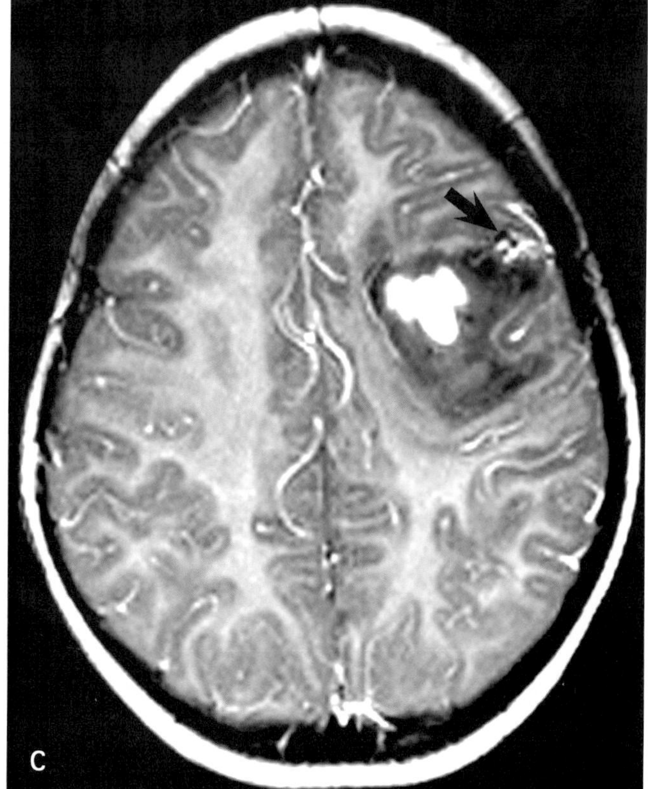

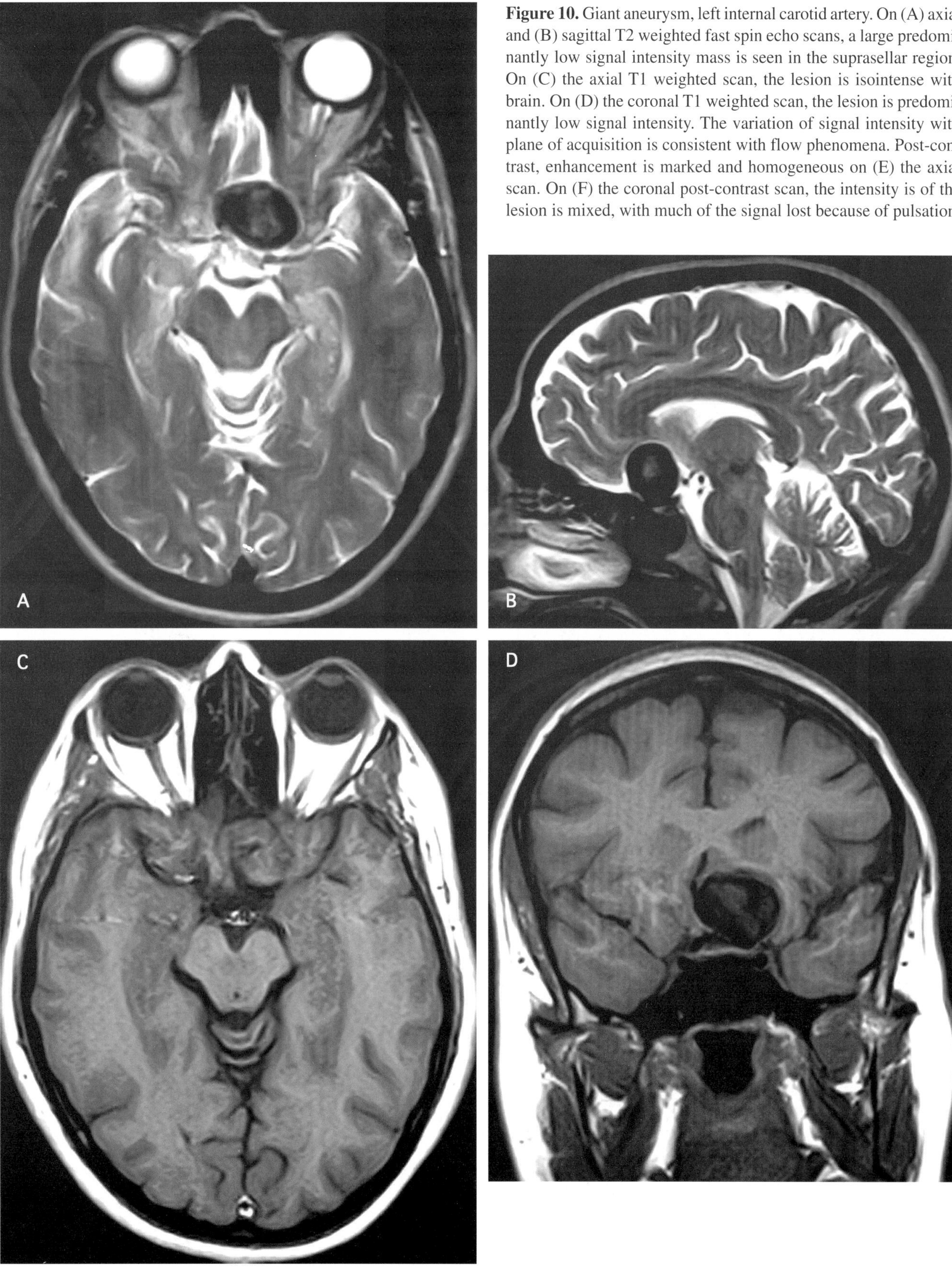

Figure 10. Giant aneurysm, left internal carotid artery. On (A) axial and (B) sagittal T2 weighted fast spin echo scans, a large predominantly low signal intensity mass is seen in the suprasellar region. On (C) the axial T1 weighted scan, the lesion is isointense with brain. On (D) the coronal T1 weighted scan, the lesion is predominantly low signal intensity. The variation of signal intensity with plane of acquisition is consistent with flow phenomena. Post-contrast, enhancement is marked and homogeneous on (E) the axial scan. On (F) the coronal post-contrast scan, the intensity is of the lesion is mixed, with much of the signal lost because of pulsation.

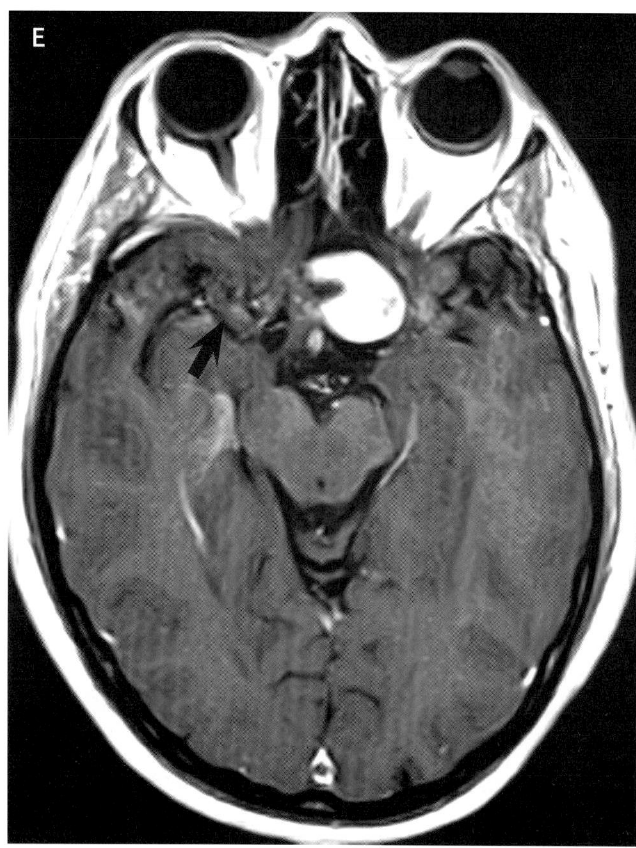

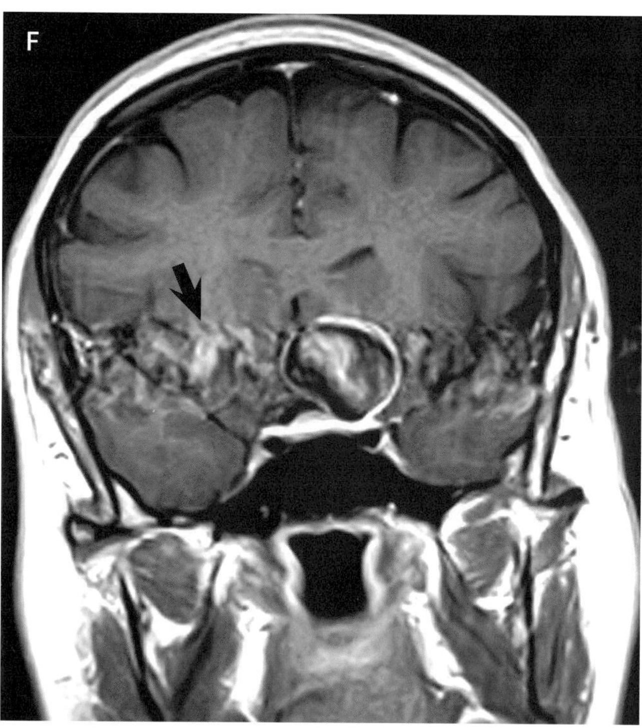

Figure 10 (*continued*). A faint pulsation artifact can be identified in (E), extending from right to left across the scan (arrow). This artifact (arrow) is greatest on the post-contrast coronal scan (F), extending from right to left and encompassing the entire height of the lesion. The imaging appearance of giant aneurysms on MR can be complex, because of the presence of both flowing blood and thrombus (which may be layered). In the current case, there is no evidence of thrombus. The presence of pulsation artifacts, often accentuated on post-contrast scans, offers a clue to the nature of the lesion.

brain barrier disruption, as may be seen in early subacute infarction.[23] Use of a gadolinium chelate in this instance can be helpful to confirm the diagnosis.

Familiarity with the arterial vascular territories of the brain is also essential for proper diagnosis. Posterior cerebral artery infarction is much less common than middle cerebral artery infarction. Anterior cerebral artery infarction is even less common (figure 19). Many practicing radiologists have little experience with such lesions, leading on occasion to misdiagnosis as neoplastic disease.

First pass studies have recently received attention for use in brain infarction.[24,25] By observing the transit of the contrast bolus through the brain, qualitative and quantitative information can be obtained concerning regional cerebral blood volume. Higher contrast dose improves the sensitivity and accuracy of first pass studies.[26] In acute infarcts, prior to the development of vasogenic edema, first pass studies also permit identification of the lesion, which may otherwise not be apparent.[27]

In lacunar infarcts, enhancement during the subacute time frame is consistently noted (figure 20). Because of the common occurrence of dilated perivascular spaces and old lacunar infarcts in the elderly patient population, identification of a new lesion that could account for current clinical symptoms can be difficult on unenhanced scans. Contrast enhancement is thus advocated in particular in older patients for identification of symptomatic lesions and for clinical correlation (figure 21).[28] MR is markedly superior to CT in the demonstration of enhancement in lacunar infarction. In one study, enhancement was noted in 4 of 9 patients on CT, as compared to 8 of 9 on MR.[29]

Familiarity with enhancement of lacunar infarcts in the subacute stage improves diagnostic accuracy. In particular, subacute pontine infarcts may mimic metastatic disease. Careful clinical correlation and recognition of characteristic involvement in a vascular territory assist diagnosis (figure 22). The pons is supplied by perforating vessels principally from the basilar artery, which enter

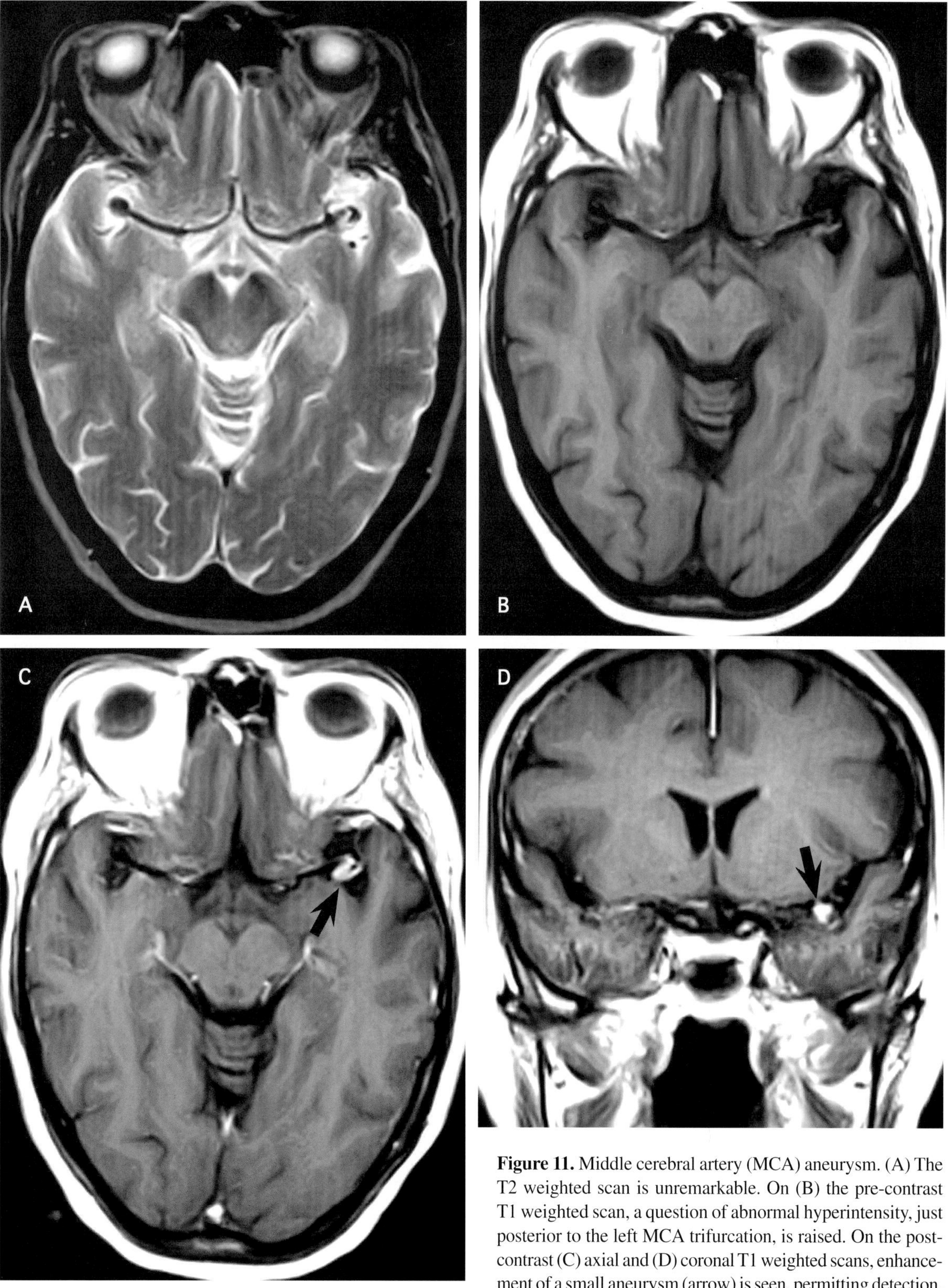

Figure 11. Middle cerebral artery (MCA) aneurysm. (A) The T2 weighted scan is unremarkable. On (B) the pre-contrast T1 weighted scan, a question of abnormal hyperintensity, just posterior to the left MCA trifurcation, is raised. On the post-contrast (C) axial and (D) coronal T1 weighted scans, enhancement of a small aneurysm (arrow) is seen, permitting detection. Slow flow within this berry aneurysm leads to marked contrast enhancement following IV gadolinium chelate administration. The lumen of the aneurysm is thus well depicted.

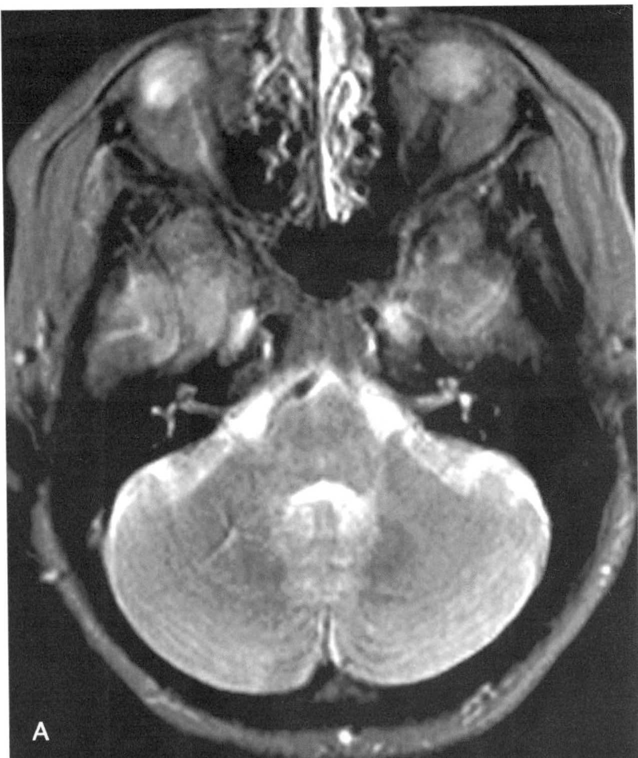

Figure 12. Venous angioma. Pre-contrast (A) T2 and (B) T1 weighted scans raise the question of a linear low signal intensity abnormality in the right cerebellar hemisphere. (C) Post-contrast, a "caput" of small draining medullary veins (arrow) is identified, which merge to form a larger transcortical vein emptying into the sigmoid sinus. IV contrast enhancement improves markedly the identification of normal and abnormal venous structures, with 30% of venous angiomas recognized only in retrospect on pre-contrast scans alone. *(From Runge VM, Brack MA, Garneau RA, Kirsch JE. Magnetic resonance imaging of the brain. Philadelphia, JB Lippincott, 1994.)*

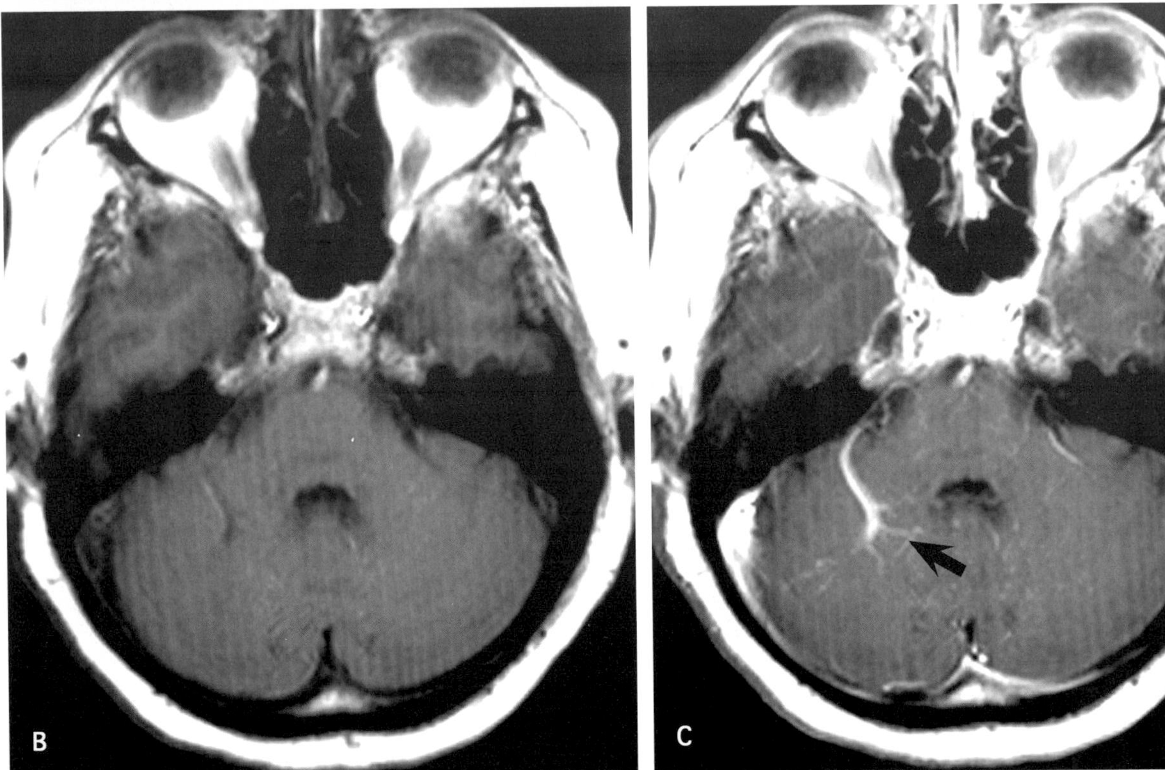

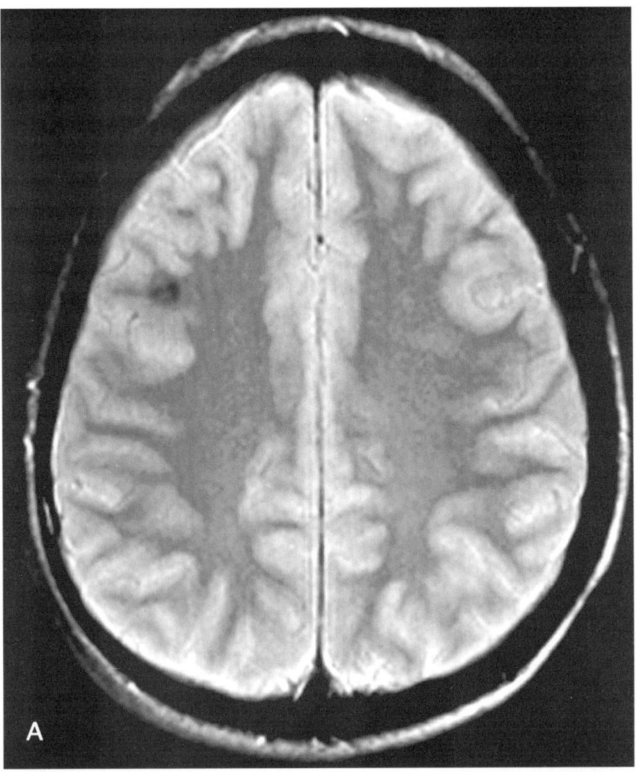

Figure 13. Cavernous angioma. A small low signal intensity abnormality is noted in the right frontal lobe on the (A) T2 weighted scan. Comparison of (B) pre- and (C) post-contrast T1 weighted scans reveals punctate enhancement (arrow) within a portion of the lesion. On histologic exam, cavernous angiomas exhibit well-defined borders and consist of a honeycomb of abnormal vascular spaces. Contrast enhancement aids in lesion characterization, by identification of the vascular component. The diagnosis was confirmed at surgery. *(From Runge VM, Brack MA, Garneau RA, Kirsch JE. Magnetic resonance imaging of the brain. Philadelphia, JB Lippincott, 1994.)*

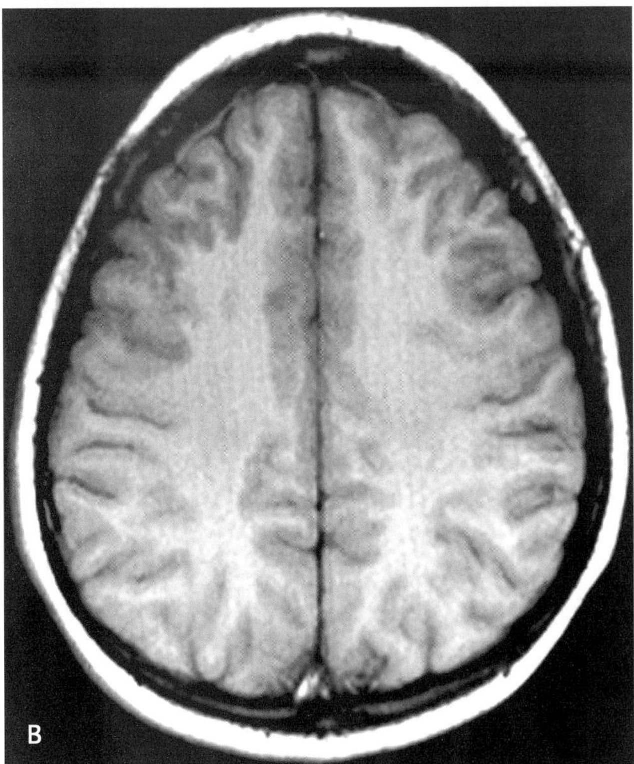

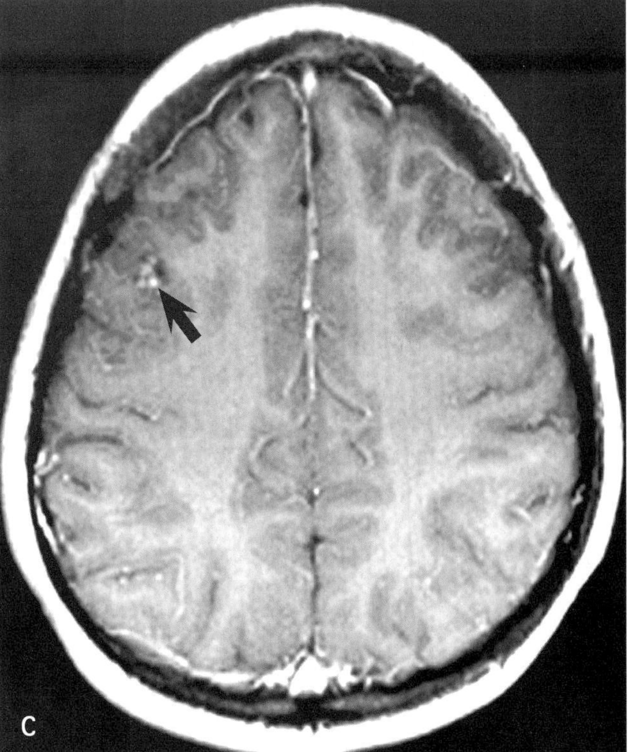

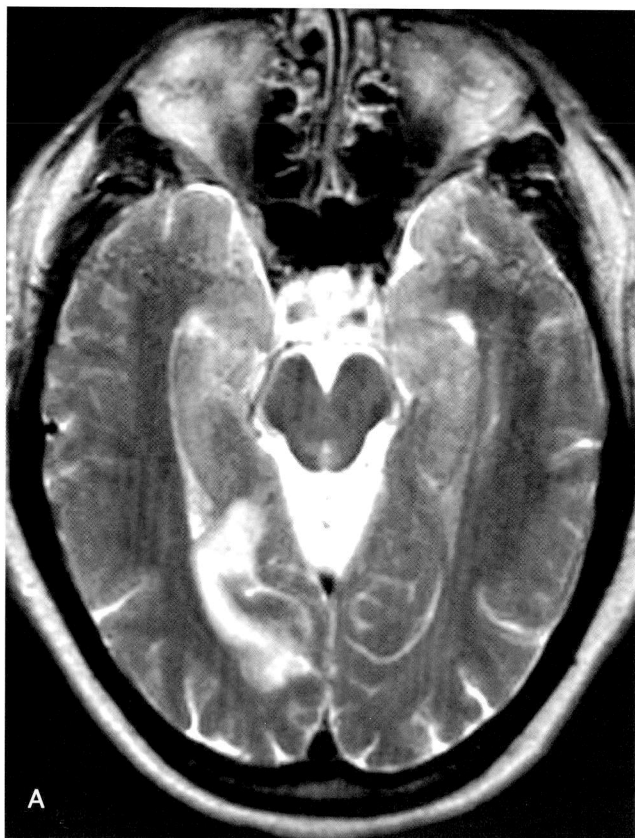

Figure 14. Acute posterior cerebral artery infarction. The patient presents with a two day history of visual problems. Abnormal high signal intensity is noted in the right posterior cerebral artery distribution on (A) the T2 weighted scan. The same area demonstrates subtle low signal intensity on (B) the T1 weighted scan. (C) Post-contrast, there is prominent intravascular enhancement in this region. This finding supports the leading diagnosis, that of cerebral infarction, and permits dating of the abnormality. Vascular enhancement is the earliest type of abnormal contrast enhancement identified on MR in cerebral infarction, and is frequently seen in one to three day old lesions.

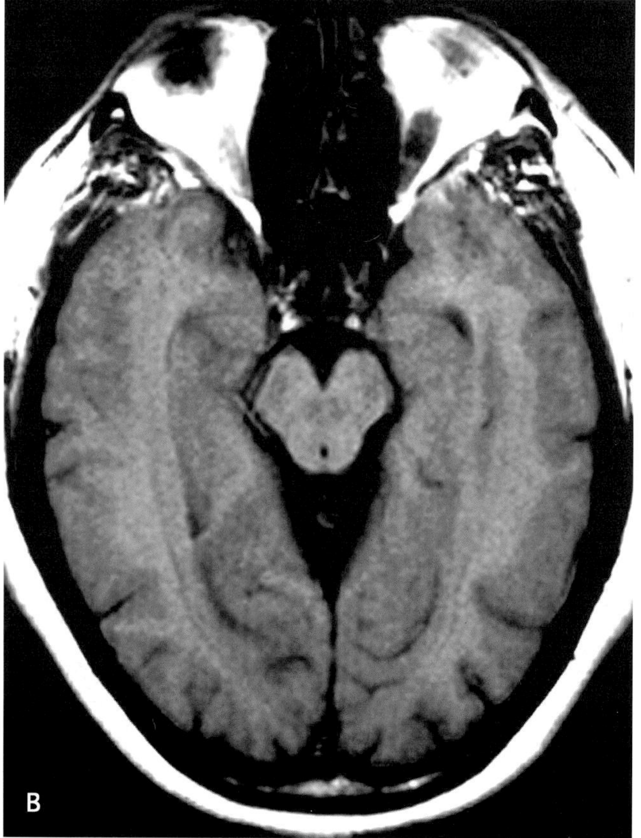

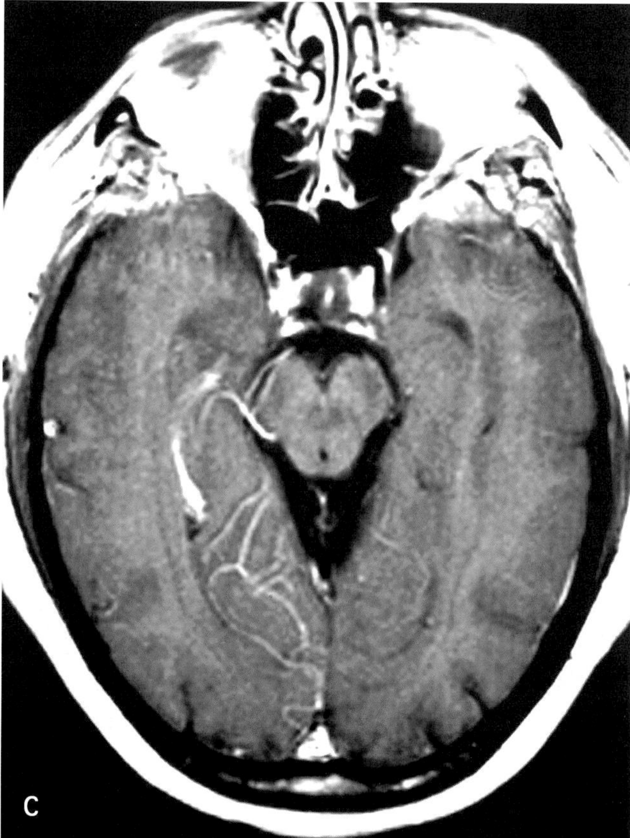

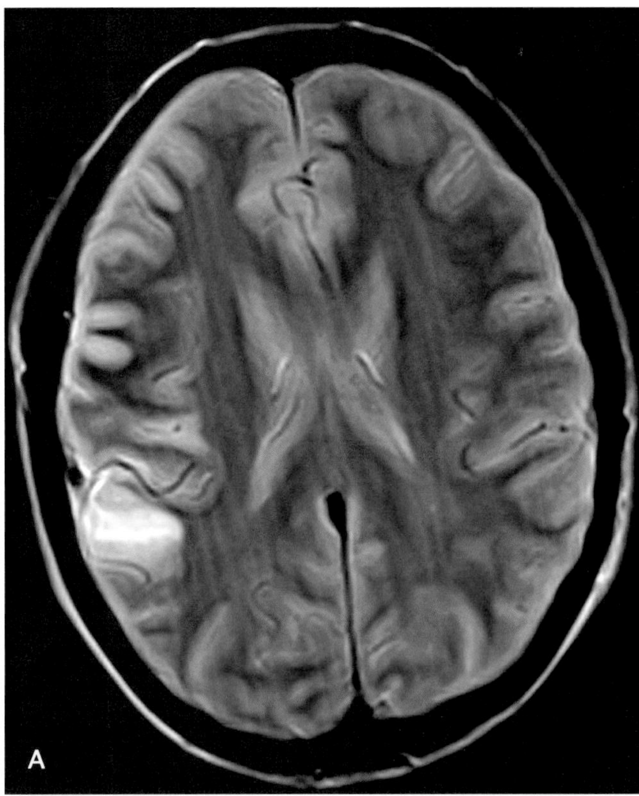

Figure 15. Meningeal enhancement in an acute middle cerebral artery infarction. On (A) the T2 weighted scan, there is abnormal high signal intensity within a posterior frontal gyrus on the patient's right side. On (B) the pre-contrast T1 weighted scan, the cortical sulci are not well visualized on the right. This finding is consistent with mass effect and suggestive of cytotoxic edema. (C) Post-contrast, there is extensive meningeal enhancement along the right hemisphere, with a single area of vascular enhancement. Meningeal enhancement adjacent to the area of damaged tissue can be seen in acute infarction. It occurs from day one to three following ictus, but is uncommon.

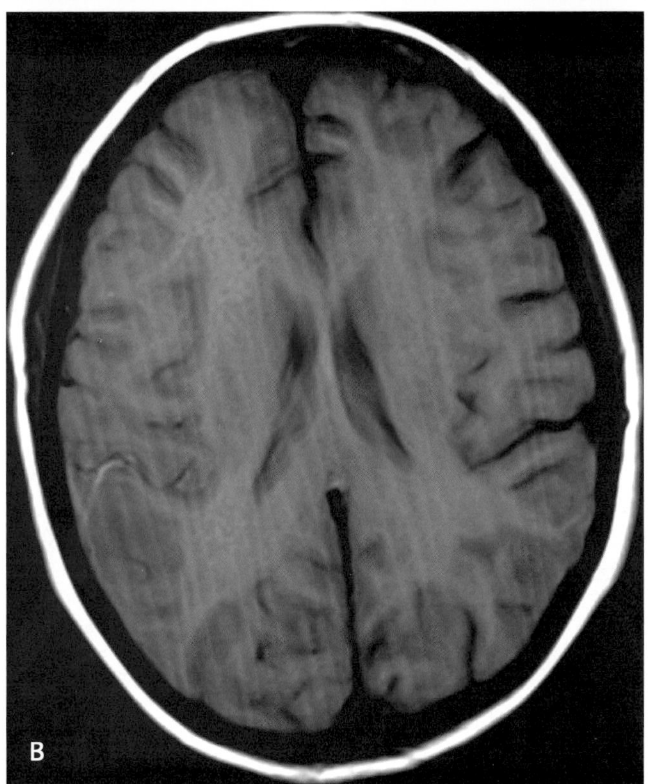

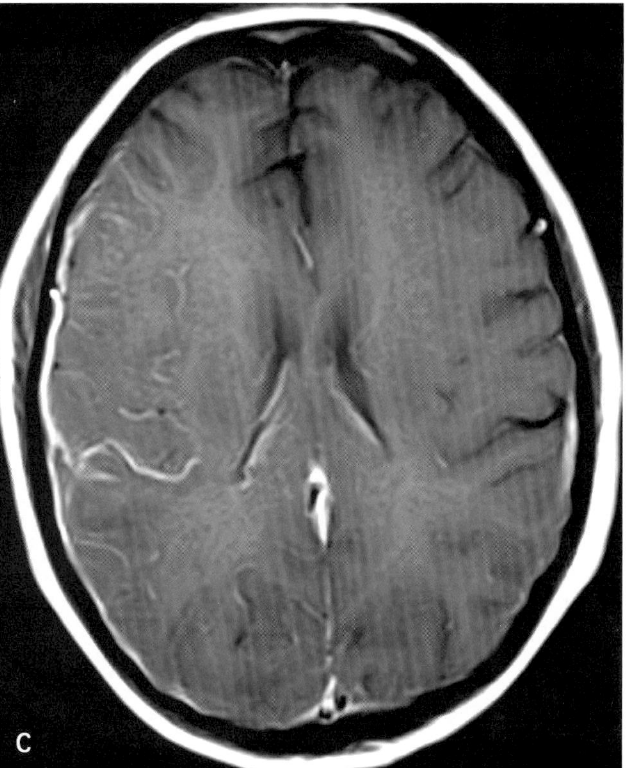

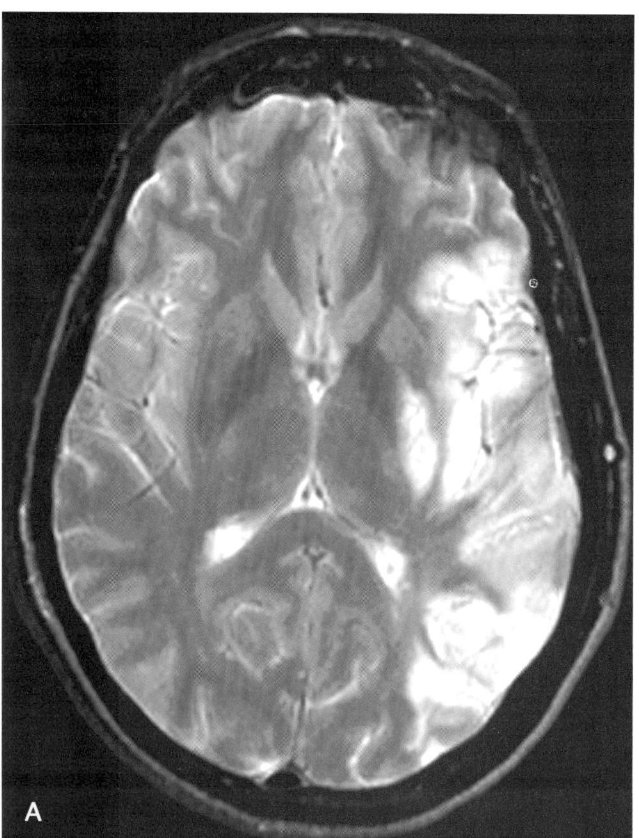

Figure 16. Subacute middle cerebral artery infarction. Images were obtained six days following ictus. On (A) the T2 weighted scan, abnormal high signal intensity is noted in the left middle cerebral artery distribution, principally involving gray matter. Comparison of (B) pre- and (C) post-contrast T1 weighted scans reveals gyriform enhancement in the posterior middle cerebral artery distribution. Meningeal enhancement is also noted overlying much of the edematous region (the latter defined by the T2 weighted scan). Parenchymal enhancement is the predominant pattern of abnormal contrast enhancement in subacute cerebral infarction. *(From Runge VM, Brack MA, Garneau RA, Kirsch JE. Magnetic resonance imaging of the brain. Philadelphia, JB Lippincott, 1994.)*

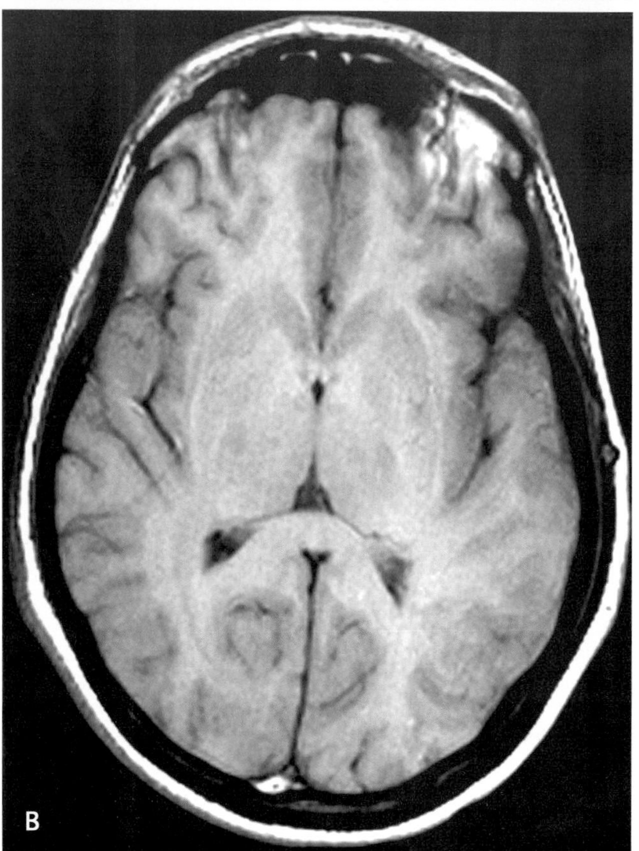

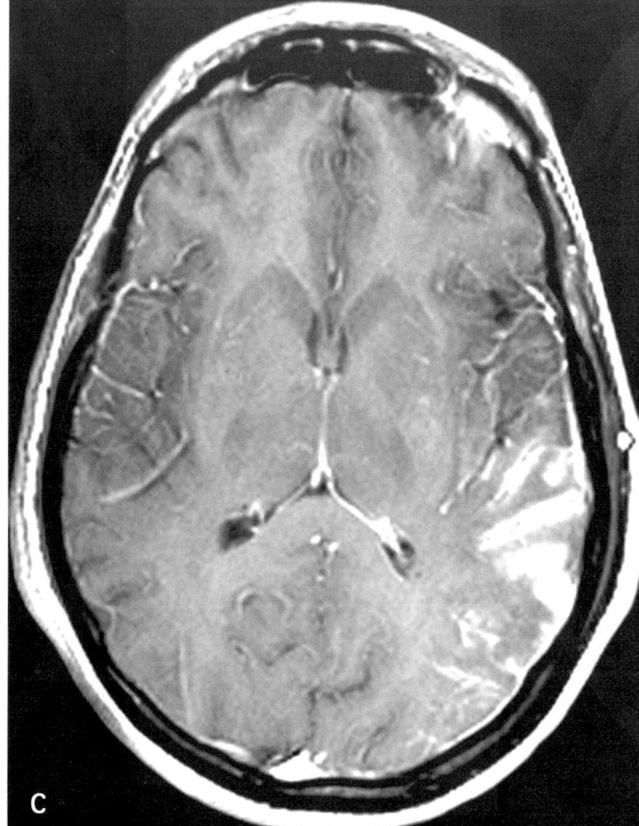

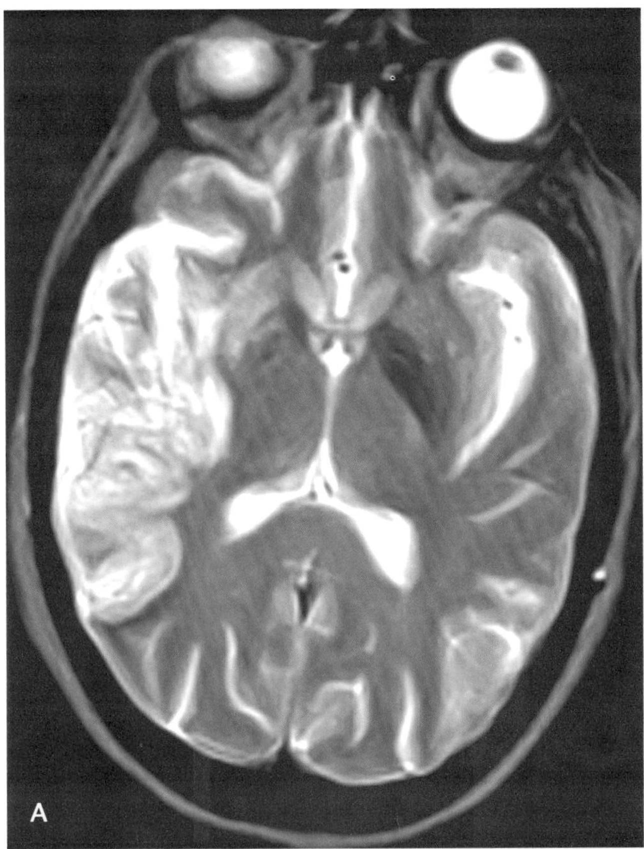

Figure 17. Parenchymal enhancement in a subacute middle cerebral artery (MCA) infarction. Gyriform high signal intensity is noted on (A) the T2 weighted scan within the right MCA distribution, reflecting vasogenic edema. Mild mass effect is noted on (B) the pre-contrast T1 weighted scan, with slight shift of the atria of the lateral ventricles and loss of visualization of cortical sulci. On (C) the post-contrast T1 weighted scan, there is intense gyriform enhancement, consistent with blood-brain barrier disruption in a subacute infarct.

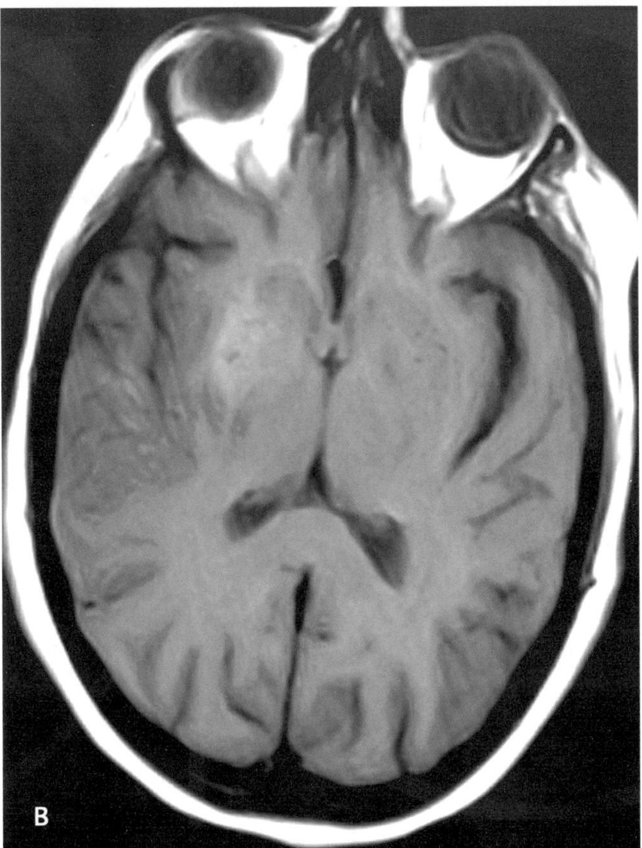

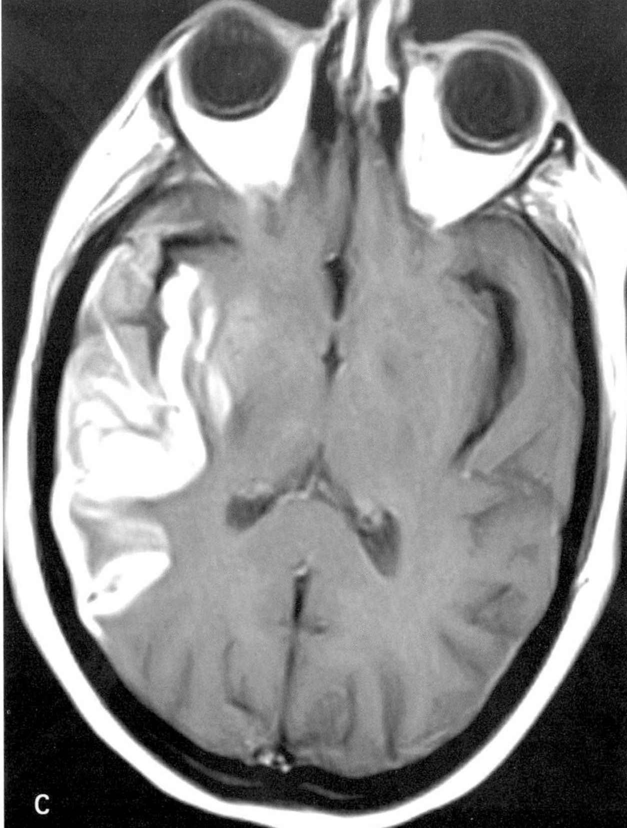

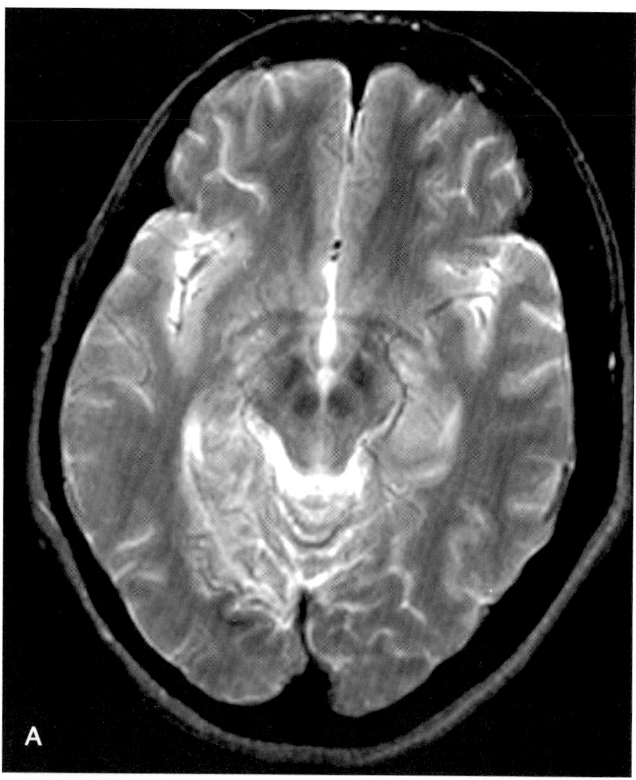

Figure 18. Isointense subacute posterior cerebral artery infarction. The MR exam was obtained 19 days following clinical presentation. Pre-contrast (A) T2 and (B) T1 weighted scans are unremarkable. (C) Post-contrast, gyriform enhancement is noted in the right posterior cerebral artery distribution. Parenchymal enhancement occurs because of blood-brain barrier disruption, identifying brain damaged by cerebral ischemia. In the subacute time frame, as with CT, there may be sufficient resolution of vasogenic edema on MR to render the lesion undetectable without IV contrast administration.

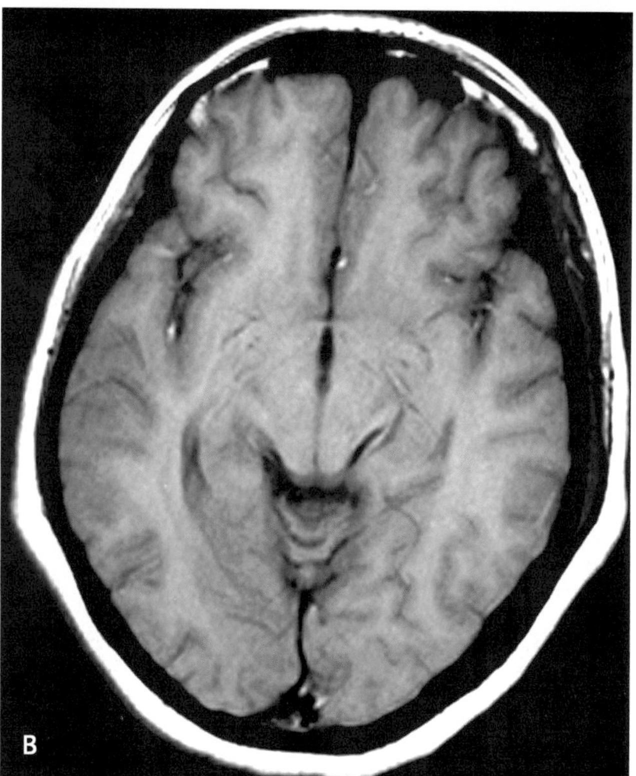

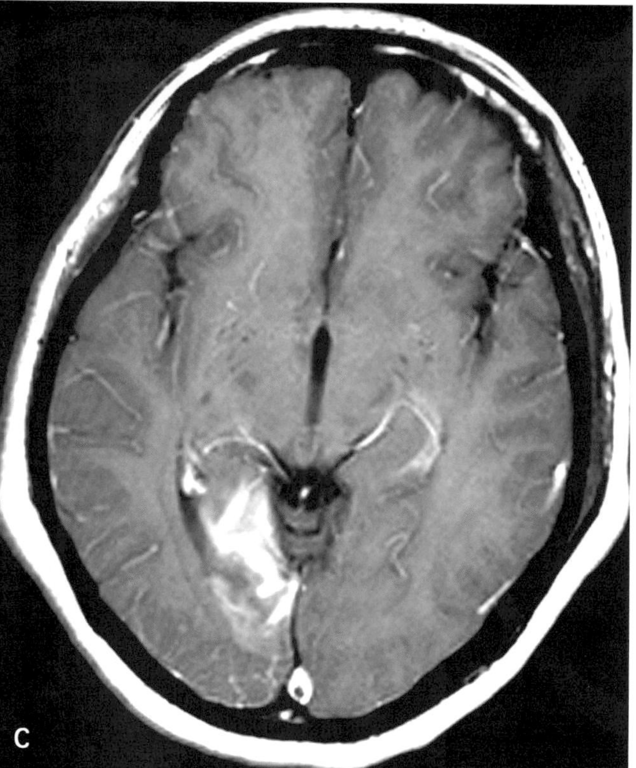

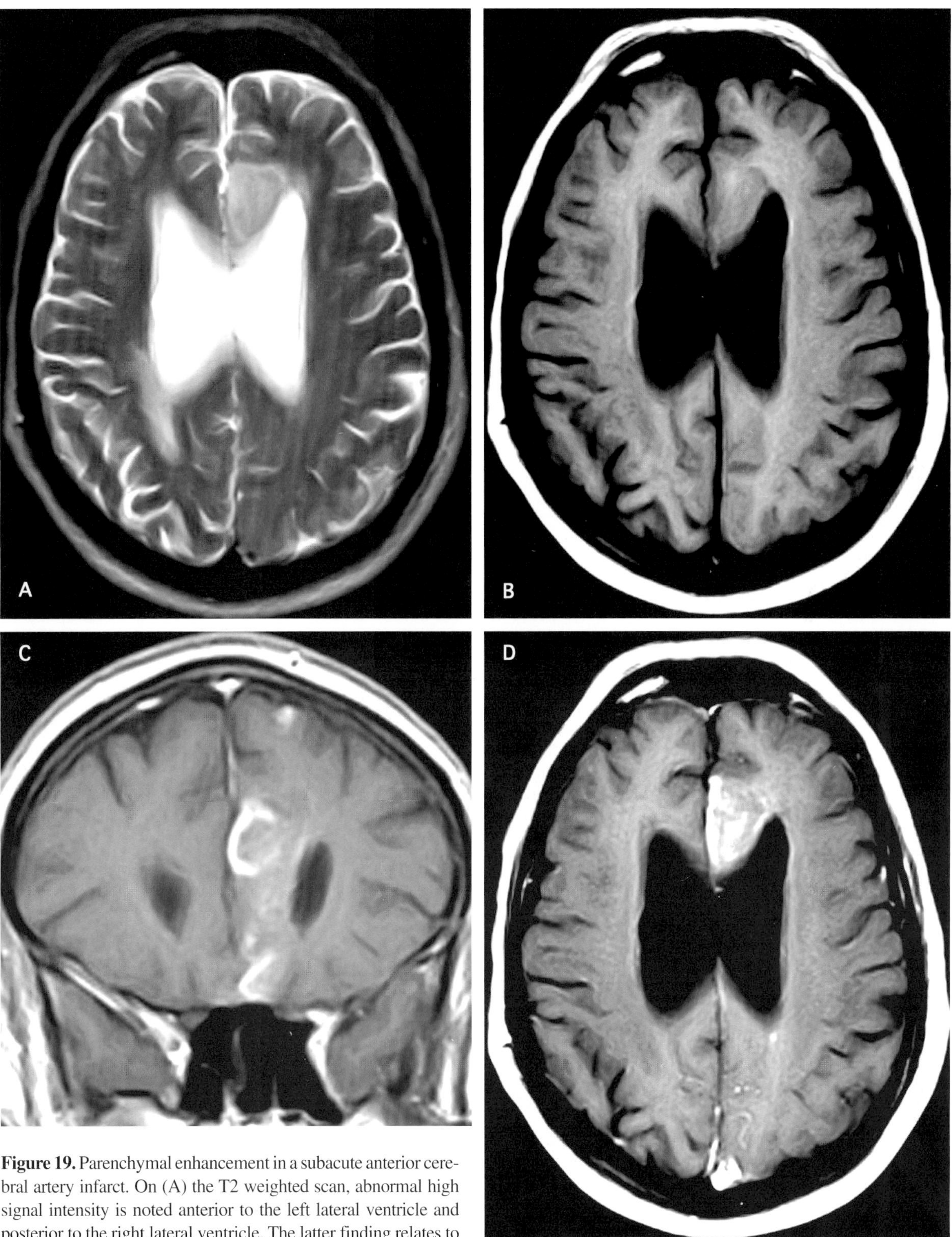

Figure 19. Parenchymal enhancement in a subacute anterior cerebral artery infarct. On (A) the T2 weighted scan, abnormal high signal intensity is noted anterior to the left lateral ventricle and posterior to the right lateral ventricle. The latter finding relates to known chronic ischemic changes. Comparing the (B) pre- and (D) post-contrast axial T1 weighted scans, abnormal contrast enhancement is noted anteriorly, matching in position the lesion on the T2 weighted scan. The (C) coronal post-contrast T1 weighted scan also identifies the abnormality. In this plane, the distribution of the lesion within a portion of the anterior cerebral artery territory is more evident. Enhancement is present because of blood-brain barrier disruption in this subacute lesion. As compared to middle and posterior cerebral artery infarcts, anterior cerebral artery infarcts are much less common. Familiarity with the arterial distribution of the vessel, and greater awareness of this entity, can markedly improve diagnosis.

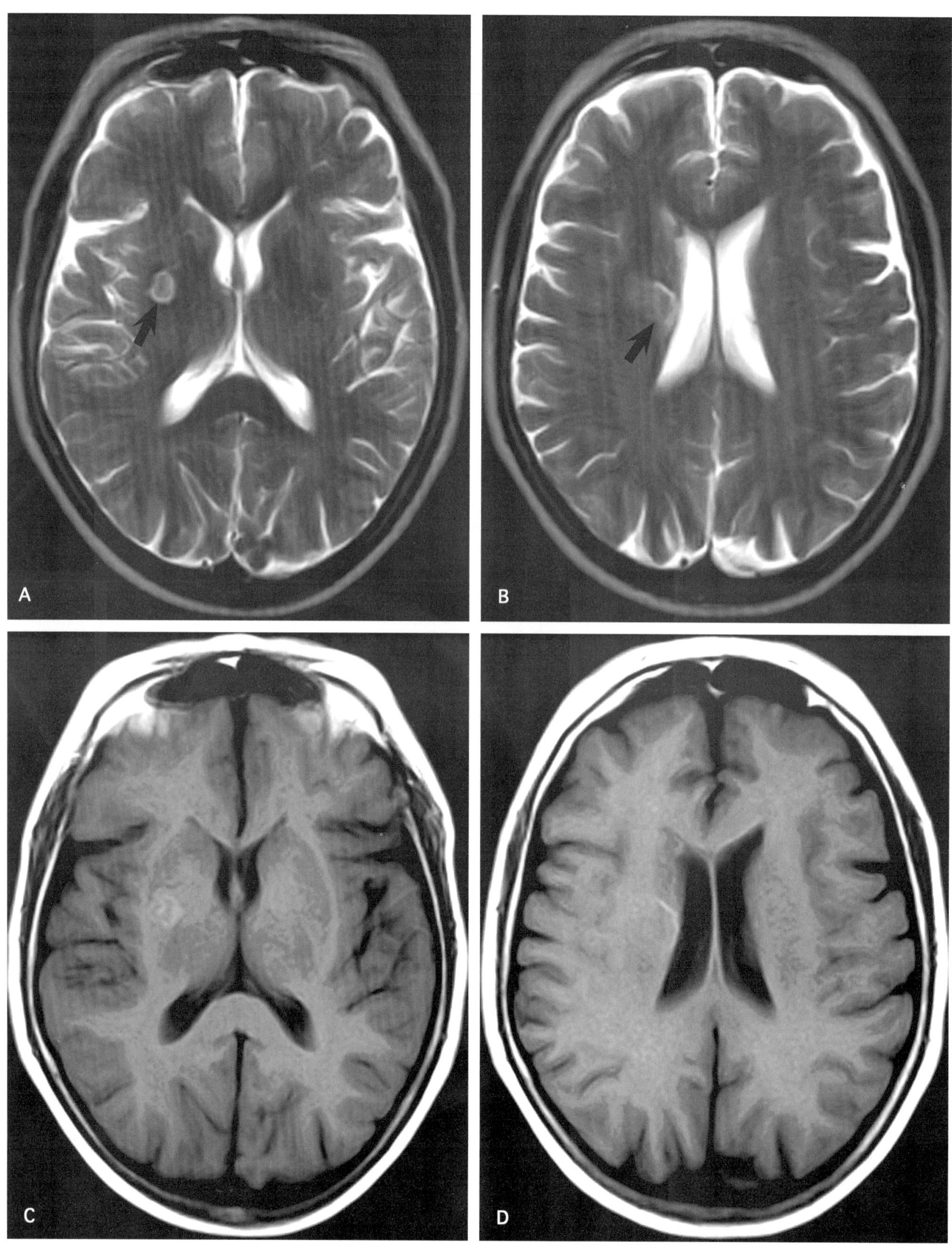
A
B
C
D

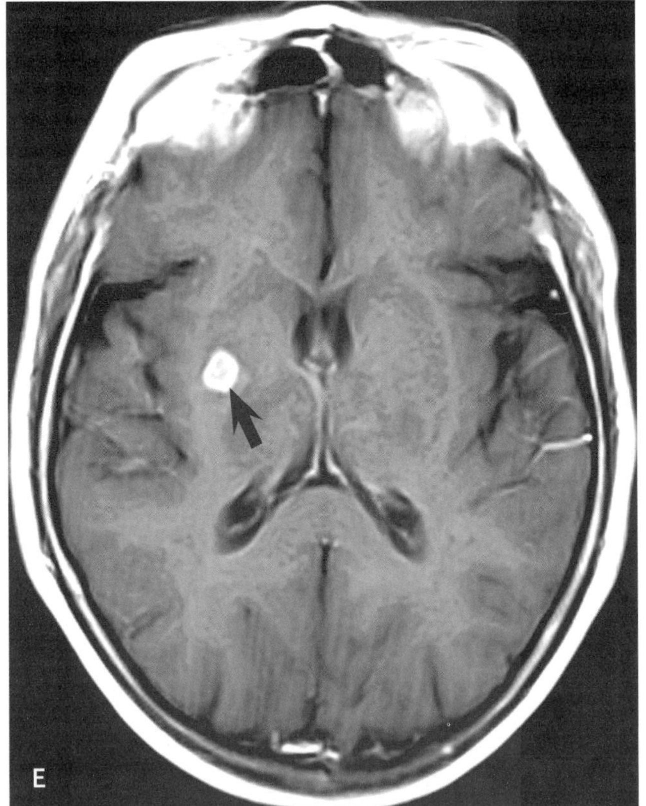

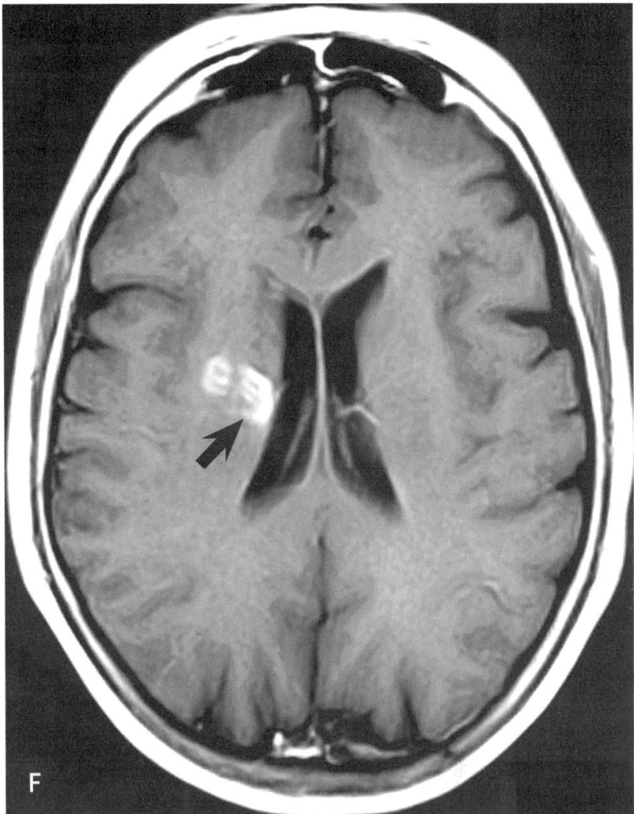

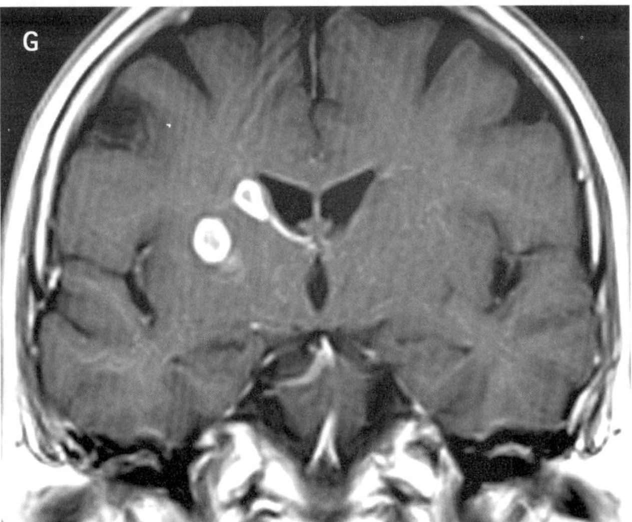

Figure 20. Subacute basal ganglia infarction. On (A, B) contiguous T2 weighted fast spin echo scans, subtle abnormal high signal intensity is noted in the globus pallidus and body of the caudate nucleus on the right (arrows). These abnormalities are much less evident on the corresponding (C, D) pre-contrast T1 weighted scans. Following contrast administration, enhancement of both lesions (arrows) is seen, well depicted on (E, F) axial and (G) coronal T1 weighted scans. Conspicuity of subacute infarcts can be markedly improved by IV contrast administration. The use of contrast also assists in dating lesions. Involvement of both the globus pallidus and caudate nucleus is not uncommon, and points to involvement of the lenticulostriate arteries. These small perforating vessels arise from the superior aspect of the proximal middle cerebral artery (M1 segment) and supply the globus pallidus, putamen, and caudate nuclei.

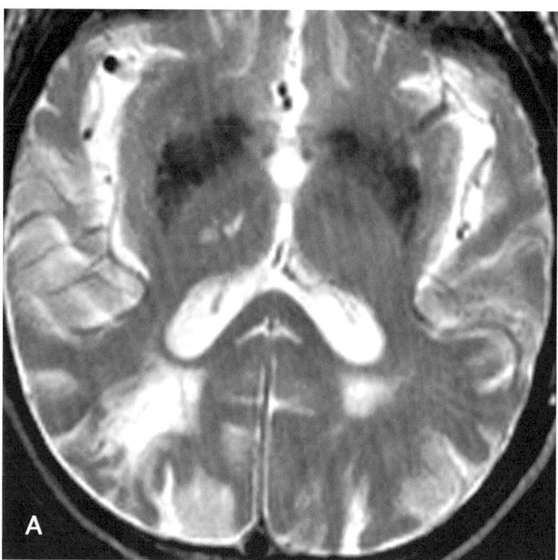

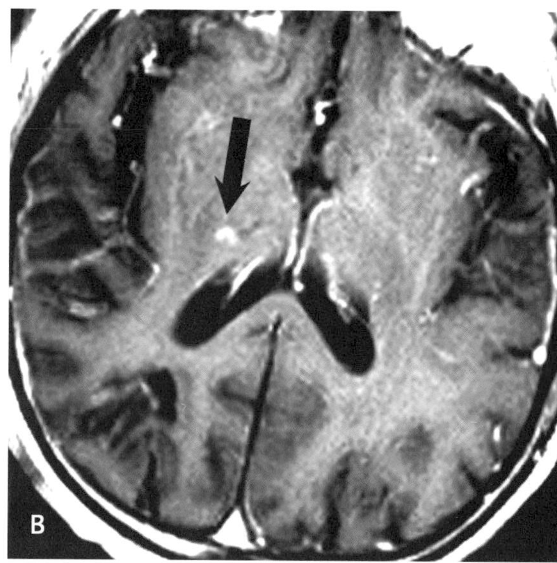

Figure 21. Subacute lacunar infarct involving the posterior limb of the internal capsule. The patient is an elderly diabetic who presents with acute hemiparesis. The MR exam was obtained 10 days following presentation, at which time the hemiparesis had resolved. Multiple high signal intensity abnormalities are noted bilaterally on (A) the T2 weighted scan. The (B) post-contrast T1 weighted scans reveals punctate enhancement (arrow) in the posterior limb of the right internal capsule. This corresponds to a high signal intensity lesion on the T2 weighted scan. By identification of abnormal contrast enhancement, this subacute infarct can be differentiated from other chronic ischemic lesions, which are incidental to the patient's current medical problems. *(From Runge VM, Brack MA, Garneau RA, Kirsch JE. Magnetic resonance imaging of the brain. Philadelphia, JB Lippincott, 1994.)*

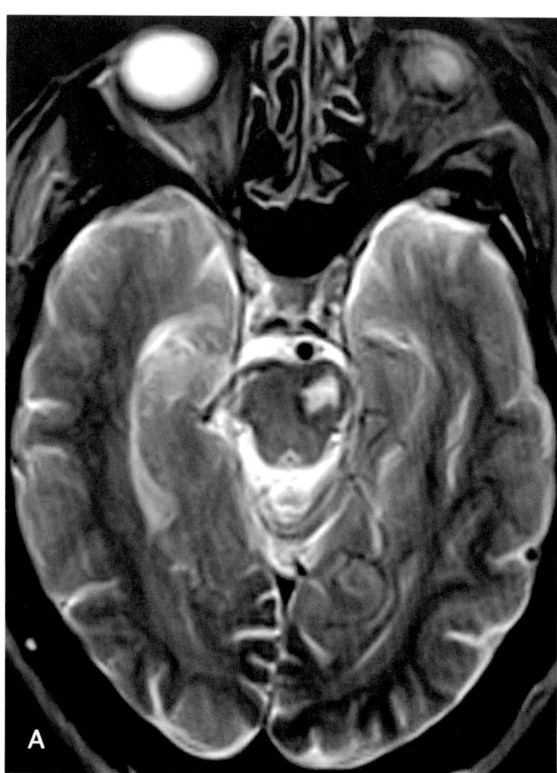

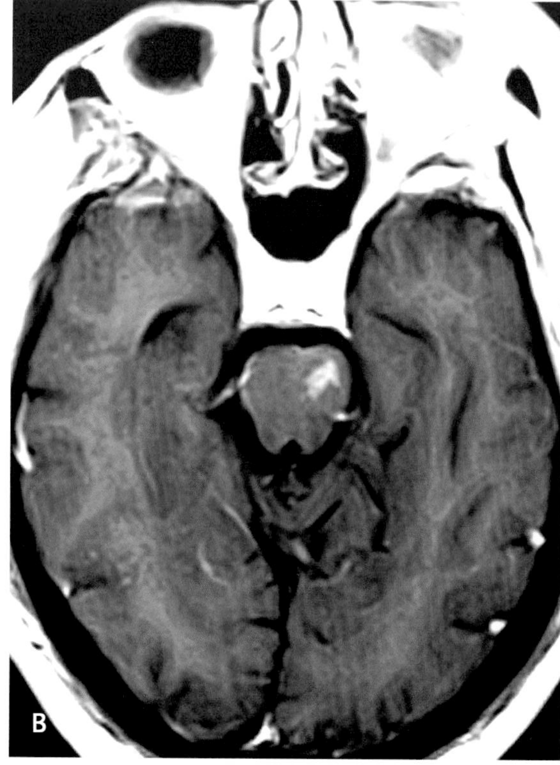

Figure 22. Subacute pontine infarction. On (A) the pre-contrast T2 weighted scan, an area of abnormal hyperintensity is noted in the left pons, with a sharp line of demarcation along the median raphe. (B) Post-contrast, on the T1 weighted scan, the bulk of the lesion enhances. As with other lacunar infarcts, pontine infarcts will consistently demonstrate contrast enhancement following gadolinium chelate administration in the subacute time period.

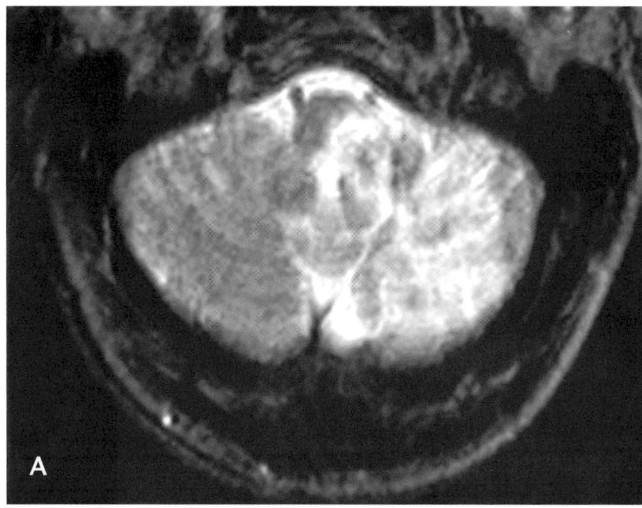

Figure 23. Posterior inferior cerebellar artery (PICA) infarction. An elderly patient presented with nausea and dizziness six days prior to the current MR exam. Abnormal high signal intensity is noted in the left cerebellar hemisphere, vermis, and medulla in the distribution of PICA on (A) the T2 weighted scan. Comparison of (B) pre- and (C) post-contrast T1 weighted scans demonstrates abnormal parenchymal enhancement, consistent with a subacute infarct. *(From Runge VM, Brack MA, Garneau RA, Kirsch JE. Magnetic resonance imaging of the brain. Philadelphia, JB Lippincott, 1994.)*

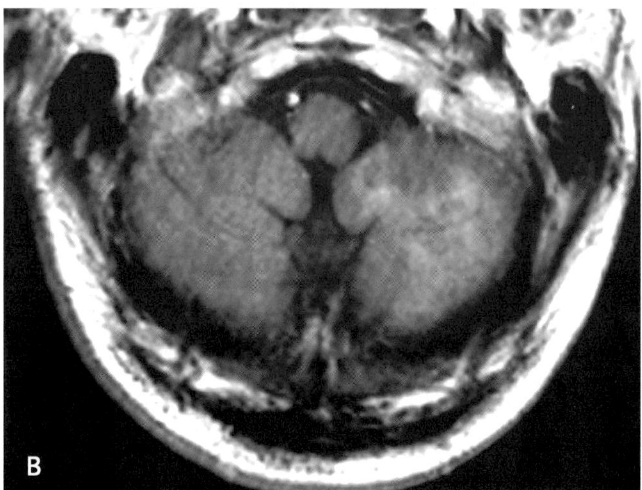

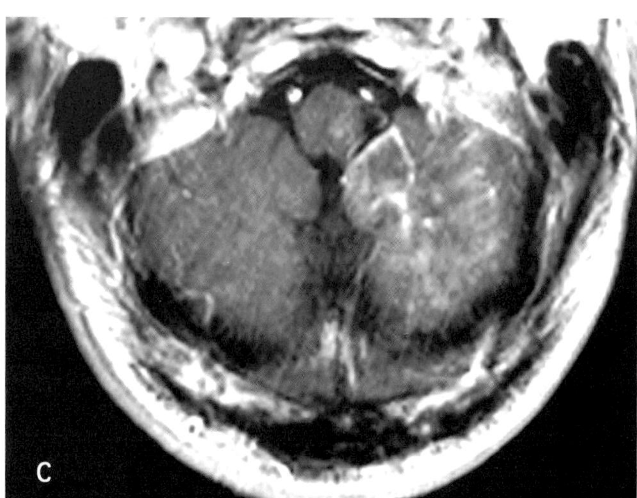

along the median raphe (basilar sulcus) and branch laterally.

In cerebellar infarcts, contrast enhancement can serve to confirm the diagnosis made from unenhanced scans. In small subacute lesions, enhancement can be punctate or linear, while in larger lesions enhancement is commonly circumferential (figure 23).

Diseases of white matter

Gadolinium chelate administration enables the assessment of lesion activity in demyelinating disease. Within this category, multiple sclerosis (MS) is the most common entity, and also the disease in which there is the most experience with contrast enhancement. In other less common entities such as acute disseminated encephalomyelitis (ADEM), contrast use should provide similar benefits.

Active lesions in MS demonstrate disruption of the BBB, and thus show enhancement post-contrast on MR (figure 24).[30,31] Although lesions are generally best identified on T2 weighted scans, on occasion a lesion will only be evident post-contrast. In an extensive serial study, four such cases were identified, with contrast enhancement preceding development of other recognizable MR abnormalities for a small number of new lesions.[32] It has been postulated that a defect in the BBB is an early, critical event in the development of new MS lesions. Enhanced MR has also been used to monitor changes in the disease process during therapy. Lesion enhancement is a transient process, with evolution from homogeneous to ring-like noted in some instances (figure 25). A short course of high dose intravenous methylprednisolone has been noted to suppress lesion enhancement, correlating with clinical improvement.[33] The rare occurrence of a giant MS plaque should be kept in mind as a diagnostic pitfall (figure 26).

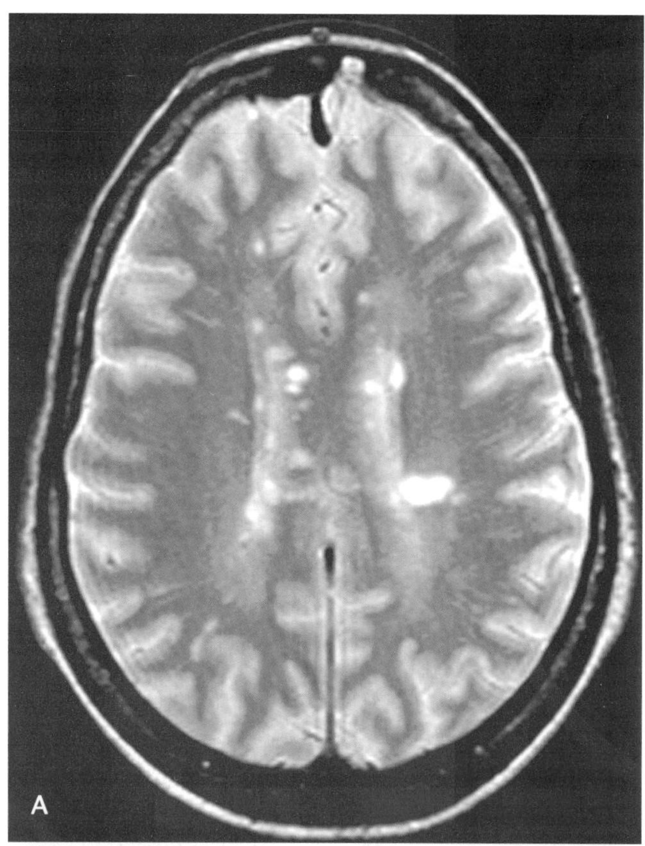

Figure 24. Multiple sclerosis, active disease. Bilateral punctate high signal intensity white matter lesions are noted in the periventricular white matter and in the body of the corpus callosum on (A) the T2 weighted scan. These findings are consistent with the diagnosis of multiple sclerosis. (B) The pre-contrast T1 weighted exam identifies only a few of these abnormalities. (C) Post-contrast, several lesions (arrows) demonstrate abnormal enhancement, signifying active disease. Contrast enhancement plays a specific role in multiple sclerosis for the demonstration of active lesions and for following response to therapy. *(From Runge VM, Brack MA, Garneau RA, Kirsch JE. Magnetic resonance imaging of the brain. Philadelphia, JB Lippincott, 1994.)*

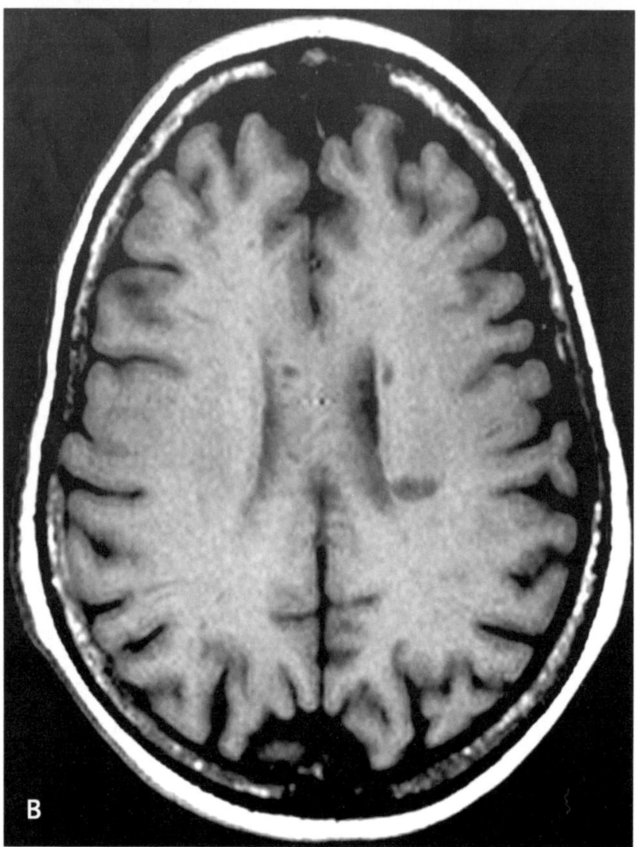

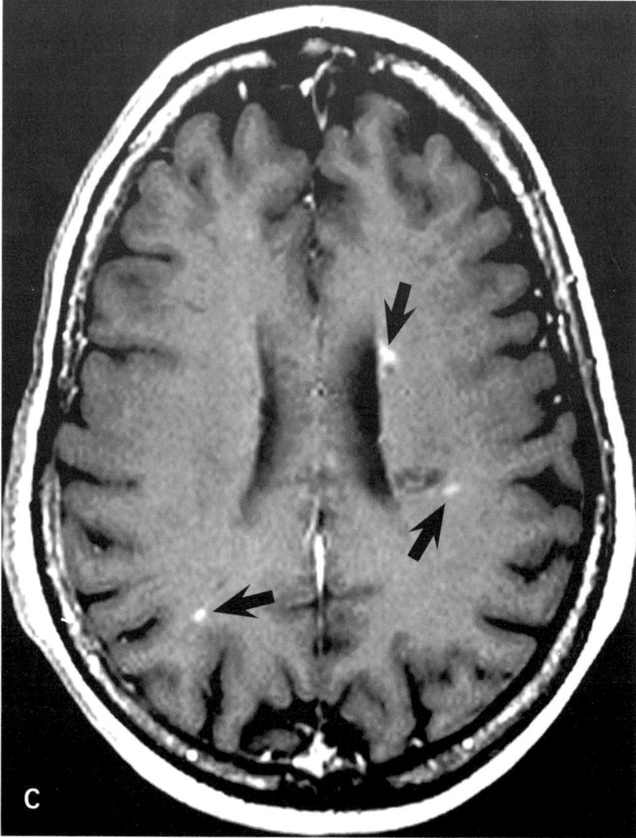

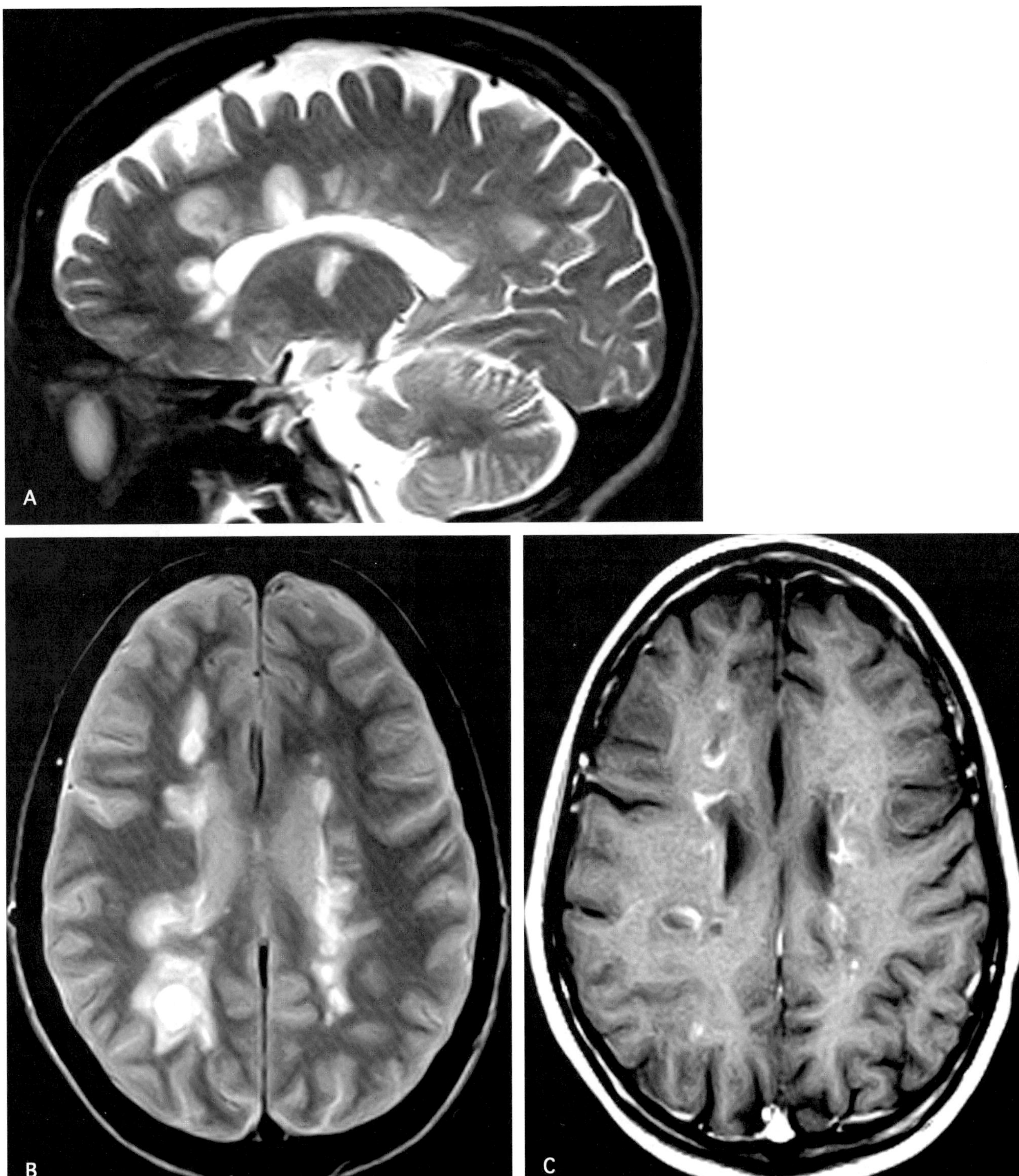

Figure 25. Multiple sclerosis (MS) mimicking metastatic disease. On (A) the sagittal heavily T2 weighted fast spin echo scan, multiple periventricular high signal intensity abnormalities are noted. Some involve the corpus callosum and have a broad base along the border of the lateral ventricle. The distribution of the lesions in the periventricular white matter is confirmed on (B) the axial scan with intermediate T2 weighting. On (C) the corresponding post-contrast T1 weighted scan, many of the lesions demonstrate ring enhancement. Focusing on the post-contrast exam alone, the multiplicity of lesions and ring enhancement could lead to an incorrect diagnosis of metastatic disease. The knowledge that MS plaques can demonstrate ring enhancement, together with recognition of the characteristic location of these lesions, leads to the proper diagnosis. The availability of pertinent clinical history is also paramount to film interpretation.

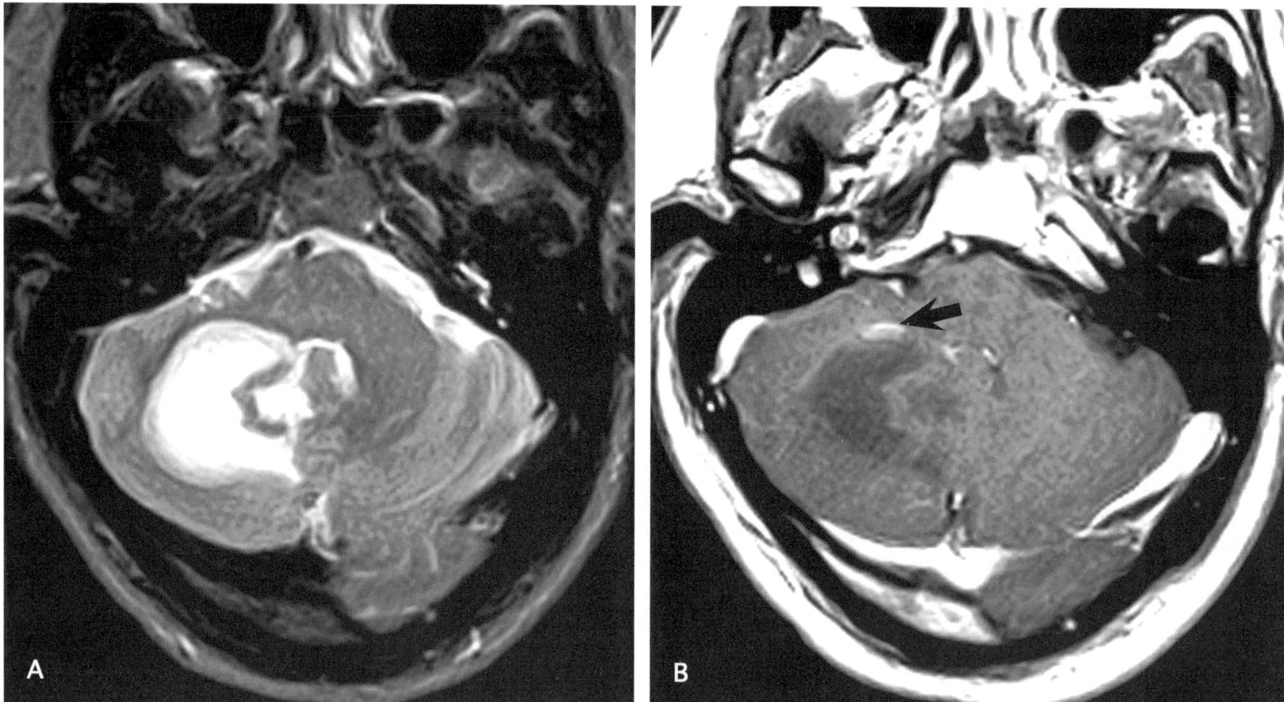

Figure 26. Multiple sclerosis (MS) mimicking primary brain tumor. On (A) the T2 weighted scan, a large lesion in the right cerebellar hemisphere is noted. White matter is principally involved. The dentate nucleus stands out, surrounded by edema. On (B) the post-contrast T1 weighted scan, mild enhancement is noted along the rim of the lesion, best seen anteriorly (arrow). The remainder of the MR head exam was normal. Misdiagnosis of a solitary giant MS plaque is a known diagnostic pitfall on CT. It is not as well known that this situation can also occur on MR. The lesion in this case was biopsied, with a subsequent exam of the spinal cord revealing additional lesions characteristic for MS.

Trauma

By five to six days following head trauma, parenchymal contrast enhancement may be observed because of damage to the blood-brain barrier (figure 27). Although not critical for lesion recognition, it is important to be familiar with this finding to avoid misdiagnosis. The use of contrast may also in the future improve our understanding of the nature and timing of underlying pathophysiologic changes.[34]

Conclusion

Since the initial clinical evaluation of contrast enhancement in neoplastic disease of the brain in the 1980s, many major new applications have emerged. Contrast administration permits improved lesion detection and differential diagnosis for non-neoplastic disease of the brain. Its use is highly recommended in infection and vascular disorders. Utility has also been demonstrated in demyelinating diseases of white matter and subacute trauma. Only in congenital disease of the brain, when acute abnormalities are not suspected clinically and neoplasia is not a consideration, are unenhanced scans alone routinely employed. The scope of applications continues to broaden with concomitant rapid development of new MR software and hardware, in particular echo planar imaging.

References

1. Ramsey R, Geremia G. CNS complications of AIDS: CT and MR findings. AJR 1988;151:449-454.

2. Balakrishnan J, Becker P, Kumar A, et al. Acquired immmunodeficiency syndrome: correlation of radiologic and pathologic findings in the brain. Radiographics 1990;10:201-215.

3. Castillo M. Brain infections in human immunodeficiency virus positive patients. Top Magn Reson Imaging 1994;6:3-10.

4. Tuite M, Ketonen L, Kieburtz K, Handy B. Efficacy of gadolinium in MR brain imaging of HIV infected patients. AJNR 1993;14:257-263.

5. Schroth G, Kretzschmar K, Gawehn J, et al. Advantage of magnetic resonance imaging in the diagnosis of cerebral infections. Neuroradiology 1987;29:120-126.

6. Lester J, Carter M, Reynolds T. Herpes encephalitis: MR monitoring of response to acyclovir therapy. J Comput Assist Tomogr 1988;12:941-943.

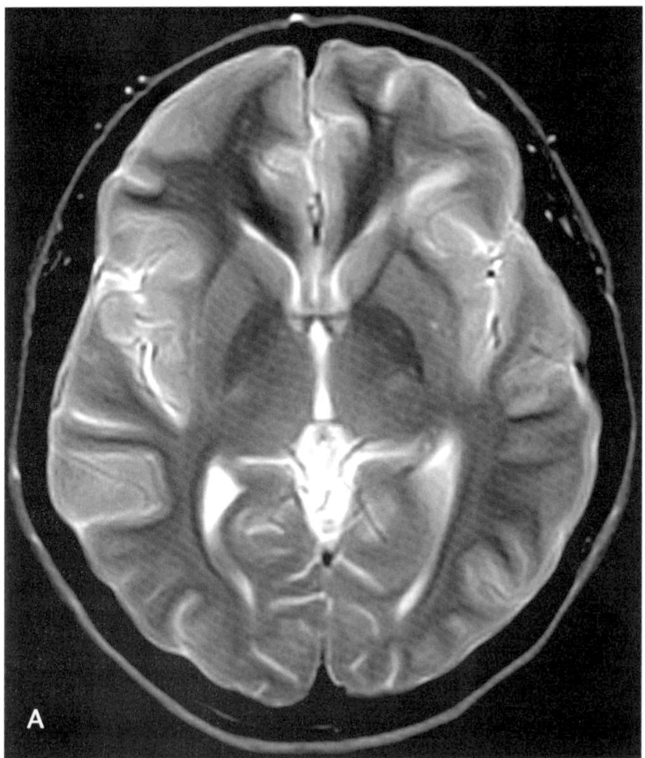

Figure 27. Cortical contusion. A young person presents several days following a severe fall down a flight of stairs. There is subtle abnormal high signal intensity within left frontal white matter on (A) the T2 weighted scan. (B) The pre-contrast T1 weighted scan is unremarkable. (C) Post-contrast, gyriform enhancement is noted in several locations, all within cortical gray matter of the frontal lobe. Contusion of the brain cortex has led to blood-brain barrier disruption, which demonstrates more accurately the degree and extent of injury than vasogenic edema, the latter visualized on the T2 weighted scan.

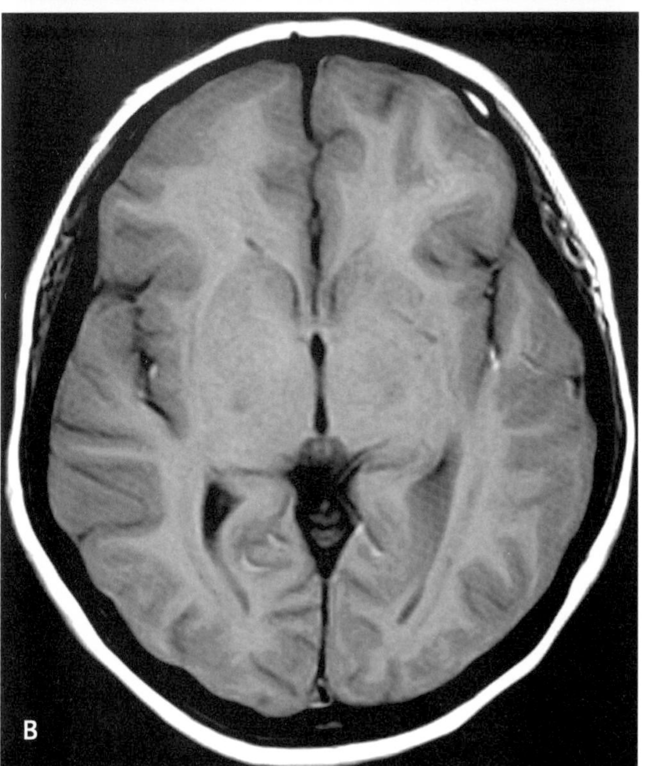

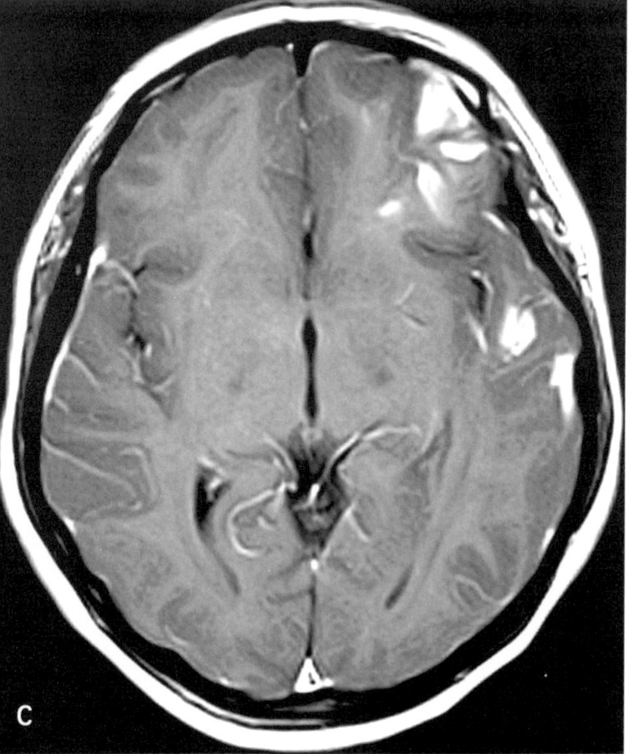

7. Demaerel P, Wilms G, Robberecht W, et al. MRI of herpes simplex encephalitis. Neuroradiology 1992;34:490-493.
8. Runge VM, Clanton JA, Price AC, et al. Evaluation of contrast enhanced MR imaging in a brain abscess model. AJNR 1985;6:139-147.
9. Mathews VP, Kuharik MA, Edwards MK, et al. Gd DTPA enhanced MR imaging of experimental bacterial meningitis: evaluation and comparison with CT. AJR 1989;152:131-136.
10. Chang KH, Han MH, Roh JK, et al. Gd DTPA enhanced MR imaging of the brain in patients with meningitis: comparison with CT. AJR 1990;154:809-816.
11. Frank JA, Girton M, Dwyer AJ, et al. Meningeal carcinomatosis in the VX2 rabbit tumor model: detection with Gd DTPA enhanced MR imaging. Radiology 1988;167:825-829.
12. Schorner W, Henkes H, Sander B, Felix R. MR demonstration of the meninges: normal and pathological findings. ROFO 1988;149:361-368.
13. Lee YY, Tien RD, Bruner JM, et al. Loculated intracranial leptomeningeal metastases: CT and MR characteristics. AJR 1990;154:351-359.
14. Burke JW, Podrasky AE, Bradley WG Jr. Meninges: benign post-operative enhancement on MR images. Radiology 1990;174:99-102.
15. Elster AD, DiPersio DA. Cranial postoperative site: assessment with contrast enhanced MR imaging. Radiology 1990;174:93-98.
16. Marchal G, Michiels J, Bosmans H, Van Hecke P. Contrast enhanced MRA of the brain. J Comput Assist Tomogr 1992;16:25-29.
17. Runge VM, Kirsch JE, Lee C. Contrast-enhanced MR angiography. J Magn Reson Imaging 1993;3:233-239.
18. Chakeres DW, Schmalbrock P, Brogan M, et al. Normal venous anatomy of the brain: demonstration with gadopentetate dimeglumine in enhanced 3-D MR angiography. AJR 1991;156:161-172.
19. Wilms G, Demaerel P, Marchal G, et al. Gadolinium enhanced MR imaging of cerebral venous angiomas with emphasis on their drainage. J Comput Assist Tomogr 1991;15:199-206.
20. Muras I, Conforti R, Scuotto A, et al. Cerebral cavernous angioma. Diagnostic considerations. J Neuroradiol 1993;20:34-41.
21. Elster AD, Moody DM. Early cerebral infarction: gadopentetate dimeglumine enhancement. Radiology 1990;177:627-632.
22. Imakita S, Nishimura T, Yamada N, et al. Magnetic resonance imaging of cerebral infarction: time course of Gd DTPA enhancement and CT comparison. Neuroradiology 1988;30:372-378.
23. Runge VM, Kirsch JE, Wells JW, et al. Visualization of blood-brain barrier disruption on MR images of cats with acute cerebral infarction: value of administering a high dose of contrast material. AJR 1994;162:431-435.
24. Edelman RR, Mattle HP, Atkinson DJ, et al. Cerebral blood flow: assessment with dynamic contrast enhanced T2*-weighted MR imaging at 1.5 T. Radiology 1990;176:211-220.
25. Warach S, Li W, Ronthal M, Edelman RR. Acute cerebral ischemia: evaluation with dynamic contrast-enhanced MR imaging and MR angiography. Radiology 1992;182:41-47.
26. Runge VM, Kirsch JE, Wells JW, Woolfolk CE. Assessment of cerebral perfusion by first-pass, dynamic, contrast-enhanced, steady-state free-precession MR imaging: an animal study. AJR 1993;160:593-600.
27. Finelli DA, Hopkins AL, Selman WR, et al. Evaluation of experimental early acute cerebral ischemia before the development of edema: use of dynamic, contrast enhanced and diffusion weighted MR scanning. Magn Reson Med 1992;27:189-197.
28. Regli L, Regli F, Maeder P, Bogousslavsky J. Magnetic resonance imaging with gadolinium contrast agent in small deep (lacunar) cerebral infarcts. Archives of Neurology 1993;50:175-180.
29. Miyashita K, Naritomi H, Sawada T, et al. Identification of recent lacunar lesions in cases of multiple small infarctions by magnetic resonance imaging. Stroke 1988;19:834-839.
30. Grossman RI, Gonzalez-Scarano F, Atlas SW, et al. Multiple sclerosis: gadolinium enhancement in MR imaging. Radiology 1986;161:721-725.
31. Miller DH, Rudge P, Johnson G, et al. Serial gadolinium enhanced magnetic resonance imaging in multiple sclerosis. Brain 1988;111:927-939.
32. Kermode AG, Thompson AJ, Tofts P, et al. Breakdown of the blood-brain barrier precedes symptoms and other MRI signs of new lesions in multiple sclerosis. Pathogenetic and clinical implications. Brain 1990;113:1477-1489.
33. Burnham JA, Wright RR, Dreisbach J, Murray RS. The effect of high dose steroids on MRI gadolinium enhancement in acute demyelinating lesions. Neurology 1991;41:1349-1354.
34. Lang DA, Hadley DM, Teasdale GM, et al. Gadolinium DTPA enhanced magnetic resonance imaging in human head injury. Acta Neurochir Suppl 1990;51:293-295.

Chapter 4

Spine: Neoplastic And Non-Neoplastic Disease

J. Randy Jinkins, M.D. and Val M. Runge, M.D.

Introduction

Magnetic resonance (MR) has permitted for the first time noninvasive, accurate delineation of the spinal cord and spinal nerve roots. The subsequent development of paramagnetic gadolinium chelates has made it possible to accurately and sensitively pinpoint disruptions or absences in the blood-central nervous system (CNS) barrier frequently associated with spinal disease.[1] This chapter outlines the use of MR contrast agents in the evaluation of disease involving the spinal column, spinal neural tissue, and spinal leptomeninges.[2]

General Principles of MR Contrast Use

Gadolinium containing contrast agents must come into close proximity with water protons in order to exert their effect and thereby enhance proton relaxation. In the CNS this can only occur if there is a disruption in the blood-CNS barrier. The blood-CNS barrier in the spine consists of the blood-cord barrier, the blood-nerve barrier, and the relative blood-leptomeningeal barrier. A breakdown in any one of these may cause leakage of a gadolinium chelate in sufficient quantities from regional blood vessels to produce enhancement on T1-weighted MR imaging. In certain slow-flow states, as may be seen in arterial occlusive disease or venous pathology affecting the CNS, advantage can also be taken of the intravascular location of the gadolinium chelate. In such cases, pathologic intravascular enhancement may be observed.

The decision whether or not to use a contrast agent in any MR examination should ideally be decided prospectively, based on adequate information from the clinical history and physical exam supplied by the referring physician. Alternatively, the decision can be made after the pre-contrast exam and largely based on imaging criteria. However, this is not ideal as it will often require patient recall in order to perform the contrast enhanced study. Considering the continuing rise in cost of medical care, it is important to attempt to make these decisions prospectively. This avoids prolonging the diagnostic work up, duplicating diagnostic procedures, and ultimately extending the period and expense of patient care.

Differential Diagnosis of Pathologic Spinal Enhancement

In order to focus the differential diagnosis, the MR examination can be used in much the same way as other CNS imaging procedures have been in the past. For instance, a different although overlapping differential diagnostic set can be generated for a disease process depending upon the spinal compartment in which gadolinium chelate enhancement is identified. Pathologic enhancement identified in the intramedullary compartment (spinal cord) will have a somewhat different differential diagnosis than will pathologic enhancement in the intradural-extramedullary or extradural spaces. This is very useful in practice because it suggests a more narrow differential diagnosis, and thereby forms an important part of pattern recognition. This principle is fundamental to all fields of diagnostic imaging.

Applications of MR Contrast Use

Hereditary and Developmental Disease

The disease processes amenable to contrast enhancement in this category will for the most part lie within the class of abnormalities known as the phacomatoses. These are heredi-

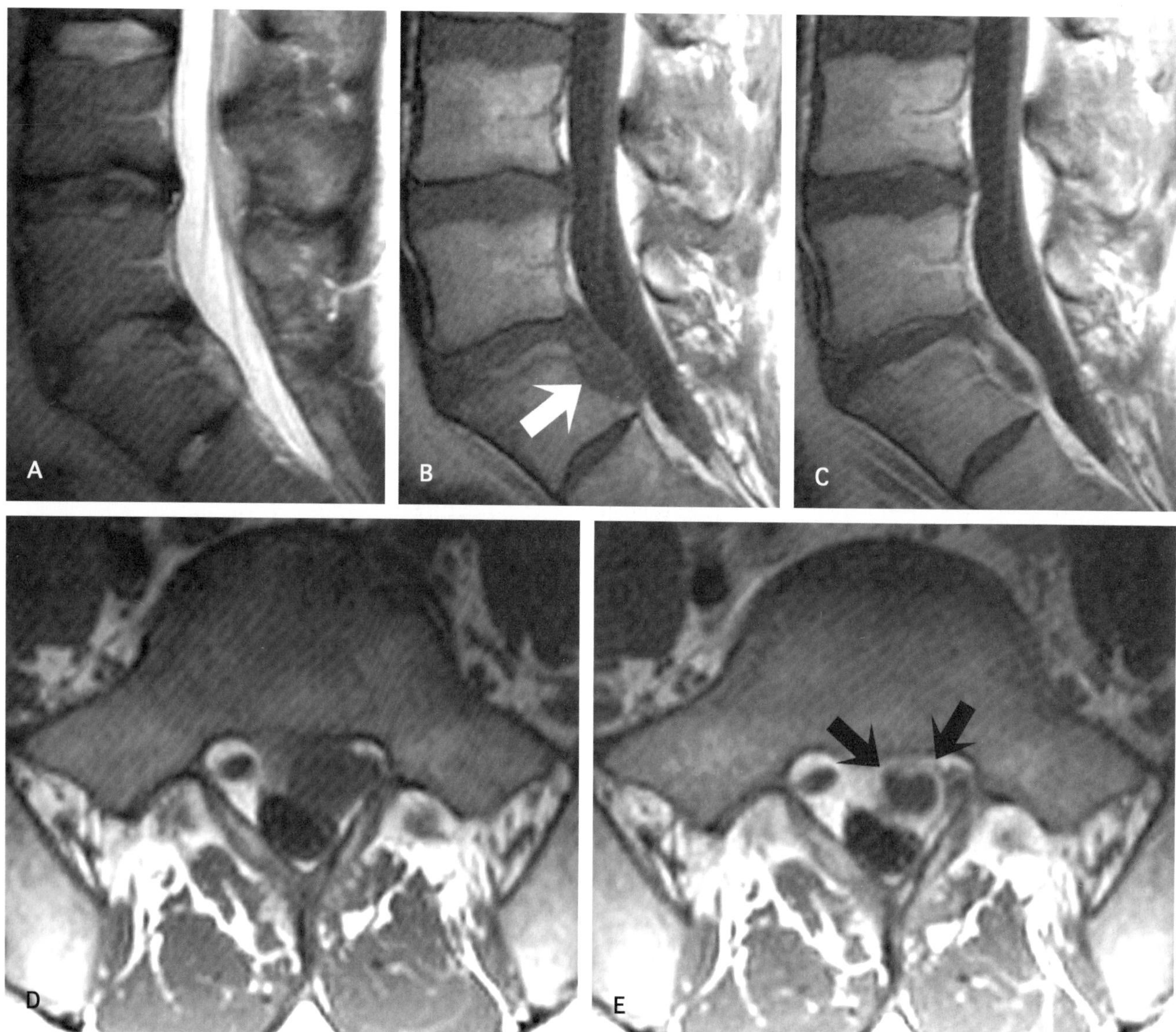

Figure 1. Free disk fragment. On (A) the T2-weighted sagittal scan, a soft tissue mass with abnormal high signal intensity is identified posterior to S1. This mass (white arrow) is isointense with the remaining disk material at the L5-S1 level on (B) the T1-weighted sagittal scan. (C) Post-contrast, the periphery of the mass enhances. Inspection of (D) pre- and (E) post-contrast axial scans through the S1 vertebral body confirm the presence of a free disk fragment. The fragment is "wrapped" by enhancing scar (arrows), deforms the thecal sac and compresses the left S1 nerve root.

tary diseases that often manifest neoplasia within the nervous system and related tissues. For example, the neurofibromatoses are neurocutaneous syndromes that typically present with multifocal neoplasms of the spinal cord, cerebrum, spinal and cranial nerves/nerve roots, and leptomeninges. In addition, gadolinium chelates have been found to be very useful for distinguishing enhancing disease, which may represent neoplasia, from nonenhancing disease, which may represent glottic or hamartomatous change.

One other pertinent example of the use of contrast media in this disease class is to search for either solid or mural enhancement (in cystic lesions) in hemangioblastomas in patients with von Hippel-Lindau disease. These tumors may be multifocal, occurring predominantly in the posterior fossa and spinal cord.

Degenerative Disease

Unenhanced MR well demonstrates degenerative and traumatic changes within the spinal cord and epidural tissues. In addition, there are major applications for the use of MR contrast agents in the study of spinal degenerative disease (figure 1).[3]

In the unoperated spine, it has been found that there is frequently a breakdown in the blood-nerve barrier associated with root pathology, for example that caused by disk

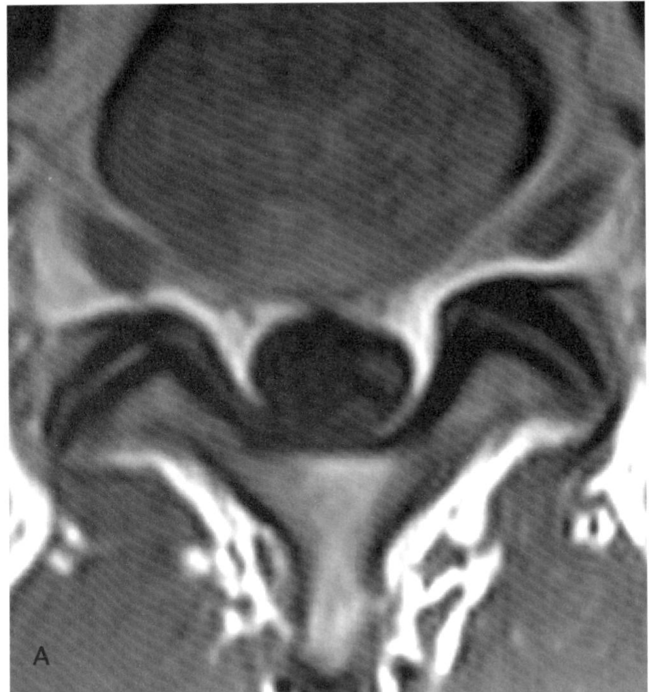

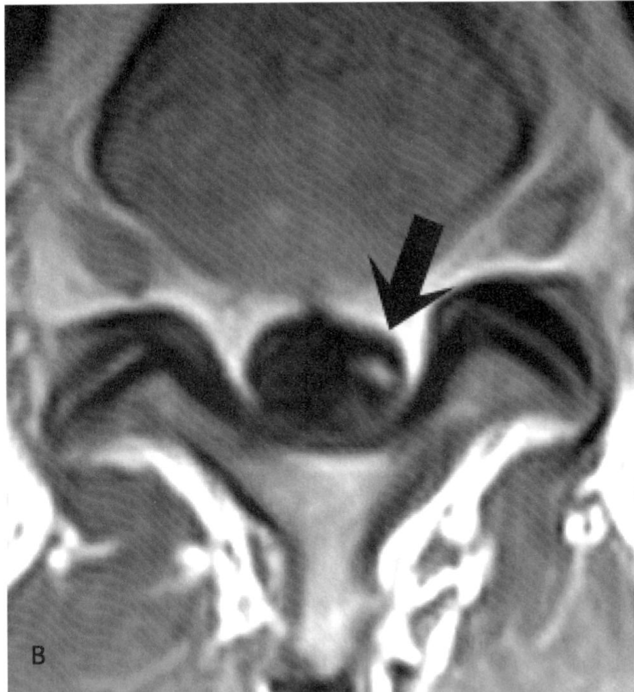

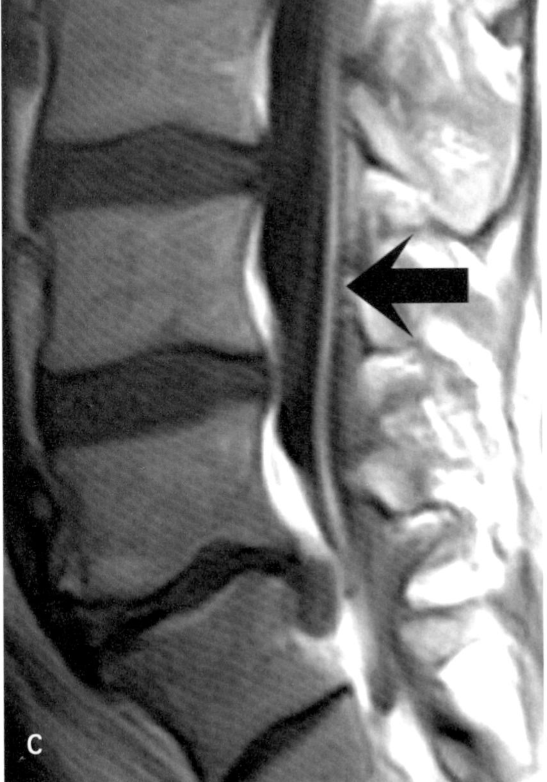

Figure 2. Enhancing nerve root, due to compression by a large free fragment. Comparison of (A) pre- and (B) post-contrast T1-weighted axial scans at the L5-S1 level reveals intense enhancement of the left S1 nerve root (arrow) within the thecal sac. This is confirmed on (C) the post-contrast T1-weighted sagittal scan (arrow), which also identifies nerve root compression by a large disk fragment. The patient was referred for a MR scan due to recent onset of a left S1 radiculopathy.

herniation.[4] Focal breakdown of the blood-nerve barrier in such instances is most certainly due to direct trauma. Nerve root enhancement remote from the site of the actual neural injury is likely due to Wallerian degeneration of the injured axons (figure 2). This remote enhancement may extend from the site of nerve injury proximally all the way to the spinal cord and distally through the neural foramen. With regeneration of the axon, the blood-nerve barrier disruption has been seen to resolve with an expected parallel resolution of enhancement.

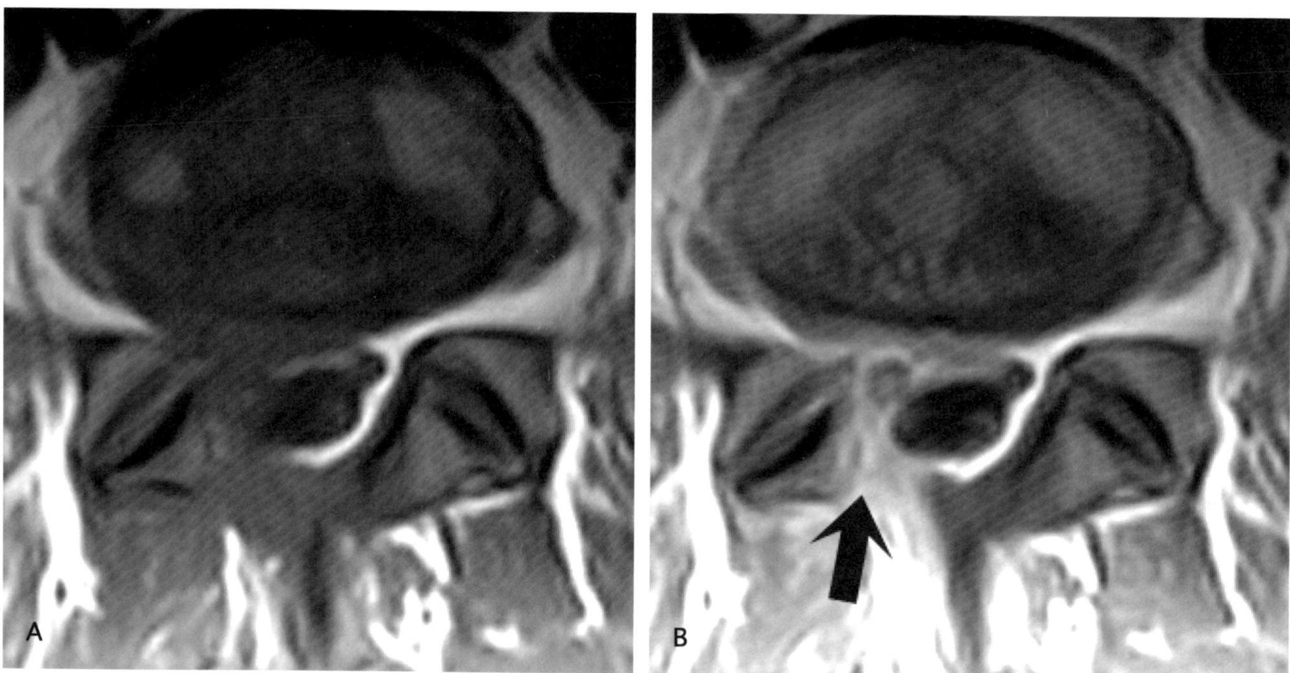

Figure 3. Post-diskectomy scar tissue. Two months following a right laminectomy and diskectomy, a soft tissue mass is identified anterior and to the right of the thecal sac on (A) the pre-contrast T1-weighted axial scan. (B) Post-contrast, there is uniform enhancement of this abnormal soft tissue (arrow), consistent with scar. The right S1 nerve root can only be identified post-contrast, surrounded by scar.

The incidence of pathologic lumbosacral nerve root enhancement in the preoperative spine associated with clinical radicular symptoms was found to be roughly 60% following intravenous administration of a standard 0.1 mmol/kg dosage of a gadolinium chelate. In this same study, the incidence of lumbosacral root enhancement rose to 100% with a dose of 0.3 mmol/kg.

The use of gadolinium chelates is an integral part of MR imaging in the postoperative spine.[5] Utilizing MR contrast agents, recurrent disk herniation can be distinguished from simple, isolated epidural fibrosis, and chronic, pathologic nerve root enhancement (sterile radiculitis) can be demonstrated (figures 3, 4).[6] Following disk surgery, the use of intravenous contrast is well justified to differentiate between scar and recurrent (or residual) disk herniation, if repeat surgery is being considered. Abnormal soft tissue impinging upon the thecal sac that enhances represents scar tissue. Disk material, which is relatively avascular, will not demonstrate enhancement on early post-contrast scans. Enhanced scans should be acquired within 20 minutes following contrast administration, since contrast can diffuse into disk material on delayed scans. Sections should be thin (less than or equal to 3 mm), to avoid partial volume imaging.

Postoperative pathologic nerve root enhancement may be seen in association with recurrent disk herniation, in the presence of epidural fibrosis or simply in an isolated form in the absence of associated pathology. Other nerve root pathology may also be revealed following contrast administration (figure 5).

The incidence of pathologic nerve root enhancement was 20% in a recent postoperative study of patients presenting with the failed back surgery syndrome.[7] During the first six to eight months following surgery, neural enhancement is an expected phenomenon, presumably representing a reparative process in the asymptomatic postoperative patient. However, the presence of nerve root enhancement was not a normal postoperative finding after eight months. The correlation of the clinical syndrome with nerve root enhancement in either the pre- or postoperative lumbosacral spine was seen to be over 90%. Although untested at present, the treatment of clinically correlative nerve root enhancement will likely be aimed at a stabilization of the axon membrane utilizing various conservative modes of therapy (e.g., bed rest, corticosteroids, or colchicine).

A recently recognized application of MR contrast agents[8] is in patients presenting with spinal or "neurogenic" claudication. A MR study in such patients found that a significant number (approximately 70%) demonstrated enhancement of spinal nerve roots in association with central stenosis of the lumbosacral spinal canal. This breakdown of the blood-nerve barrier was apparently caused by direct neural trauma engendered by the central spinal stenosis coupled with extensive Wallerian degeneration. From a practical standpoint, vascular claudication cannot always be easily distinguished

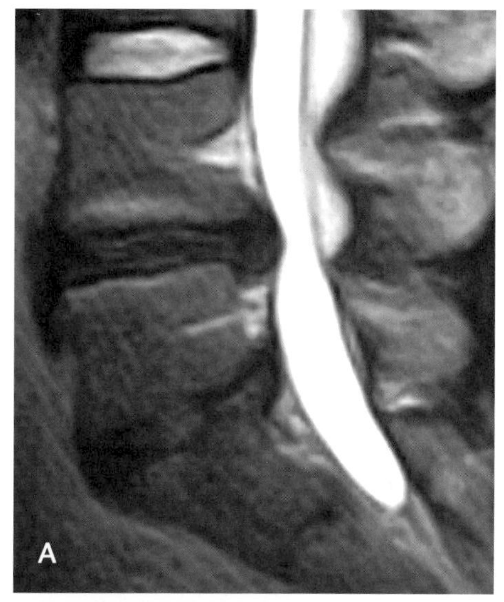

Figure 4. Post-diskectomy recurrent disk extrusion. (A) T2 and (B) T1-weighted midline sagittal scans reveal abnormal soft tissue anterior to the thecal sac at the L4-5 and L5-S1 levels. Two previous percutaneous diskectomies had been performed. (C) Post-contrast, the majority of abnormal soft tissue at each level does not enhance. Enhancing soft tissue (arrows, C) above and below the L4-5 disk space level corresponds to dilated epidural venous plexus. Comparison of (D) pre- and (E) post-contrast T1-weighted axial scans at the L4-5 level confirms the presence of a recurrent disk herniation (arrow), with a small amount of surrounding enhancing granulation tissue. Lumbar microdiskectomy was subsequently performed.

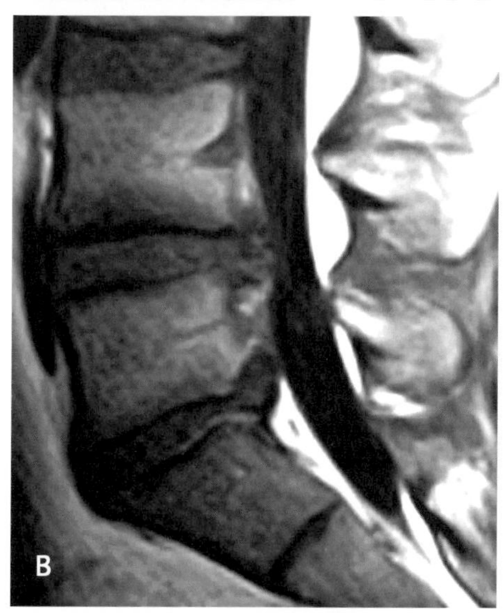

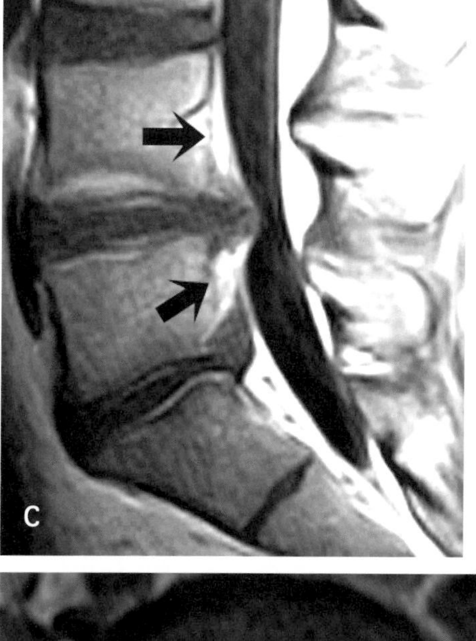

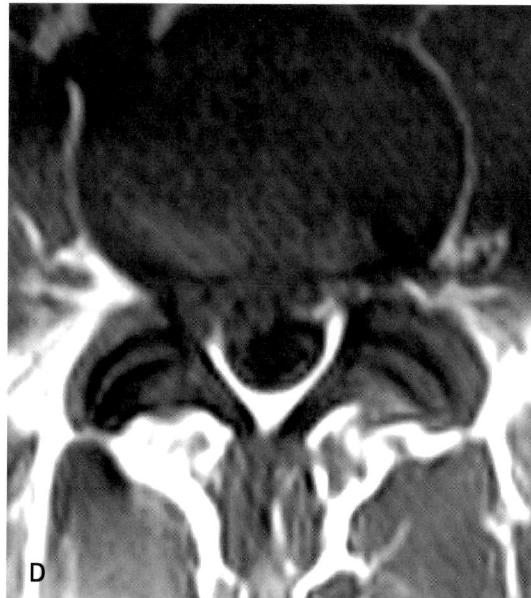

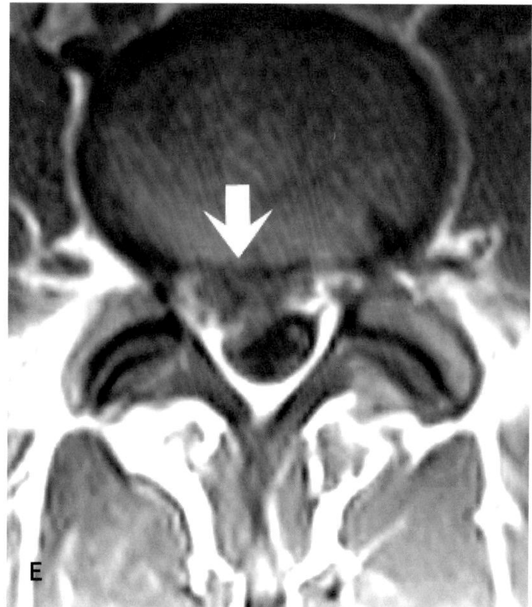

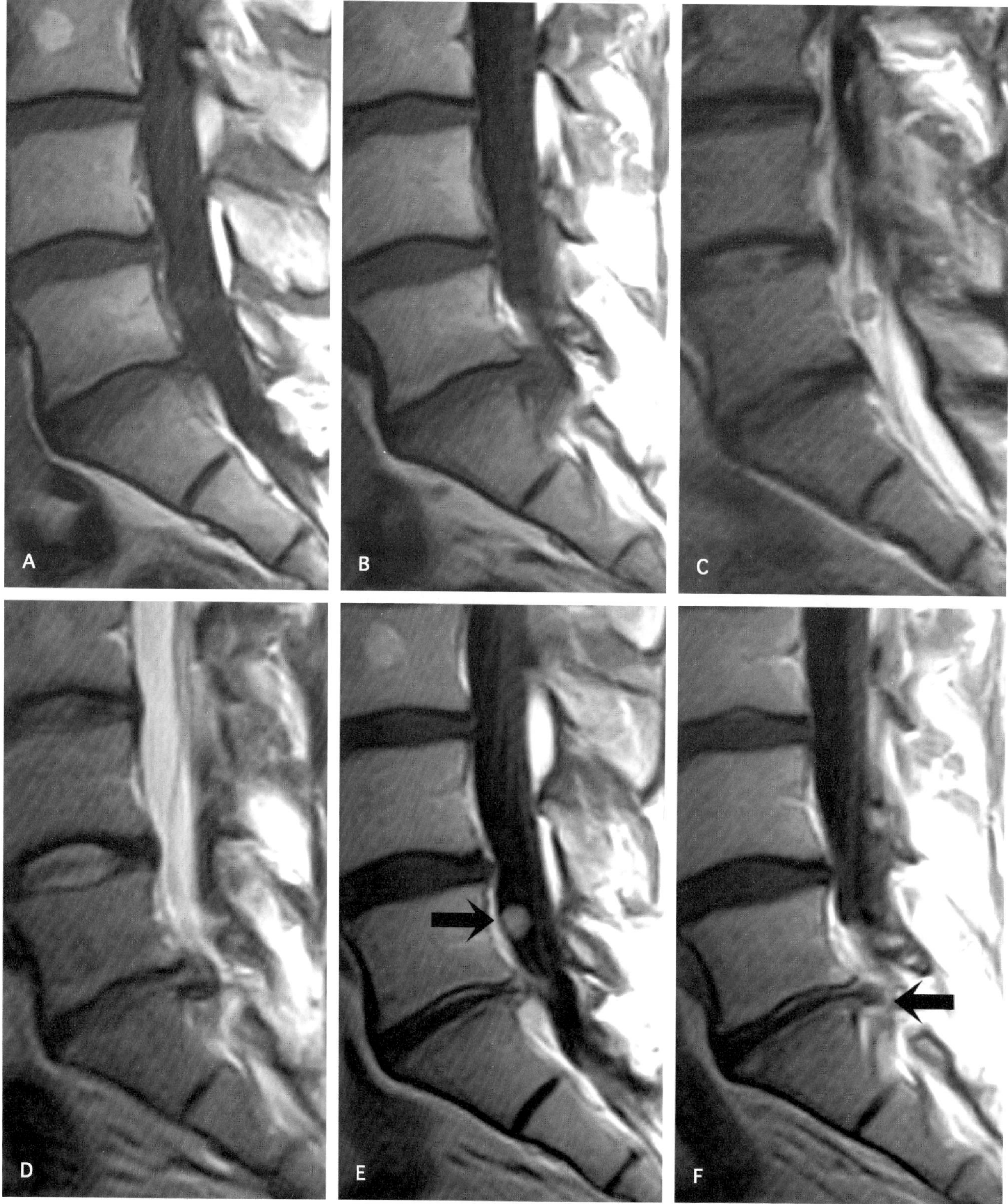

Figure 5. Recurrent disk (two years after surgery) and lumbar nerve root schwannoma. (A, B) T1 pre-contrast, (C, D) T2 and (E, F) T1 post-contrast images are presented. Soft tissue extrudes posteriorly at L5-S1, well seen in B and D. Administration of contrast identifies non-enhancing central disk material, "wrapped" with enhancing scar (arrow, F). An "incidental" schwannoma (arrow, E) is well seen following contrast administration.

from neurogenic claudication in the elderly patient. If neural enhancement following intravenous gadolinium chelate administration is identified in such patients, some component of the clinical syndrome can be attributed to central stenosis. In this way, the observation of nerve root enhancement can influence patient treatment.

If there is non-bony compression of the thecal sac, and the diagnosis (or extent of disease) remains unclear despite the pre-contrast MR, intravenous contrast plays an important role. Patients fall into two categories, those with disk disease and those with metastatic involvement.

Contrast use in the non-operated spine has received less attention than that post-operatively. We believe, however, that this is an important area for contrast use when applied conservatively, a stance supported by the literature. In the non-operated spine, contrast enhancement is seen in dilated epidural veins and de novo scar. Improved recognition and delineation of disk herniation are seen post-contrast. For intravenous contrast to be employed in this instance, the clinical symptoms should be that of disk disease and the patient should be a candidate for surgery. Extruded disks are one area for application. The reader should also be familiar with nerve root enhancement (as previously noted), which serves as a marker of root pathology both pre- and post-operatively, often with excellent clinical correlation.

In difficult cervical spine MR cases, contrast use can increase diagnostic confidence.[9] Congestion of the epidural venous plexus can be particularly prominent in the cervical spine (figure 6). Contrast use has also been commented upon in the thoracic spine.[10] Enhancement improves the recognition of disk disease in this hard to image area of the body (figure 7).

Infection

MR imaging of infection in the spine is clearly assisted by the use of gadolinium chelates (figure 8).[11] Hematogenous spread of infectious disease to the spinal column and its contents may be manifested in extensive and complex ways (figure 9). Unchecked focal vertebral osteomyelitis and discitis will eventually extend into the paraspinous soft tissues and epidural space. Contrast use improves delineation of epidural infection (figure 10), increases diagnostic confidence, localizes regions likely to provide positive biopsy, and enables differentiation of active infection from a response to antibiotics.

The majority of spinal infections are predominantly phlegmonous, or solid in nature. However, many of these infections eventually evolve into semi-fluid abscesses. These two inflammatory processes differ on imaging in that solid soft tissue infection will enhance uniformly, while abscess formation will leave pockets of nonenhancing tissue (i.e., pus). The latter occurs because the gadolinium chelate does not penetrate into fluid, pus filled cavities, except on occasion on delayed scans. For the same reasons, in many instances the periphery of the infected disk may enhance after gadolinium chelate administration, while the central portion of the infected disk may not. This implies that the vascular supply of the infected granulation tissue has not yet reached the otherwise nonvascularized internal structure of the disk.

Problematic cases arise where peridiscal or osseous enhancement is identified after intravenous gadolinium chelate administration in patients presenting with back pain. It is not clear from an imaging standpoint whether or not this enhancement may represent a low grade infection, or if this is simply enhancement within sterile, fibrovascular peridiscal degenerative change. There is no simple solution for this problem on the basis of imaging. Percutaneous needle biopsy may be necessary to settle the question in the proper clinical situation (i.e., recent onset of low back pain with fever).

In many cases, infection of the leptomeninges and nerve roots traversing the subarachnoid space can only be identified following intravenous gadolinium chelate administration. For example, cytomegalovirus infection presenting with a lumbosacral polyradiculopathy or the cauda equina syndrome is not uncommon in patients with advanced AIDS. Unenhanced images may be subtly abnormal or within normal limits. After intravenous gadolinium chelate administration, however, the nerve roots are frequently seen to brightly enhance. It should be noted that this enhancement is not a specific finding, since neoplastic meningitis or even sterile arachnoiditis may have an identical appearance on enhanced MR.[12]

Infections of the spinal cord itself are rare, although occasionally parenchymal infectious deposits may be observed. Intramedullary infectious disease will present clinically with a spinal cord syndrome that relates to the level and side of the pathologic process. If the infection is not checked, the clinical syndrome will progress to a complete transverse myelopathy. By demonstrating the area(s) of enhancement, contrast can be used to direct the surgeon to the site of biopsy in order to make a specific microbiologic diagnosis. It must be reiterated that such hematogenously borne deposits cannot be distinguished from those of a neoplastic nature on imaging alone, and thus histologic diagnosis is mandatory. The specific infectious agent can on occasion be isolated and/or cultured from CSF or peripheral blood specimens. However, direct spinal cord biopsy may be required in some cases.

Vascular Disease

MR is a means of evaluation that is noninvasive as well as relatively free of discomfort for the patient with signs and symptoms of cord ischemia/infarction. Shortly after the vascular incident and clinical exacerbation, the affected segment(s) of spinal cord may be swollen and of relatively

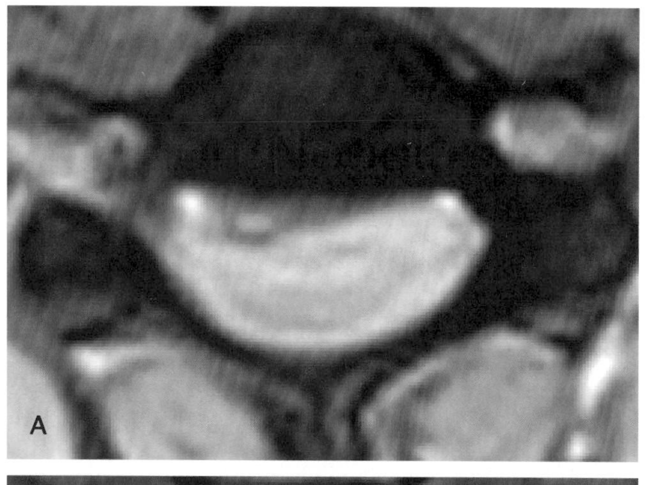

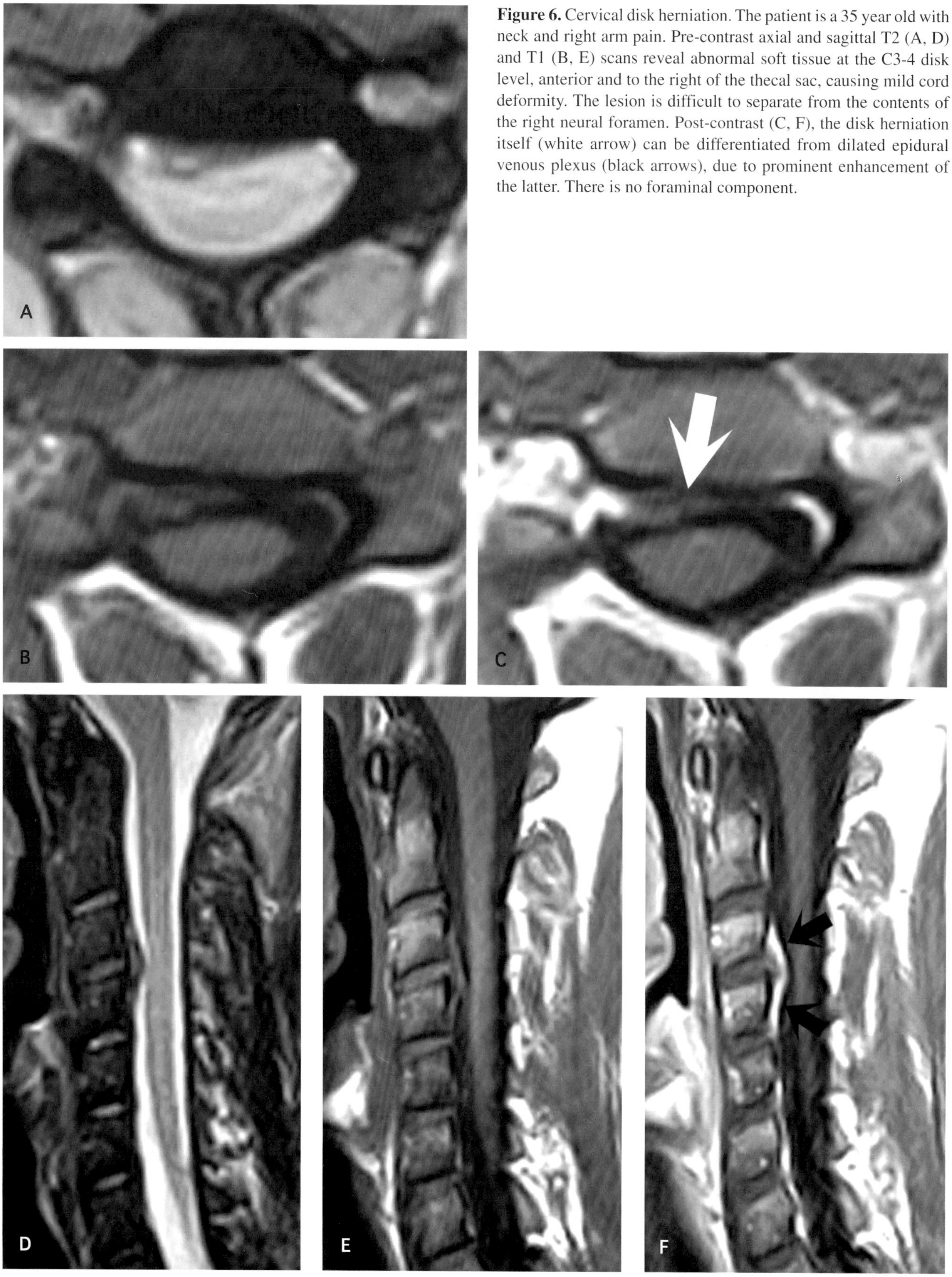

Figure 6. Cervical disk herniation. The patient is a 35 year old with neck and right arm pain. Pre-contrast axial and sagittal T2 (A, D) and T1 (B, E) scans reveal abnormal soft tissue at the C3-4 disk level, anterior and to the right of the thecal sac, causing mild cord deformity. The lesion is difficult to separate from the contents of the right neural foramen. Post-contrast (C, F), the disk herniation itself (white arrow) can be differentiated from dilated epidural venous plexus (black arrows), due to prominent enhancement of the latter. There is no foraminal component.

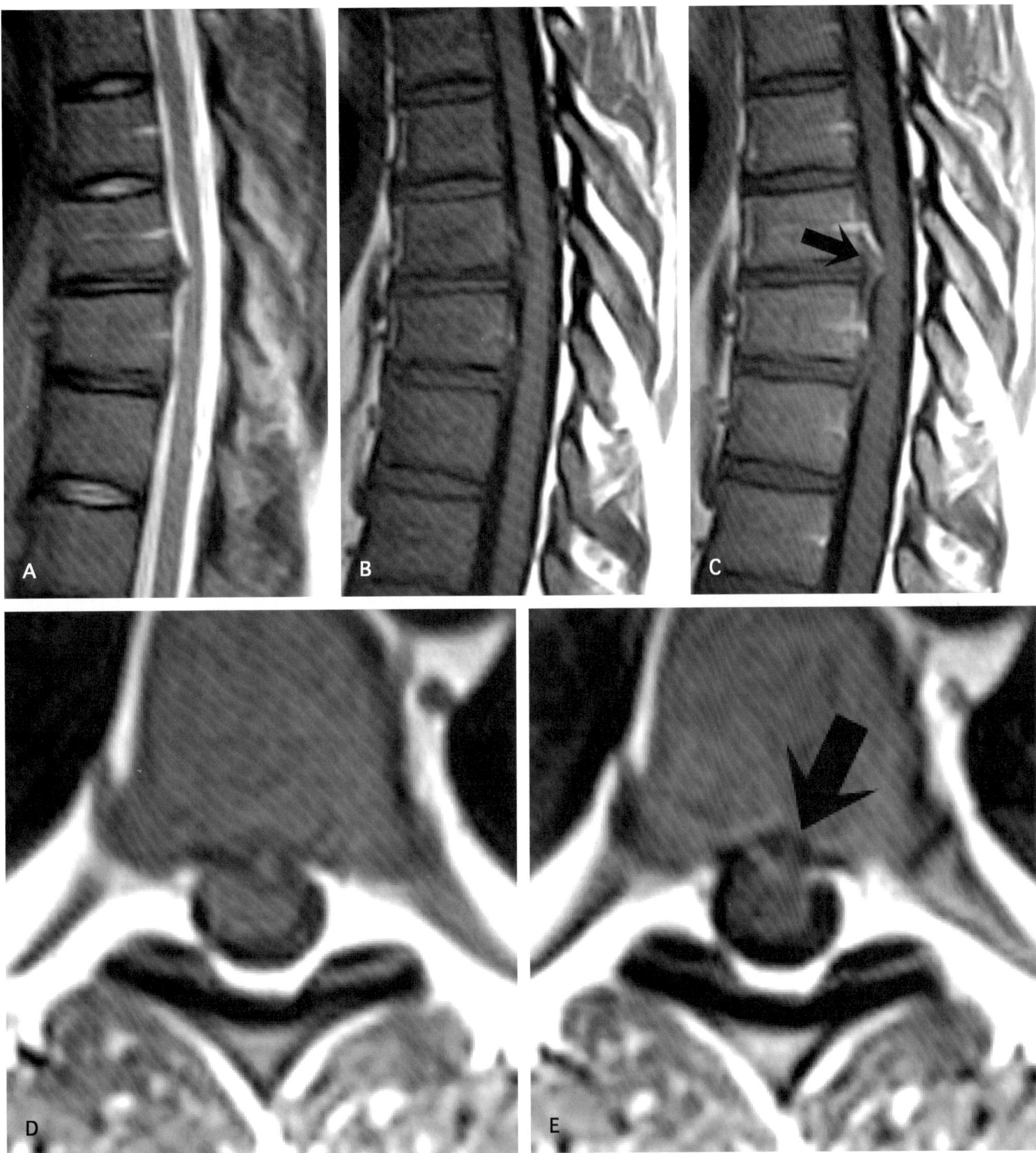

Figure 7. Thoracic disk herniation. The patient is a 31 year old individual with band-like paresthesias in the mid-thorax following a car accident. The (A) T2-weighted sagittal scan reveals anterior compression of the thecal sac at T7-8. Abnormal soft tissue can be noted on both the T2 and the pre-contrast (B) T1-weighted scans. (C) Contrast use permits identification of enhancing dilated epidural venous plexus and granulation tissue surrounding the disk (arrow). In comparing the (D) pre- and (E) post-contrast axial scans, enhancement aids in identification of the interface between the disk (arrow) and the thecal sac.

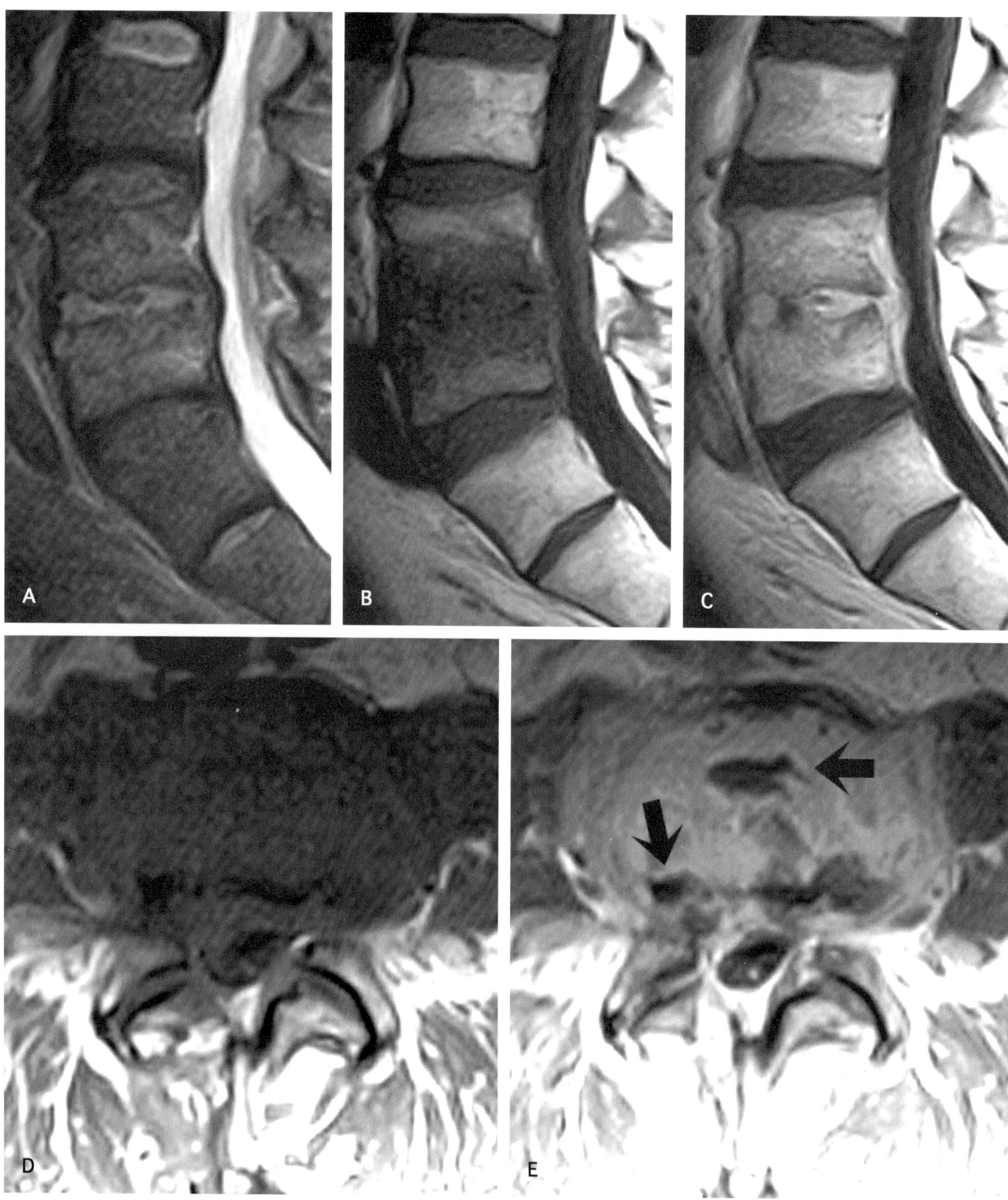

Figure 8. Post-operative disk infection. Pre-contrast on (A) the T2-weighted sagittal scan, diffuse abnormal high signal intensity (SI) is noted within the marrow of the L4 and L5 vertebral bodies. The disk is reduced in height, irregular, and of abnormal high SI. On (B) the pre-contrast T1-weighted scan, the L4-5 disk is difficult to identify. Also noted is abnormal low SI within the lower half of L4 and the upper half of L5, paralleling the disk. (C) Post-contrast, abnormal enhancement of the disk space is noted, together with a soft tissue mass that compresses the thecal sac. Comparison of (D) pre- and (E) post-contrast T1-weighted axial scans at the disk level reveals a paraspinous mass with enhancement. There is abnormal enhancement of the disk as well, permitting identification of fluid pockets that remain low SI (arrows).

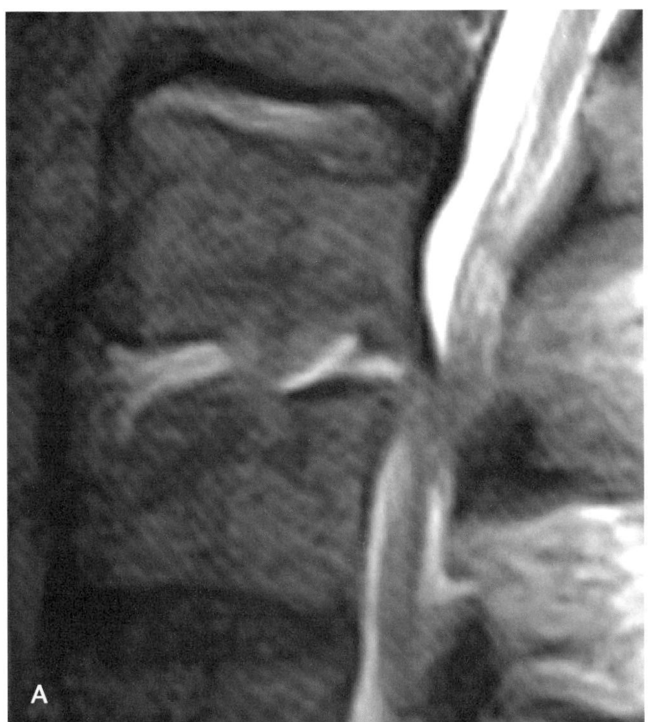

Figure 9. Discitis, hematogenous. On (A) the T2-weighted scan, the L2-3 disk is high signal intensity (which by itself could be normal), yet irregular in contour. There is absence of the normal intranuclear cleft. The thecal sac is narrowed at the L2-3 level. On (B) the pre-contrast T1-weighted scan, both the L2 and L3 vertebral bodies are of abnormal low signal intensity. There is loss of definition between the L2-3 disk and the adjacent vertebral endplates. On (C) the post-contrast T1-weighted scan, there is enhancement of the L2 and L3 marrow space, with irregular enhancement along the disk margin and residual low signal intensity (non-enhancing) soft tissue within the disk space. The latter corresponds in position to the high signal intensity noted on the T2-weighted scan, and represents inflammatory exudates. The basis for thecal sac narrowing is now evident, with abnormal paraspinal enhancing soft tissue. In the adult patient, non-iatrogenic disk space infection is usually the result of hematogenous seeding to soft tissue or the subchondral portion of the vertebral body.

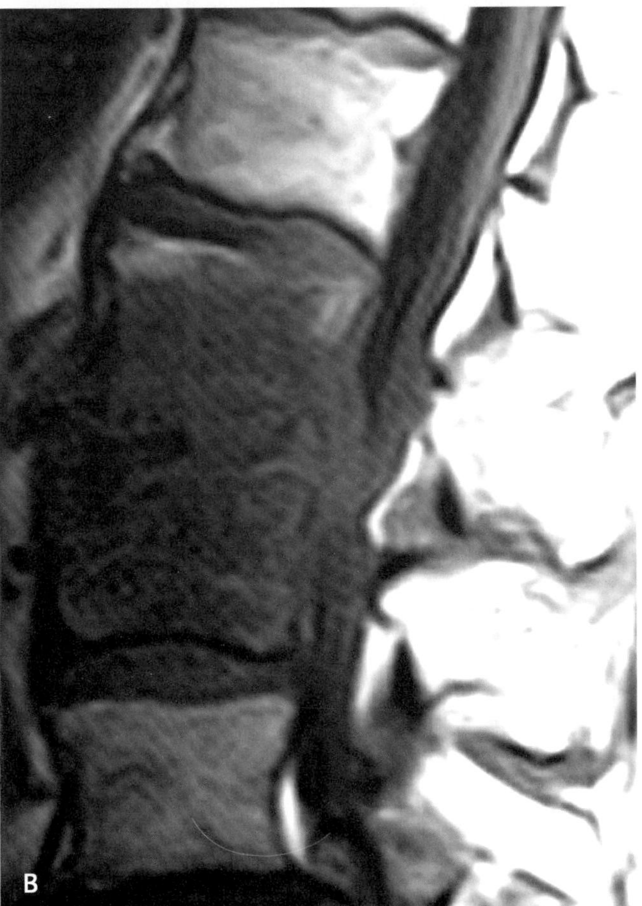

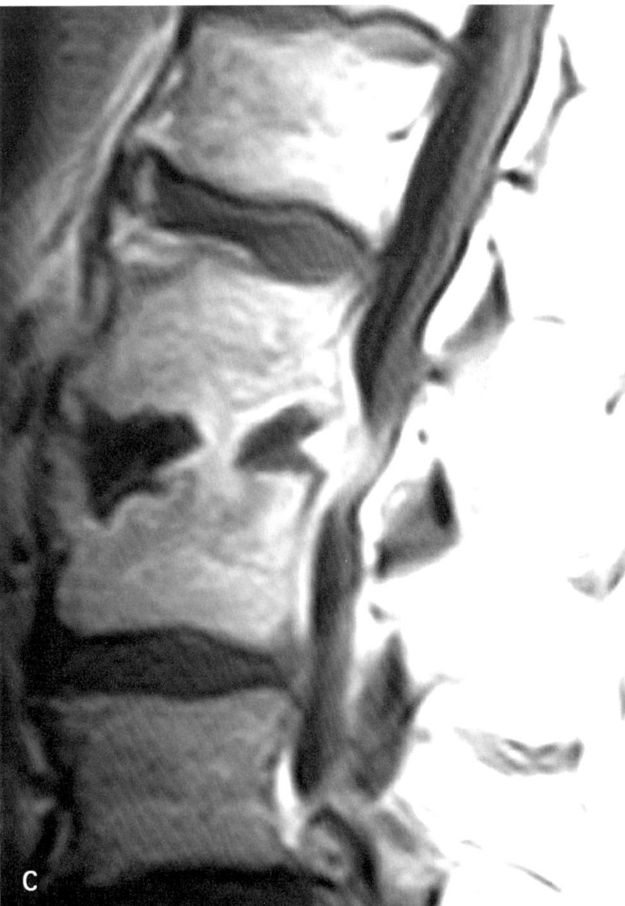

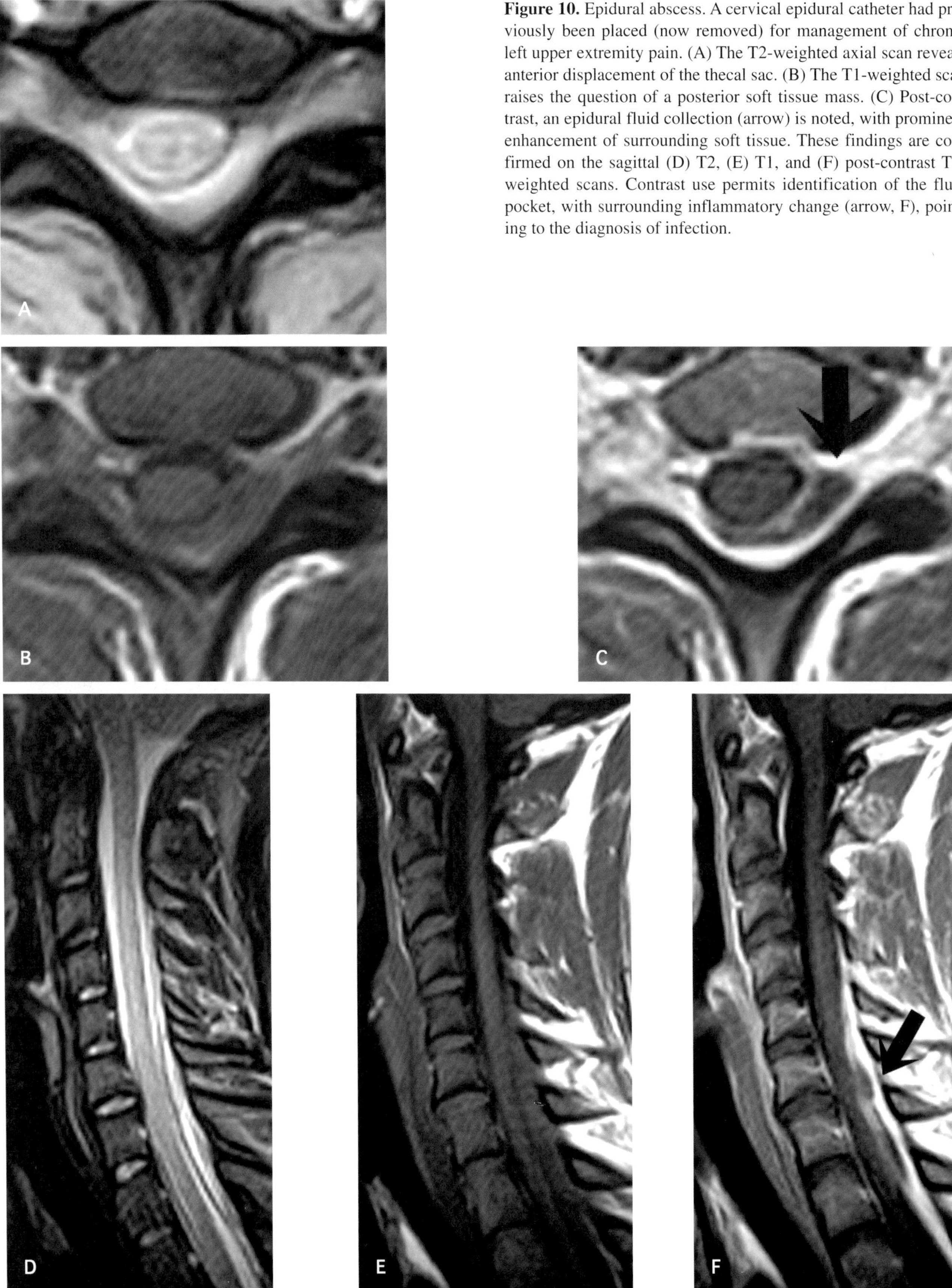

Figure 10. Epidural abscess. A cervical epidural catheter had previously been placed (now removed) for management of chronic left upper extremity pain. (A) The T2-weighted axial scan reveals anterior displacement of the thecal sac. (B) The T1-weighted scan raises the question of a posterior soft tissue mass. (C) Post-contrast, an epidural fluid collection (arrow) is noted, with prominent enhancement of surrounding soft tissue. These findings are confirmed on the sagittal (D) T2, (E) T1, and (F) post-contrast T1-weighted scans. Contrast use permits identification of the fluid pocket, with surrounding inflammatory change (arrow, F), pointing to the diagnosis of infection.

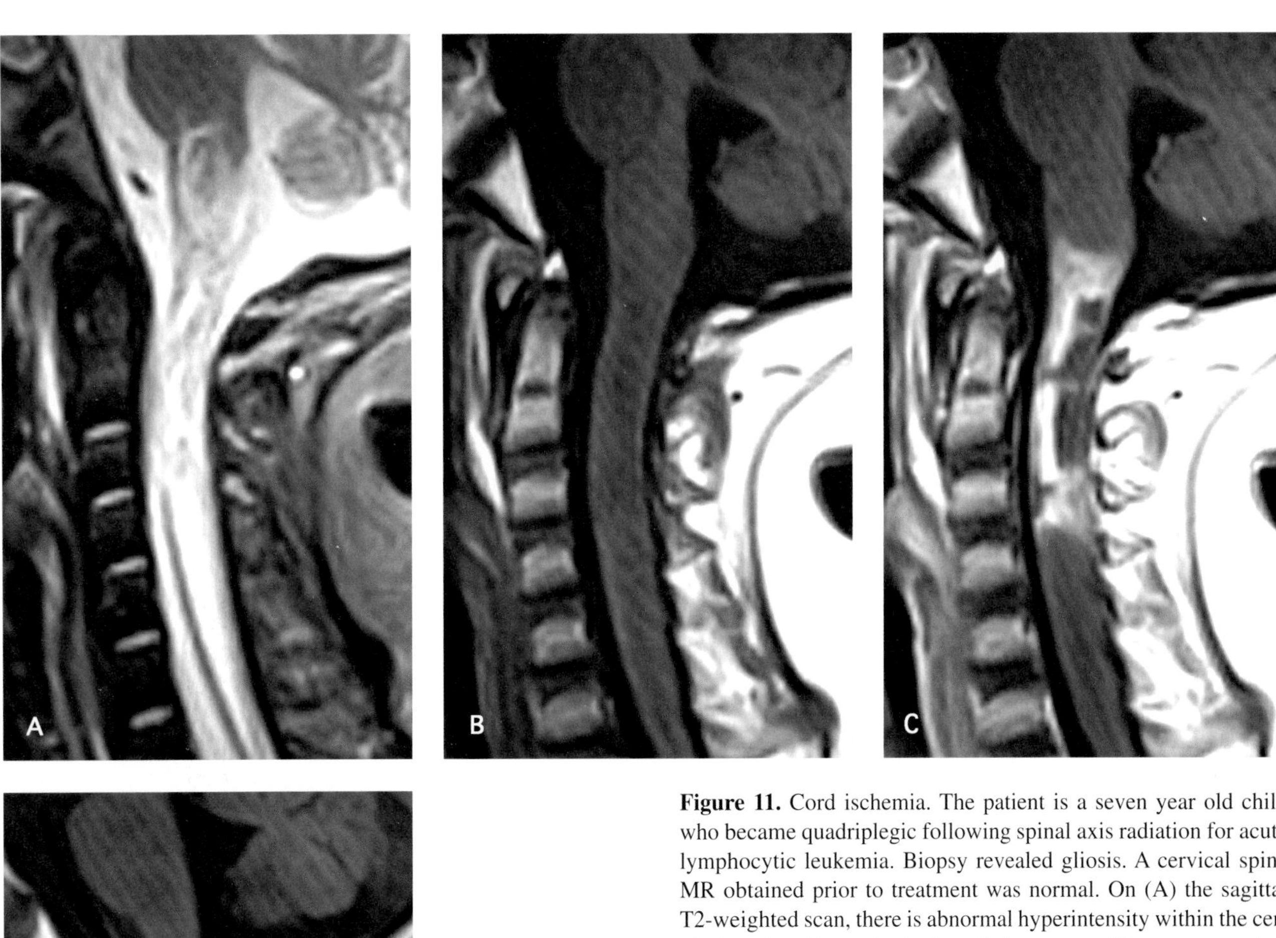

Figure 11. Cord ischemia. The patient is a seven year old child who became quadriplegic following spinal axis radiation for acute lymphocytic leukemia. Biopsy revealed gliosis. A cervical spine MR obtained prior to treatment was normal. On (A) the sagittal T2-weighted scan, there is abnormal hyperintensity within the cervical cord and lower brainstem. Enlargement of the upper cervical cord is best visualized on (B) the pre-contrast T1-weighted scan. Comparison of (B) pre- and (C) post-contrast sagittal T1-weighted scans reveals marked abnormal enhancement within the upper cervical cord. The MR exam was repeated five months later, with (D) the sagittal T1-weighted scan shown. At that time, only atrophy of the upper cervical cord was noted. There was no abnormal contrast enhancement.

low signal intensity on T1-weighted imaging as compared to normal areas of the cord remote from the region of ischemia. On T2-weighted imaging, the signal intensity of the abnormal cord areas typically becomes hyperintense. Multisegmental enhancement of the spinal cord may be identified if frank infarction of the spinal cord has occurred. Enhancement of the ischemic/infarcted cord may persist for months. Frank cord atrophy involving the affected segments is often the final result. With dural arteriovenous fistulas, venous stasis can result in ischemia and/or infarction. Other etiologies, including therapeutic radiation, may also lead to cord ischemia (figure 11).

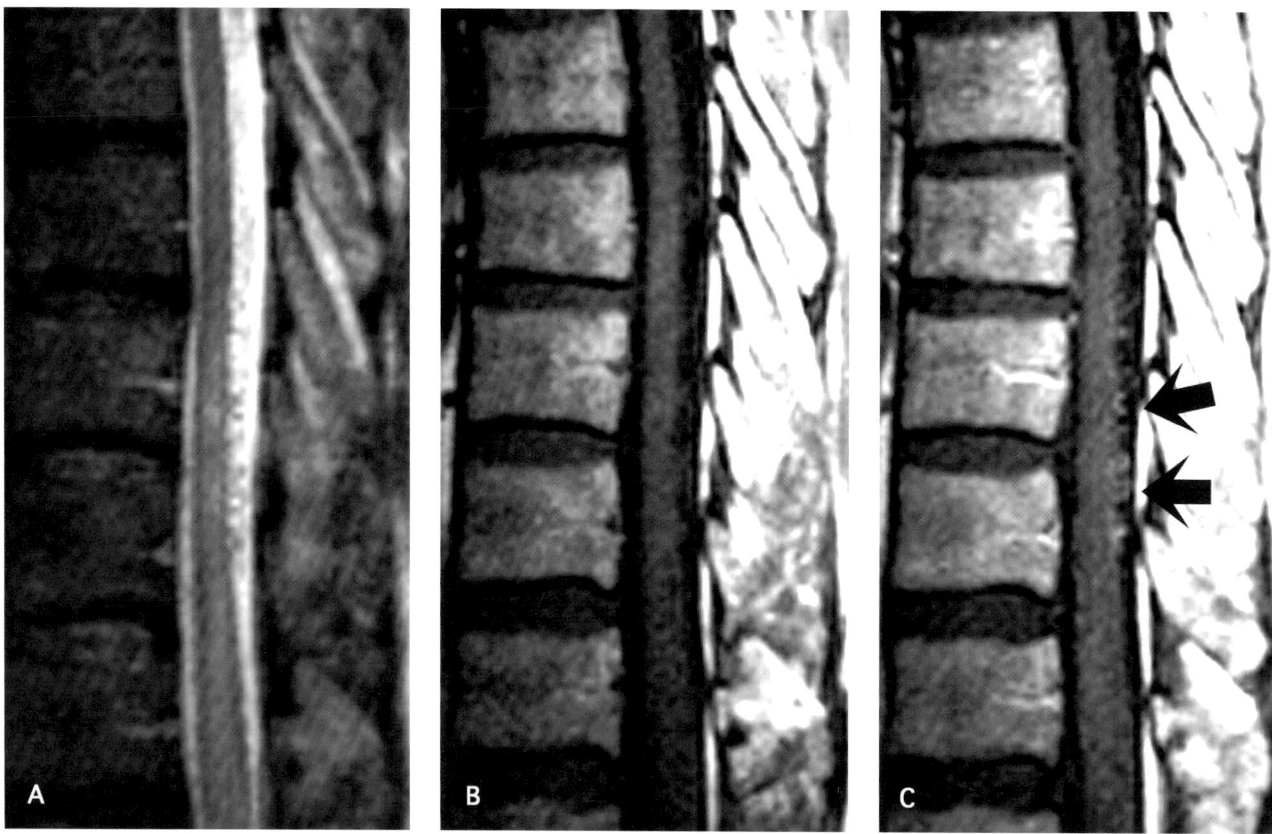

Figure 12. Dural spinal arteriovenous fistula. On (A) the sagittal midline T2-weighted image, the question of abnormal hyperintensity within the lower cord and conus is raised. Immediately posterior to the cord, multiple small serpiginous signal voids are identified, spanning at least two vertebral segments. (B) The pre-contrast T1-weighted image is normal. (C) Post-contrast, abnormal enhancement (arrows) is noted along the dorsal aspect of the cord, confirming the presence of enlarged draining veins. By enhancement of flow within dilated veins, contrast administration improves visualization of spinal arteriovenous malformations and fistulae.

Although infarction of the spinal cord can be due to atherosclerosis of the vessels supplying the cord parenchyma, such insults can also be seen after surgery on the thoracoabdominal aorta, or following spinal/paraspinal surgery that inadvertently injures or ligates major radiculospinal arteries. Spinal vascular malformations are another significant source of cord ischemia.[13] While all types may induce cord symptoms in practice, dural arteriovenous fistulae are not uncommonly encountered. Vascular malformations may be revealed by the presence of longitudinal, serpentine or cross-sectional signal voids. This assumes that the blood flow through the abnormal vessels is sufficiently rapid to create a flow void. However, the vascular flow may be slow in some situations, especially in the case of dural arteriovenous fistula. The presence of the vascular abnormality in this setting can only be seen clearly after the administration of a gadolinium chelate, resulting in enhancement of blood within the abnormal vessels (figure 12).[14] The clinical syndrome should guide the imaging physician as to whether the patient warrants contrast administration, especially in the face of a negative or equivocal unenhanced MR examination. Trauma should also be noted as a cause of cord ischemia and contrast enhancement on MR (figure 13).

Neoplastic Disease

The study of oncological disease affecting the spinal column, leptomeninges and neural tissue is one of the primary applications of contrast agents in MR of the spine. MR imaging is equally good for the evaluation of primary as well as metastatic disease to these tissues.[15,16,17] Gadolinium chelates are employed to visualize areas of breakdown in the blood-CNS barrier associated with primary neoplasia and to direct the surgeon for biopsy or resection (figure 14).[18] Parenchymal neoplasia of the spinal cord may be solid in nature or cavitary/necrotic. Cystic or necrotic areas do not demonstrate enhancement after gadolinium chelate administration.

Intravenous contrast should be routinely given when an intramedullary abnormality is noted pre-contrast, except for a benign syrinx or cord atrophy. If there is a high clinical suspicion of an intramedullary lesion (or a lesion along the

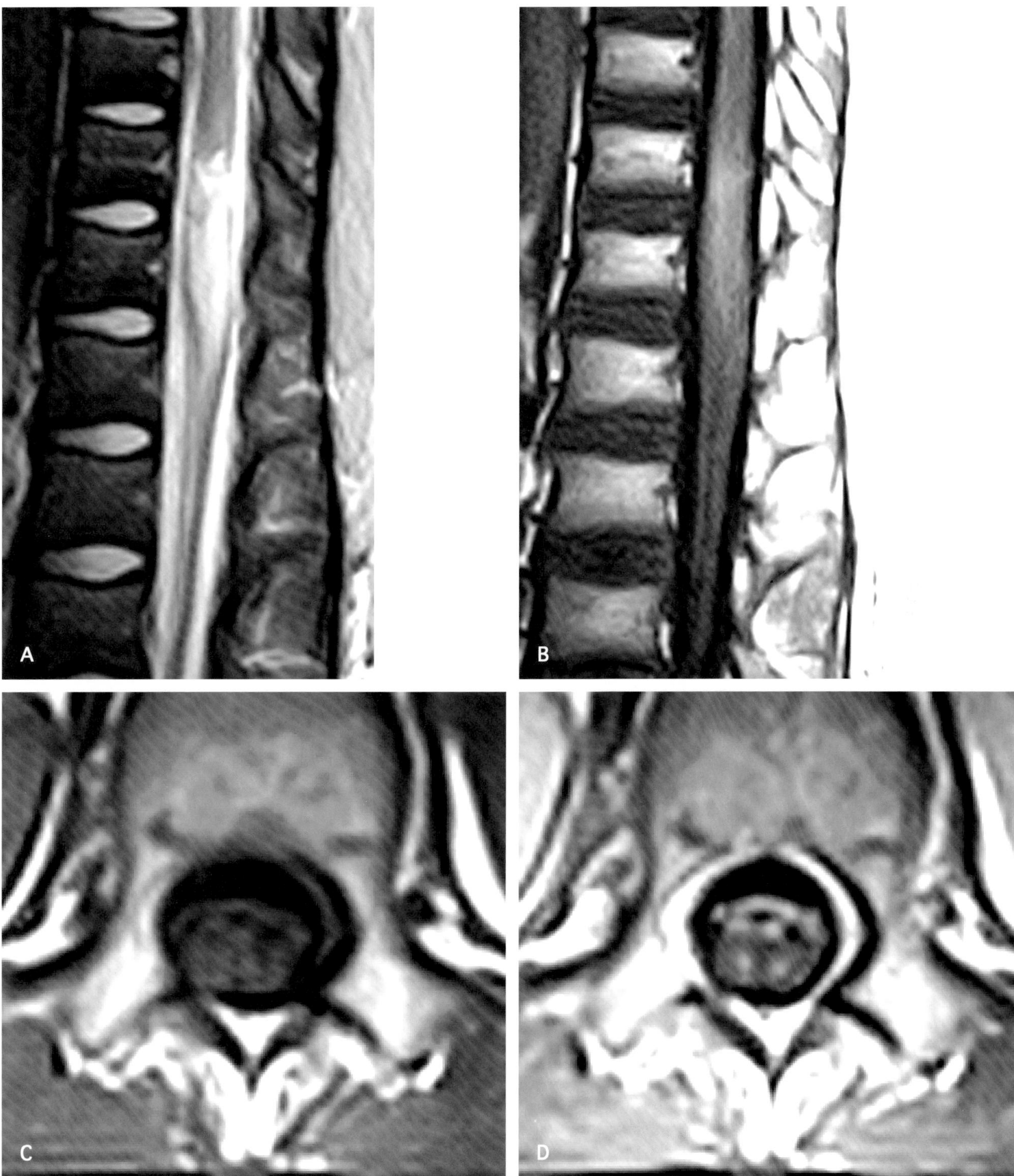

Figure 13. Traumatic cord injury. The patient is a nine year old child with loss of lower extremity sensation and motor function following an auto accident. Scans were obtained two weeks later. On (A) the sagittal T2-weighted image, there is abnormal hyperintensity within the conus. Slight hyperintensity, suggestive of petechial hemorrhage, is present in the same area on (B) the sagittal pre-contrast T1-weighted scan. Comparing (C) pre- and (D) post-contrast axial T1-weighted scans at the level of the conus, there is abnormal enhancement of multiple anterior nerve roots, as well as within the cord substance. Enhancement can occur in the subacute time period following trauma due to ischemia and disruption of the blood-spinal cord barrier. This should not be confused with enhancement due to other tissue pathology.

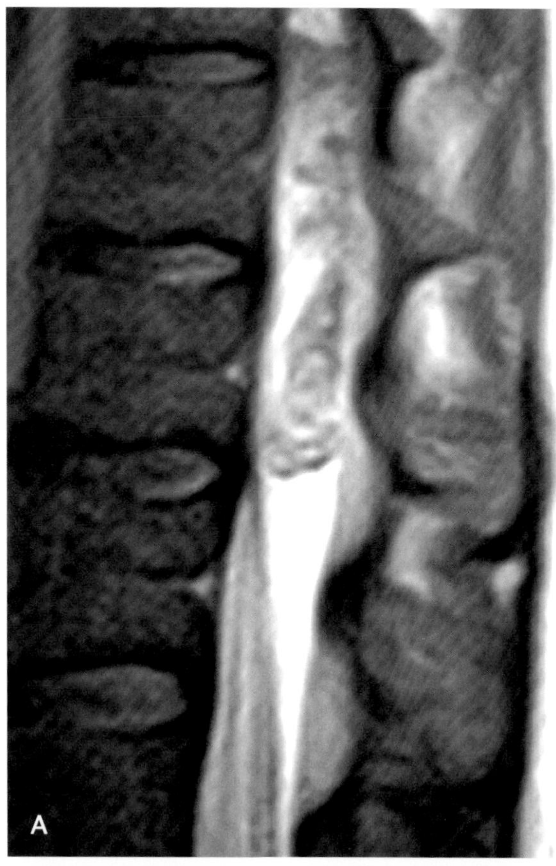

Figure 14. Mixed papillary ependymoma of the conus medullaris. On (A) the sagittal T2-weighted scan, an intradural extramedullary soft tissue mass is noted. The spinal cord is displaced anteriorly and flattened. On (B) the axial T2-weighted scan, the mass is seen posteriorly and to the right, with severe compression of the cord. On (C) the post-contrast T1-weighted scan, there is heterogeneous enhancement of the mass (arrows), greater peripherally and less centrally. The cord itself is thinned, and lies anterior and slightly to the left. The patient presented with slowly increasing low back pain and left lower extremity weakness. Virtually all ependymomas demonstrate strong enhancement following intravenous contrast injection on MR.

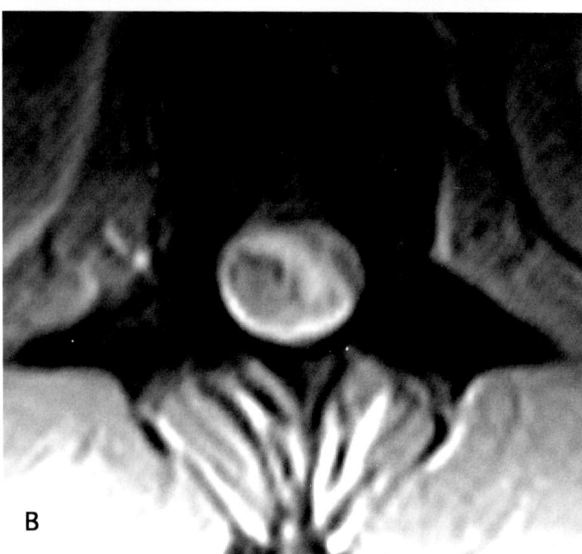

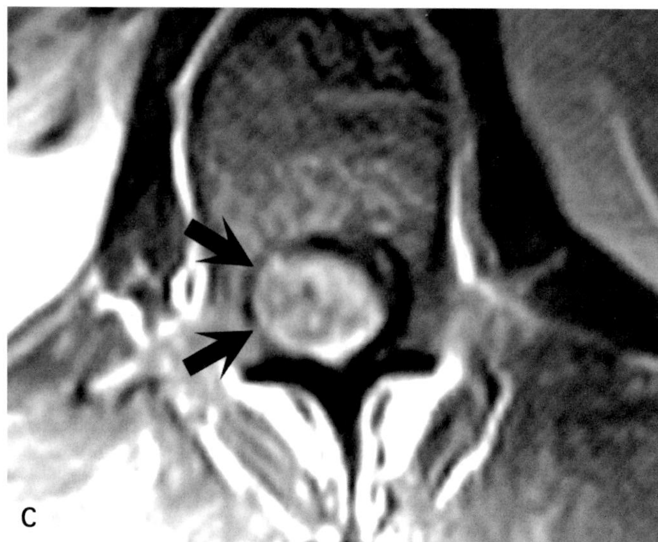

surface of the cord), then contrast should also be given (figure 15). Four of thirteen intramedullary tumors in one study[18] were identified only post-contrast. Contrast is of great use for improved lesion delineation and characterization (figure 16).

Contrast can pinpoint the nidus of a tumor, suggest regions for biopsy, differentiate benign processes from tumor (in the case of hemorrhage), and identify active disease. Tumor can be differentiated from a syrinx cavity or gliosis. Post-operatively, contrast aids in the differentiation of residual or recurrent tumor from scar (figure 17). If lesion enhancement is not seen on immediate post-contrast images, delayed imaging (45-60 minutes) should be considered. Delayed enhancement has been noted in cord astrocytomas.

In the absence of a Chiari malformation (i.e. tonsillar ectopia with hydromyelia), the search for possible enhance-

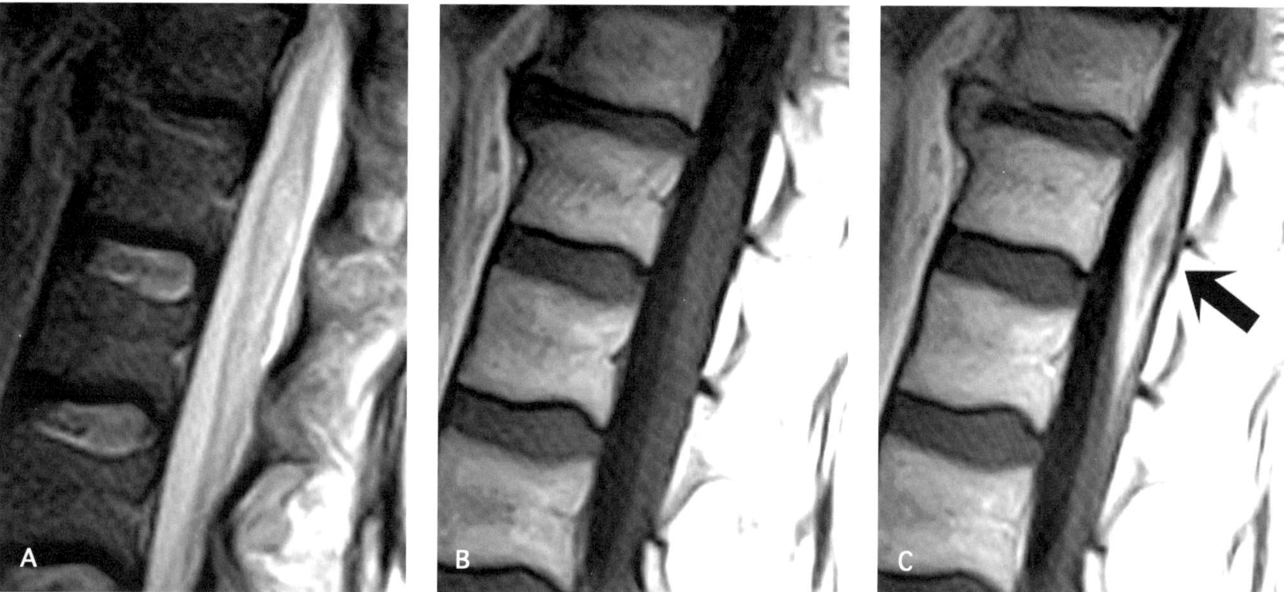

Figure 15. Ependymoma of the conus medullaris, with improved conspicuity on post-contrast scans. On the pre-contrast (A) T2-weighted sagittal scan, the conus is slightly hyperintense compared to the more proximal cord, raising the possibility of an intrinsic lesion. (B) The pre-contrast T1-weighted scan is normal. (C) Post-contrast, an enhancing conus lesion is identified (arrow). In neoplastic disease that involves the cord, contrast administration commonly improves lesion demarcation and conspicuity.

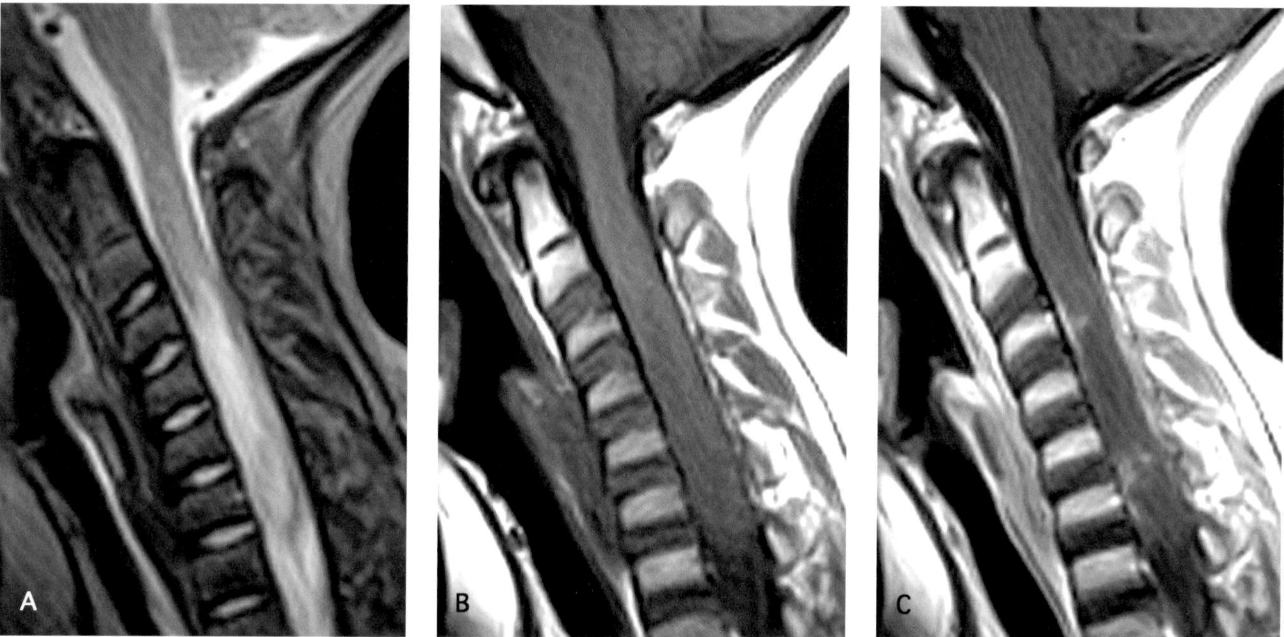

Figure 16. Astrocytoma of the cervical cord. On (A) the pre-contrast T2-weighted sagittal scan, a hyperintense cord lesion is noted which extends from C3 to C7. (B) The pre-contrast T1-weighted scan reveals marked cord enlargement. (C) Post-contrast, there is mottled abnormal enhancement within portions of the lesion. Although not all cord astrocytomas demonstrate enhancement post-contrast on MR, when present, this finding improves differential diagnosis and provides guidance for biopsy. Administration of contrast is particularly important in the presence of a syrinx, if a neoplastic origin is in question.

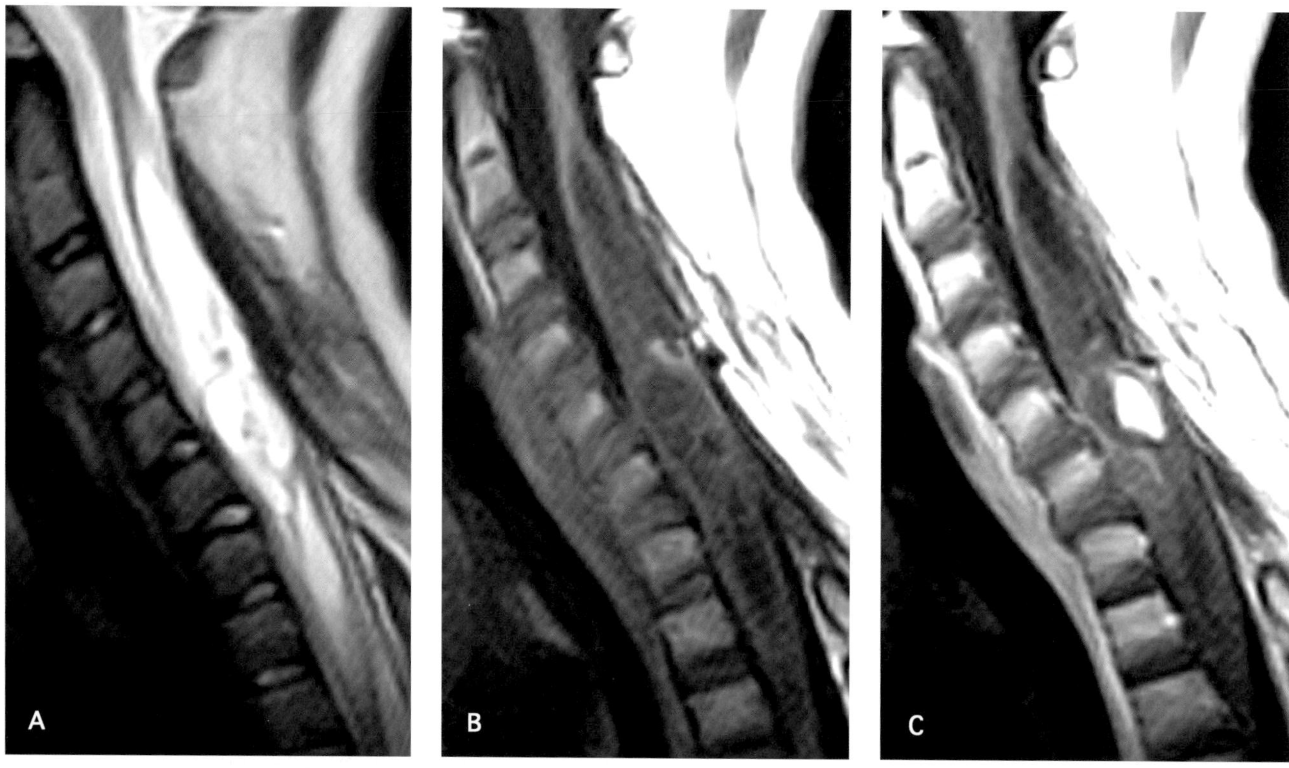

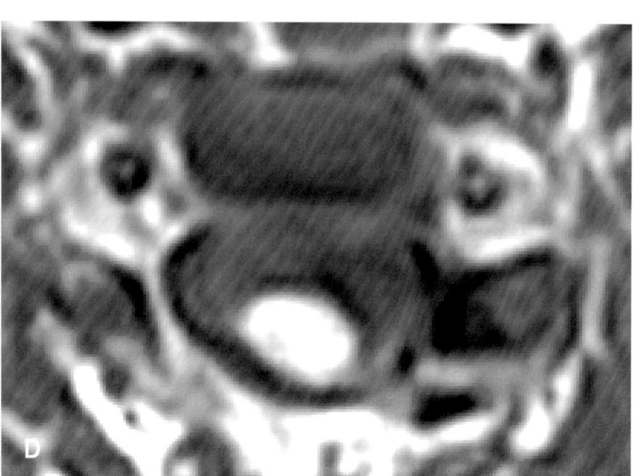

Figure 17. Recurrent astrocytoma. The MR exam was performed several years following an extensive laminectomy for removal of a spinal cord astrocytoma. Examining the sagittal pre-contrast (A) T2 and (B) T1-weighted scans, a syrinx cavity is noted that expands the cord and extends from C2 to T2. The signal intensity characteristics of the syrinx differ from that of cerebrospinal fluid, suggesting a neoplastic origin. On the (C) sagittal and (D) axial post-contrast T1-weighted scans, there is abnormal enhancement of a large soft tissue nidus within the syrinx at the C5-6 level. This finding was new from the prior MR exam, and represents recurrent tumor. Post-contrast scans in the spine are particularly valuable for detection of recurrent intramedullary neoplastic disease. Such lesions are often difficult to detect without contrast administration, due to the distortion of normal structures and the isointensity of the lesion to surrounding soft tissue.

ment within the wall of a cystic lesion discovered within the spinal cord is mandatory. Proper surgical planning can only be accomplished in this situation by challenging the blood-cord barrier with a paramagnetic contrast agent. Primary tumors may also affect the nerve roots or spinal nerves (e.g., schwannomas or neurofibromas) (figure 18), the leptomeninges (e.g. meningiomas) (figures 19, 20), or the spinal column itself (e.g. sarcomas).[19]

Contrast administration improves the demarcation of lesions from surrounding soft tissue and aids in the differentiation of disk disease from tumor (figure 21). As with intradural neoplasia, enhanced scans are important for improved differential diagnosis for lesions in the extradural space (figure 22). Contrast use also pinpoints areas for biopsy (identifying active disease) and improves the assessment of spinal canal invasion (figure 23) and tumor response to therapy.

All spinal compartments (extradural, intradural extramedullary, and intramedullary) may harbor metastatic disease to the spine. With regard to the spinal column itself, images should always first be obtained prior to the administration of a gadolinium chelate. Abnormal enhancement may bring the signal intensity of an abnormal vertebral body up to that of the normal surrounding fatty marrow. Vertebral metastatic disease may therefore be masked if unenhanced images are not obtained.[20] However, contrast agents in this circumstance are not necessarily given to demonstrate bony

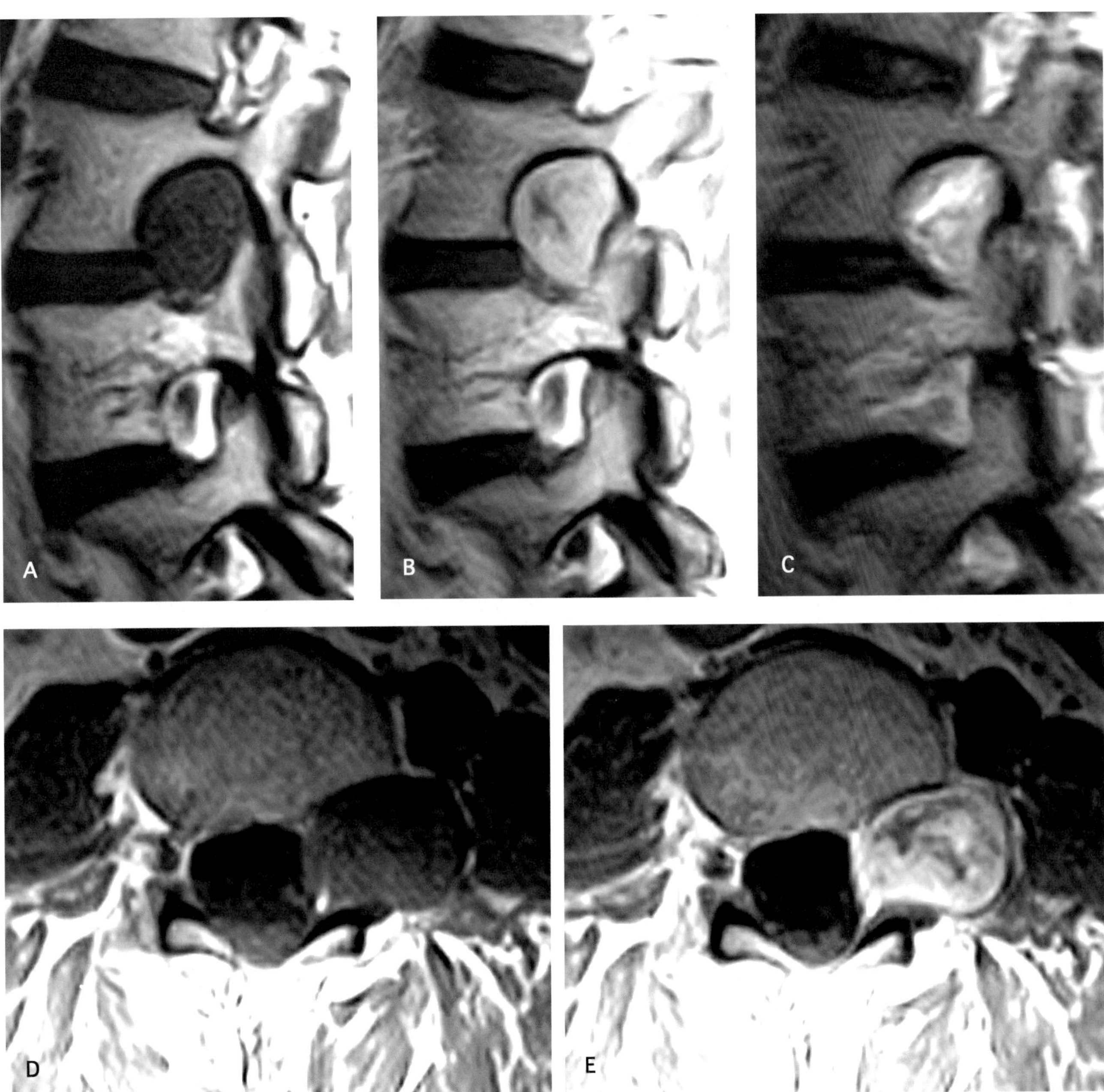

Figure 18. Neurofibroma. The patient is a 66 year old veteran with neurofibromatosis. (A) Pre-contrast and (B) post-contrast sagittal T1-weighted scans reveal a large enhancing soft tissue mass in the left L3-4 neural foramen. The mass is of high signal intensity on (C) the T2-weighted scan. Comparison of (D) pre- and (E) post-contrast axial T1-weighted scans reveals a smoothly marginated enhancing lesion, which has expanded the foramen. Contrast enhancement of the mass favors a neural origin, and improves lesion demarcation from surrounding soft tissue. Schwannomas tend to enhance in a heterogeneous fashion, often more intense peripherally. Neurofibromas typically demonstrate homogeneous contrast enhancement.

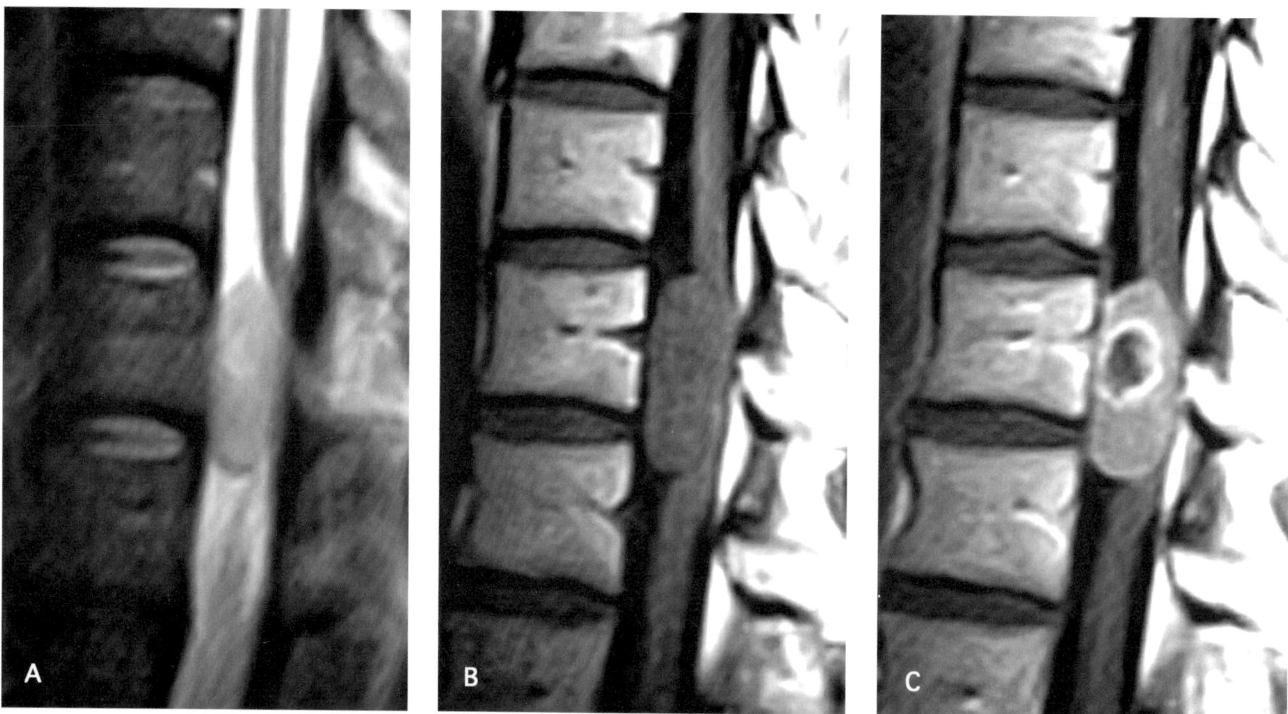

Figure 19. Thoracic meningioma. On pre-contrast (A) T2 and (B) T1-weighted sagittal scans, a mass is noted within the thecal sac, outlined by cerebrospinal fluid. The flattening and displacement of the cord favor an intradural extramedullary location. Intense enhancement (C) post-contrast improves demarcation of the lesion and places a meningioma first on the list of differential diagnoses. This 48 year old woman presented with paraplegia and progressive back pain. The lesion was surgically removed.

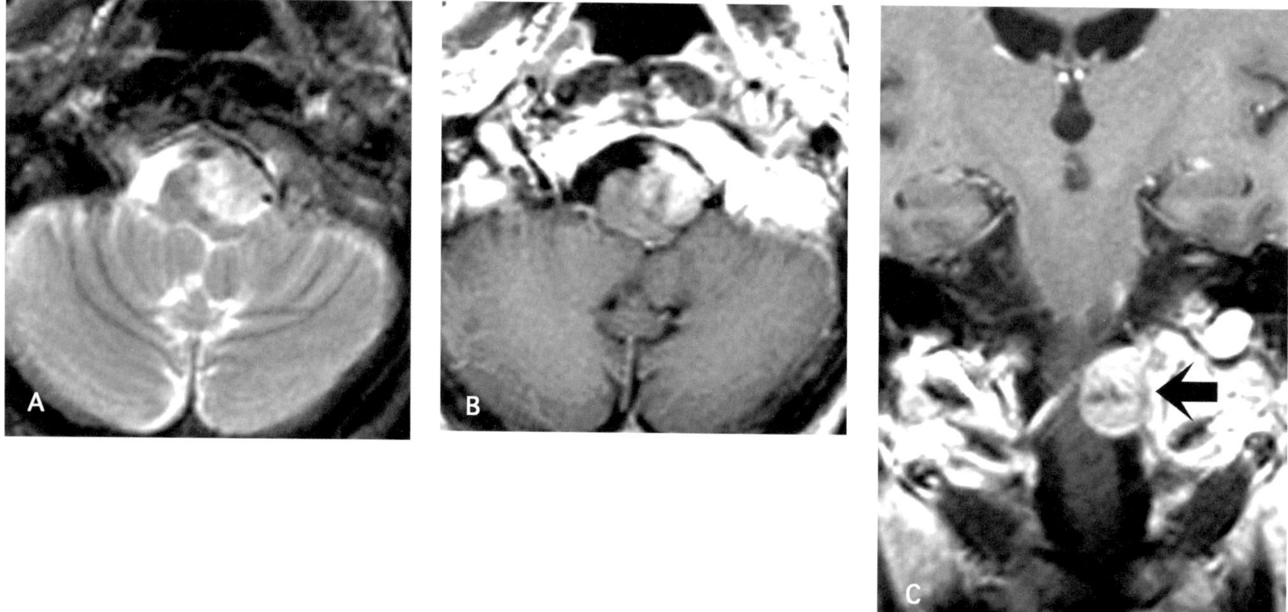

Figure 20. Foramen magnum meningioma. On the pre-contrast (A) T2-weighted axial image, a mass is seen at the level of the foramen magnum. There is substantial deformity of the medulla. (B) Axial and (C) coronal post-contrast images demonstrate intense lesion enhancement (arrow, C). The dural based origin of the lesion, questioned on the basis of pre-contrast scans, is confirmed post-contrast.

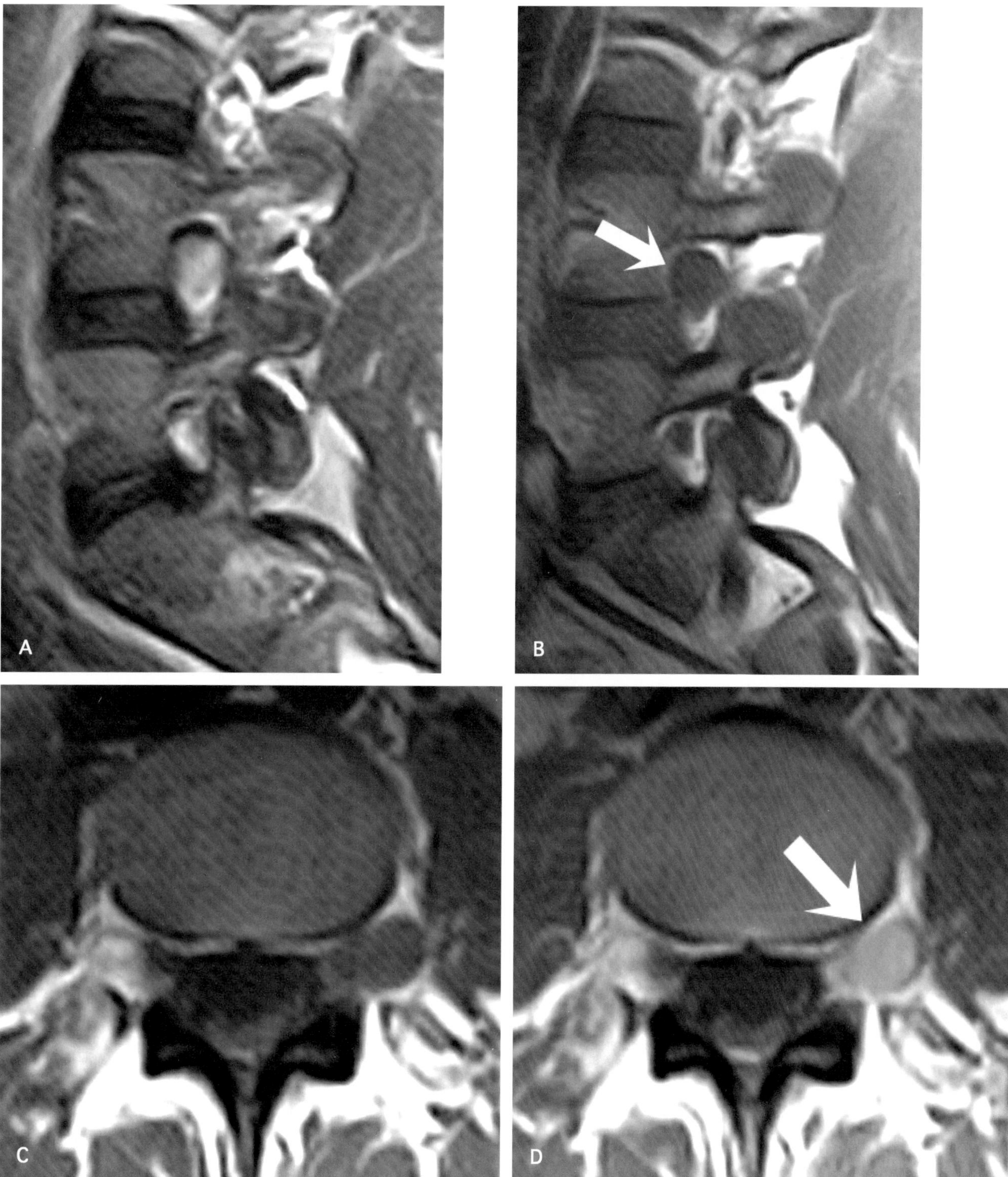

Figure 21. Neurofibroma. Parasagittal (A) T2 and (B) T1-weighted images reveal a soft tissue mass (arrow, B) in the left L4-5 neural foramen. The L4 nerve root is not identified. Comparison of (C) pre- and (D) post-contrast axial T1-weighted scans reveals homogeneous enhancement of the mass (arrow, D). Contrast enhancement in this instance provides important information for differential diagnosis, eliminating from consideration a free disk fragment. *(From Runge VM, Awh MH, Bittner DF, Kirsch JE. Magnetic resonance imaging of the spine. Philadelphia, JB Lippincott, 1995).*

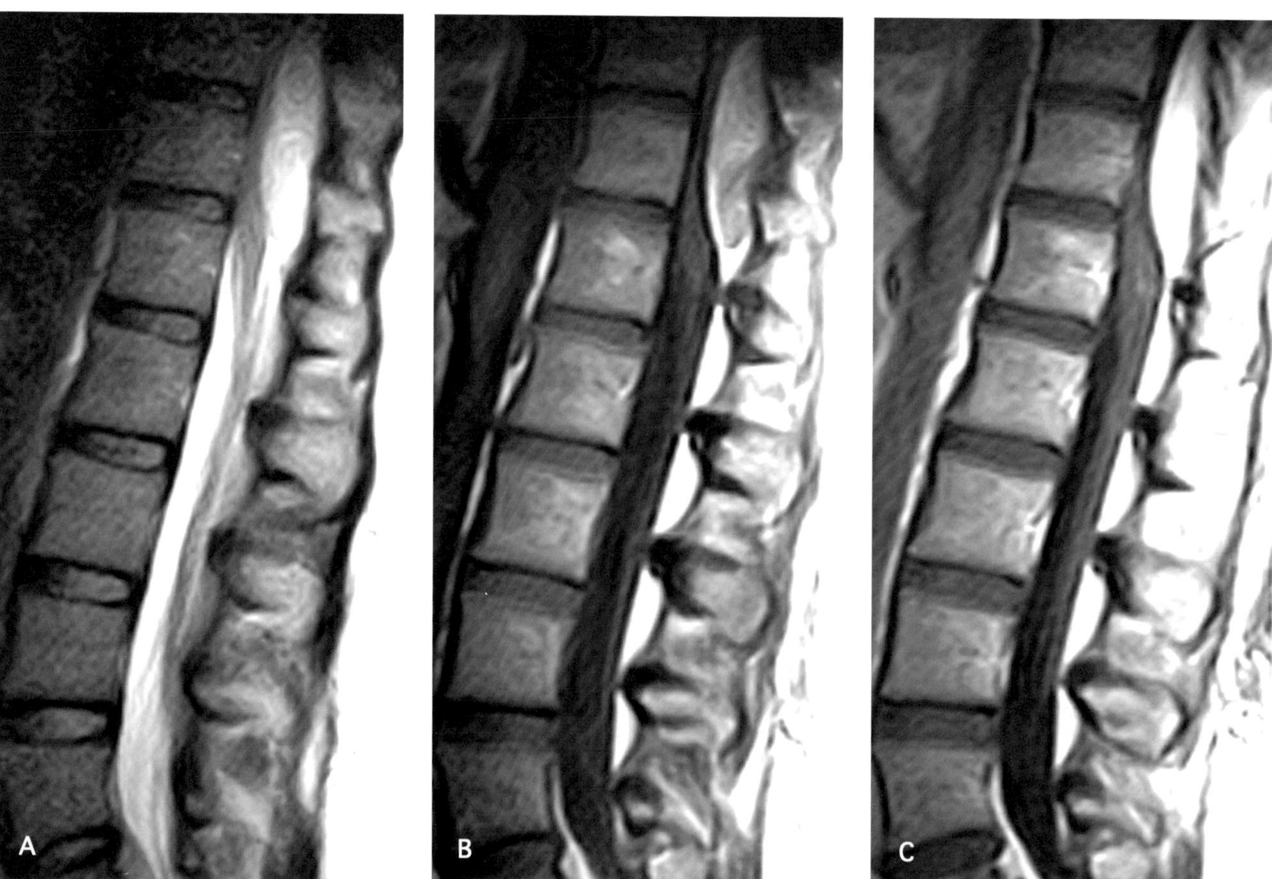

Figure 22. Angiolipoma. On (A) the T2-weighted scan, the conus is displaced anteriorly, but a soft tissue mass is not clearly identified. (B) The pre-contrast T1-weighted scan reveals a posterior epidural mass, extending from T11 to L1, with mixed high signal intensity. On (C) the post-contrast T1-weighted scan, the abnormality is noted to enhance to isointensity with fat. Although the lesion is similar in signal intensity to fat, it is heterogenous and displays abnormal contrast enhancement. These characteristics suggest a neoplastic origin. Angiolipomas are rare benign tumors, composed of lipocytes and abnormal blood vessels. These tumors are epidural in location, occur most commonly in the mid-thoracic region, and can cause cord compression.

metastatic disease. Contrast media is commonly administered in cases of known or suspected spinal column metastases in order to evaluate for intraspinal extension. Subarachnoid space obliteration and compression of neural tissue can often best be delineated following gadolinium chelate administration (figure 24). The MR examination may suffice to replace invasive studies such as myelography in this setting. Gadolinium chelate enhanced MR can usually accurately localize the intraspinal extension of metastatic disease, determine in which compartment(s) the metastatic disease lies, and demonstrate the longitudinal extent of disease. In these ways, enhanced MR directs radiation or surgical treatment plans, and improves the assessment of disease response following treatment.

Subarachnoid dissemination of malignant disease is commonly referred to as neoplastic (carcinomatous or sarcomatous) meningitis. Gadolinium chelate administration in the symptomatic patient with leptomeningeal tumor spread often reveals enhancement of the meningeal surfaces and nerve roots (figure 25).[21] Nonenhancement in the face of actual neoplastic dissemination of disease within the subarachnoid pathways (i.e. false negative enhanced MR) is known. One explanation may be that because the leptomeningeal deposits initially receive their nutrients via the CSF. They may not have a blood supply and therefore administration of contrast cannot produce enhancement of these small lesions. Noninvasive MR evaluation of patients with known oncological disease presenting with symptoms related to the spine should nevertheless be undertaken first. A positive exam can shorten the work up and lead to the cancellation of invasive diagnostic procedures, thereby facilitating timely patient triage.

The parenchyma of the spinal cord itself is not a common focus of neoplastic metastatic spread, probably because the tenuous blood supply to the spinal cord delivers a reduced tumor load to the cord. However, intravenous con-

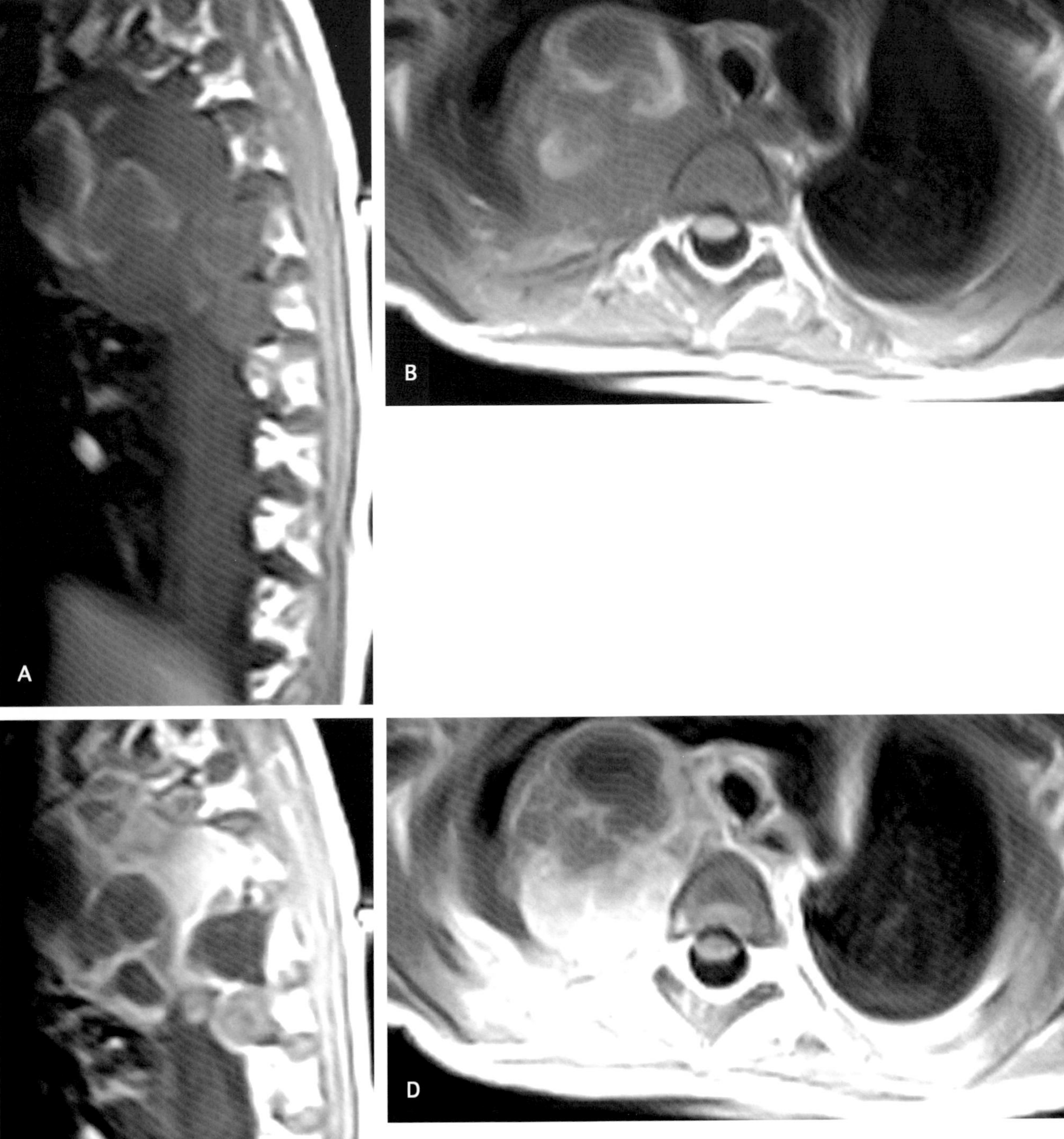

Figure 23. Ganglioneuroma. On pre-contrast (A) sagittal and (B) axial T1-weighted scans, a large paraspinal soft tissue mass is noted. Portions of the mass display marked contrast enhancement following intravenous gadolinium chelate administration (C, D). Cystic and necrotic parts of the lesion remain intermediate signal intensity. The tumors that arise from primitive sympathetic neuroblasts are distinguished by degree of cellular maturation. The most malignant is neuroblastoma, the least ganglioneuroma, with ganglioneuroblastoma falling in between.

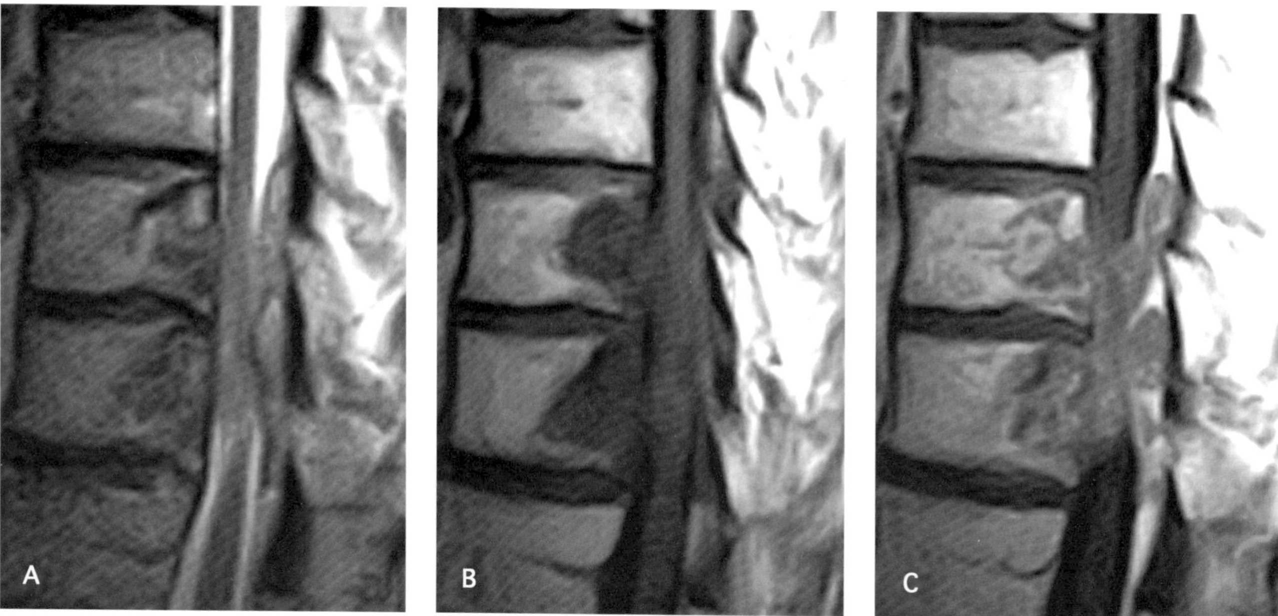

Figure 24. Vertebral body metastases, with spinal cord compression. There is replacement of normal marrow by metastatic disease in the posterior half of two lower thoracic vertebral bodies. This finding is evident on the pre-contrast (A) T2 and (B) T1-weighted sagittal scans. The spinal canal is narrowed posteriorly by abnormal soft tissue, which is well seen on the T2-weighted scan. The CSF space both anterior and posterior to the cord tapers and is absent at the level of involvement. The degree of canal compromise is best assessed on (C) the post-contrast T1-weighted scan. The identification of tumor involvement within the marrow space is poor post-contrast. However, the depiction of spinal canal compromise, in this instance a total block, by tumor both anteriorly and posteriorly is improved, due to enhancement of abnormal soft tissue. *(From Runge VM, Awh MH, Bittner DF, Kirsch JE. Magnetic resonance imaging of the spine. Philadelphia, JB Lippincott, 1995).*

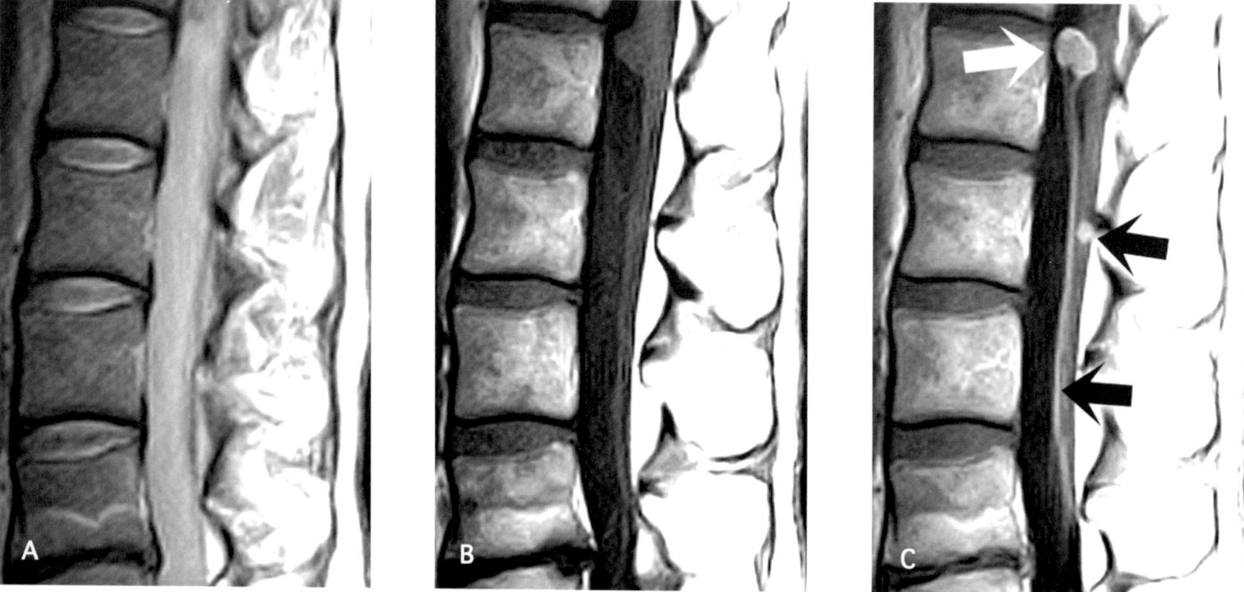

Figure 25. Leptomeningeal metastases. The presence of an intradural soft tissue mass at T12-L1 is questioned on the basis of pre-contrast sagittal (A) T2 and (B) T1-weighted scans. (C) Post-contrast, the lesion is confirmed due to intense enhancement (white arrow). Also noted post-contrast is an enhancing nerve root within the filum terminale, and a second smaller mass within the thecal sac at the L2 level (black arrows). Leptomeningeal metastases are best identified post-contrast, with enhancement in this case permitting diagnosis. This elderly individual with lung carcinoma presented six months prior to the current exam with brain metastases. *(From Runge VM, Awh MH, Bittner DF, Kirsch JE. Magnetic resonance imaging of the spine. Philadelphia, JB Lippincott, 1995).*

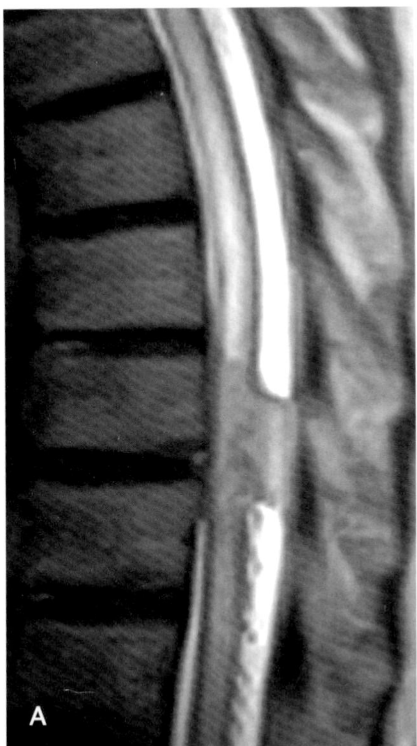

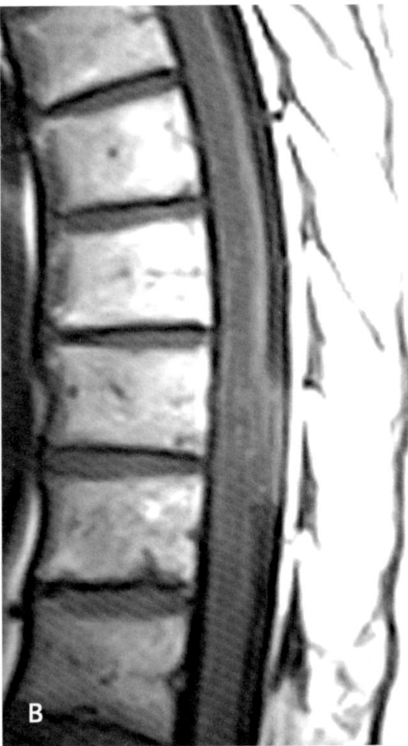

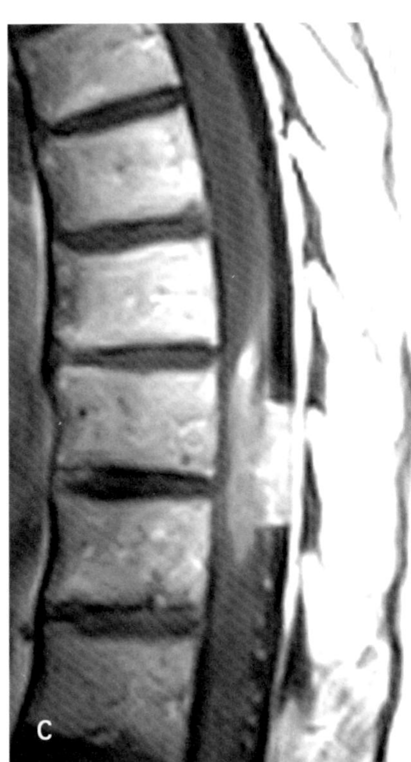

Figure 26. Intramedullary cord metastasis. On pre-contrast (A) T2 and (B) T1-weighted scans, abnormal soft tissue adjacent and posterior to the cord is noted at the T10 level. Superior and inferior to this mass, there is abnormal high signal intensity on the T2-weighted scan (and corresponding low signal intensity on the T1-weighted scan) within the cord substance. This finding could represent either a tumor syrinx or edema. On (C) the post-contrast T1-weighted scan, the mass at the T10 level enhances, and now abnormal tissue both within the cord substance and along its surface is evident. Even when large, metastases to the cord substance are often best appreciated on post-contrast scans.

trast administration can also be of use in this instance (figure 26). The presence of a metastatic deposit within the cord in a patient with known oncological disease is not one that usually requires a surgical approach.

In many cases, patients do not manifest a discrete clinical syndrome that is specific for a particular spinal compartment. For this reason one of the most important missions of the medical imager is to determine the spinal compartment of metastatic disease involvement. This will then direct a specific therapeutic approach. For instance, a patient may have metastatic disease in the epidural space, the subarachnoid space, within the spinal cord itself, or a combination of these locations. These compartments may each carry with them a different clinical therapeutic approach (surgical, medical, or radiotherapeutic), and thus the accurate compartmental definition is of practical importance.

Demyelinating Disease

An important pathologic process deserving discussion in disease of the spine, and the utility of contrast media in magnetic resonance imaging, is multiple sclerosis (MS). When MS affects the spinal cord, multiple hyperintense areas may be seen on T2-weighted studies. Images acquired in the sagittal plane often best demonstrate these MS plaques. On T2-weighted imaging, the hyperintense areas identified may represent either active or quiescent MS plaques. MS plaques undergo change in a phasic manner that is dispersed both temporally as well as spatially within the central nervous system. For these reasons, at any given time some MS plaques may be in the inflammatory phase, the demyelinative phase, the quiescent phase, or some combination of these overlapping phases. During the inflammatory phase there is a breakdown in the blood-cord barrier associated with MS plaques (figure 27). It is believed by some clinicians that the administration of contrast agents may be helpful in directing medical therapy. This may be particularly true in the use of the newer beta-interferon therapeutic agents. The treatment regimens employed in clinical practice locally will determine whether or not patients with known or suspected MS receive intravenous contrast. Although the enhancement pattern may be subtle or absent in some MS plaques of the CNS in an individual patient, the enhancement of MS plaques in other areas or in other individuals can be quite striking.[22]

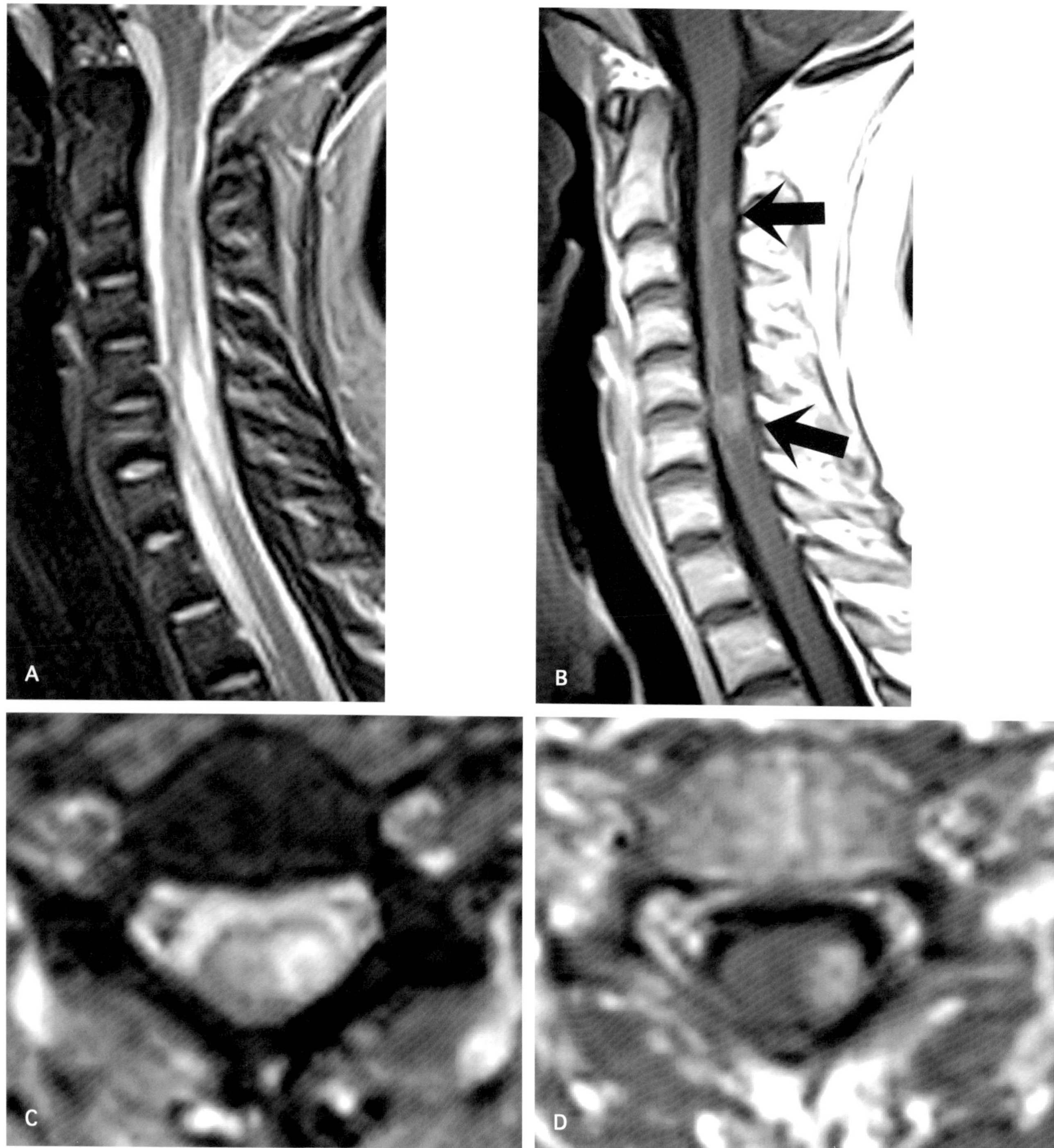

Figure 27. Multiple sclerosis, with active spinal cord plaques. On (A) the T2-weighted midline sagittal scan, two intramedullary lesions are noted, at C2-3 and C5-6, with the latter larger and exhibiting a flame-like pattern of edema extending superiorly and inferiorly. On (B) the post-contrast T1-weighted midline sagittal scan, faint lesion enhancement (arrows) is identified at both levels. Axial (C) T2-weighted gradient echo (FISP) and (D) post-contrast T1-weighted spin echo scans confirm the lower lesion, which is eccentrically located, causes focal cord enlargement, and demonstrates prominent enhancement. *(From Runge VM, Awh MH, Bittner DF, Kirsch JE. Magnetic resonance imaging of the spine. Philadelphia, JB Lippincott, 1995).*

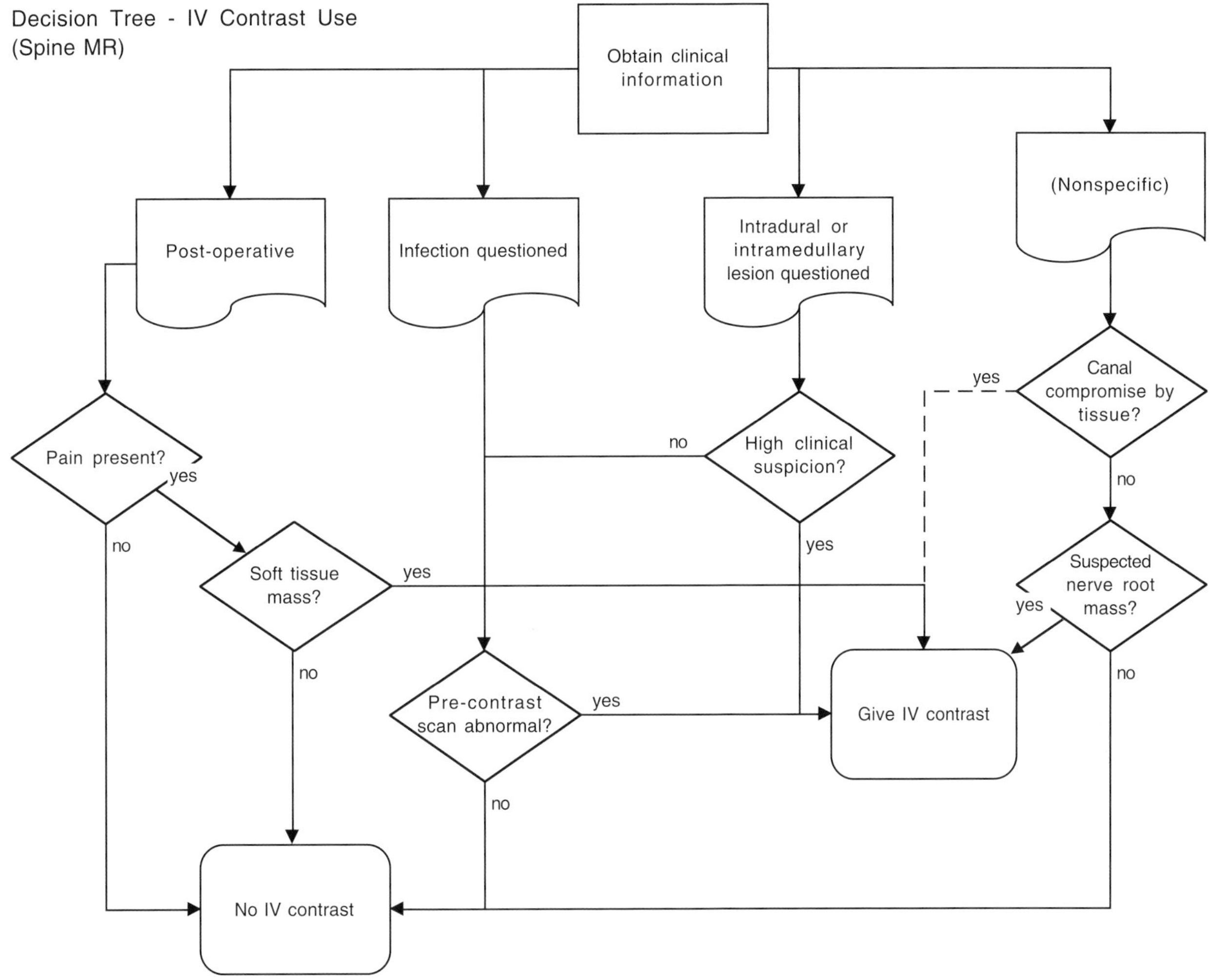

Figure 28. Recommendations for intravenous contrast use in spine MR. A guide for the use of gadolinium chelates is provided as a decision tree.

The diagnosis of MS may be complicated in patients presenting for the first time with enhancing spinal cord lesions on MR. A simple technique to employ in such situations is to subsequently scan the patient's cranium. There will often be concomitant MS plaque formation in intracranial tissue. Differential diagnostic problems can in part be resolved by demonstrating that certain abnormal areas identified on T2-weighted images enhance, while other regions of hyperintensity seen on T2-weighted images do not enhance after gadolinium administration. Such a scenario can constitute a classic MR diagnosis of phasic MS.

Conclusion

While applications of contrast media in MR evaluation of clinically suspected spinal disease appear obvious when demonstrating proven cases, in common practice the efficacious triage of patients is somewhat more complicated. Some general suggestions for when to consider the use of a gadolinium contrast agent are helpful. First, the application of a contrast agent may be necessary when the unenhanced MR examination does not clearly explain the cause of presenting clinical signs and symptoms. A contrast agent in this situation can reveal the presence of enhancing pathology associated with an absent or disrupted blood-CNS barrier that was missed on the unenhanced MR examination. Second, the use of a contrast agent can be helpful in determining the focus and extent of enhancing disease in instances where the unenhanced imaging examination is abnormal. This may assist in directing initial patient therapy and in following disease states in patients undergoing therapy. Third, contrast agents can be used to further characterize a disease process that has been identified on prior unenhanced images. The configuration (or complete absence) of pathologic enhancement forms an important part of pattern recognition and therefore is an integral part of diagnostic imaging. The recognition of patterns of enhancement both within single lesions and between lesions in the same patient can be used to further refine the differential diagnosis. A flow chart to guide the decision making process in the use of contrast media for spine MR is provided (figure 28). Although MR is quite sensitive to disruptions in the blood-CNS barrier, nevertheless, pathologic enhancement following intravenous gadolinium administration remains largely nonspecific in its nature. Histologic and/or microbiologic proof remains mandatory in most initial evaluations.

In summary, MR has been shown to be one of the most sensitive modalities in all of medical imaging with regard to pathologic change of the CNS. Contrast agents form an integral part of MR imaging with regard to their capacity to detect disruption in the blood-CNS barrier. By determining the presence of enhancing pathologic change, the extent of enhancing disease, the pattern of enhancing pathologic change, and the spinal compartment of pathologic enhancement, a more focused differential diagnosis can be generated. In this manner, the appropriate treatment can be planned and the response followed with greatest efficacy.

References

1. Breger RK, Williams AL, Daniels DL, et al. Contrast enhancement in spinal MR imaging. AJNR 1989;10:633-637.
2. Valk J. Gd-DTPA in MR of spinal lesions. AJR 1988;150:1163-1168.
3. Beale SM, Pathria MN, Masaryk TJ. Magnetic resonance imaging of spinal trauma. Top Magn Reson Imaging 1988;1:53-62.
4. Jinkins JR. MR of nerve root enhancement in the unoperated lumbosacral spine. AJNR 1993;14:193-202.
5. Hueftle MG, Modic MT, Ross JS, et al. Lumbar spine: postoperative MR imaging with Gd-DTPA. Radiology 1988;167:817-824.
6. Ross JS, Delamarter R, Hueftle MG, et al. Gadolinium-DTPA-enhanced MR imaging of the postoperative lumbar spine: time course and mechanism of enhancement. AJNR 1989;10:37-46.
7. Jinkins JR, Osborn AG, Garrett D, et al. Spinal nerve enhancement with Gd-DTPA: MR correlation with the postoperative lumbosacral spine. AJNR 1993;14:383-394.
8. Jinkins JR. Gd-DTPA enhanced MR of the lumbar spinal canal in patients with claudication. J Comput Assist Tomogr 1993;17:555-562.
9. Ross JS, Modic MT, Masaryk TJ, et al. Assessment of extradural degenerative disease with Gd DTPA enhanced MR imaging: correlation with surgical and pathologic findings. AJR 1990;154:151-157.
10. Parizel PM, Rodesch G, Baleriaux D, et al. Gd DTPA enhanced MR in thoracic disc herniations. Neurorad 1989;31:75-79.
11. Post MJ, Sze G, Quencer RM, et al. Gadolinium enhanced MR in spinal infection. J Comput Assist Tomogr 1990;14:721-729.
12. Johnson CE, Sze G. Benign lumbar arachnoiditis: MR imaging with gadopentetate dimeglumine. AJNR 1990;11:763-770.
13. Larsson E-M, Desai P, Hardin C, Jinkins JR. Venous infarction of the spinal cord resulting from dural arteriovenous fistula: MR imaging findings. AJNR 1991;12:739-743.
14. Terwey B, Becker H, Thron AK, Vahldiek G. Gadolinium-DTPA enhanced MR imaging of spinal dural arteriovenous fistulas. J Comput Assist Tomogr 1989;13:30-37.
15. Sze G, Krol G, Zimmerman RD, Deck MDF. Malignant extradural spinal tumors: MR imaging with Gd-DTPA. Radiology 1988;167:217-223.
16. Sze G, Abramson A, Krol G, et al. Gadolinium-DTPA in the evaluation of intradural extramedullary spinal disease. AJR 1988;150:911-921.
17. Sze G, Krol G, Zimmerman RD, Deck MDF. Intramedullary disease of the spine: diagnosis using gadolinium-DTPA-enhanced MR imaging. AJR 1988;151:1193-1204.
18. Dillon WP, Norman D, Newton TH, et al. Intradural spinal cord lesions: Gd-DTPA-enhanced MR imaging. Radiology 1989;170:229-237.
19. Parizel PM, Baleriaux D, Rodesch G, et al. Gd-DTPA-enhanced MR imaging of spinal tumors. AJR 1989;152:1087-1096.
20. Yuh WTC, Zachar CK, Barloon TJ, et al. Vertebral compression fractures: distinction between benign and malignant causes with MR imaging. Radiology 1989;172:215-218.
21. Lim V, Sobel DF, Zyroff J. Spinal cord pial metastases: MR imaging with gadopentetate dimeglumine. AJNR 1990;11:975-982.
22. Larsson E-M, Holtas S, Nilsson O. Gd DTPA enhanced MR of suspected spinal multiple sclerosis. AJNR 1989;10:1071-1076.

Chapter 5

Body Applications

Val M. Runge, M.D.

Introduction

The use of magnetic resonance (MR) contrast media in the head and spine dominates today's clinical applications, with experience and indications lagging in the body. Broad indications for intravenous gadolinium chelate use have been established in the central nervous system (CNS). However, the role of contrast media is less certain in body imaging. This situation can be attributed to two factors. First, the development of clinical MR initially focused on head imaging, and then subsequently expanded to include the spine. Today, body applications, regardless of the application of contrast media, still constitute a small proportion of all clinical scans. Only musculoskeletal (sports medicine) studies are performed in any substantial number. Second, the distribution of the gadolinium chelates is quite different in the CNS as opposed to the rest of the body. In the brain and spinal cord, these agents are largely confined to an intravascular distribution, due to the existence of the blood-brain and blood-spinal cord barriers. When these barriers are disrupted, gadolinium chelates play a valuable role, marking such disease. However, in the rest of the body, there is no equivalent barrier. Outside the CNS, gadolinium chelates are distributed throughout the extracellular space, in a nonspecific manner. However, if attention is paid to the manner of contrast administration (for example, bolus injection), the timing of scan acquisition, and contrast dose, valuable information can be obtained.

In spite of these problems, indications have been established for the use of MR contrast media in the body. Not inconsequential in this process has been the rapid advance in machine design during the past ten years. Breathhold MR imaging of the upper abdomen has now become routine, opening broad avenues for clinical use. Body CT developed similarly. Now, years later, applications for extracellular iodinated agents are well established. Dynamic imaging, with acquisition times in the seconds, is also now a routine option on current generation MR scanners. Advances in pharmaceutical development have paralleled those in instrumentation, with contrast media in two new classes, reticuloendothelial cell and hepatobiliary, in or near clinical use.

Consistent with the intention of the text overall, emphasis is placed in this chapter on current clinical applications. The reader is referred to chapter six for a more in depth look at contrast media in pre-clinical and clinical development. The use of contrast media in MR of the body has also been the subject of several recent reviews, to which the reader is directed.[1,2,3]

Contrast Media

Three extracellular gadolinium chelates (gadoteridol, gadopentetate dimeglumine, and gadodiamide) are currently available for clinical use in the US. When applied at a dose of 0.1 mmol/kg, these agents cannot be distinguished in terms of lesion enhancement.

Intravenous iron oxide particles hold promise for use as reticuloendothelial agents. However, severe hypotension was encountered in early clinical trials, requiring reformulation. These agents are yet to be approved for clinical use.

Hepatobiliary gadolinium chelates have recently been evaluated in clinical trials in Europe. The first to reach the US, Gd BOPTA, is currently in its second round of clinical trials here. In addition to its hepatobiliary uptake, Gd BOPTA also binds weakly to proteins, leading to its evaluation in the brain and spine as well as in the liver.

A variety of oral agents have been evaluated in clinical trials, with opacification of the gut important for MR exams of the abdomen and pelvis. Although oral formulations of various gadolinium chelates, manganese chloride, and iron oxide particles have all been evaluated, no agent is yet in widespread clinical use.

Imaging Technique

The choice of imaging technique is critical for successful MR studies of the body with both intravenous and oral contrast media. For example, an early observation was that T1-weighted sequences displayed well the effect of intravenous gadolinium chelate administration, while T2-weighted sequences did not. The basis for this finding is now clearly understood. Paramagnetic agents decrease both T1 and T2. The decrease in T1 leads to an increase in signal intensity, which is pronounced on T1-weighted sequences. The decrease in T2 leads to a decrease in signal intensity, which is typically only observed at very high concentration or on heavily T2-weighted scans. In most tissues, at the contrast doses typically employed, an increase in signal intensity is observed on T1-weighted scans in areas of gadolinium chelate accumulation. However, in the renal pelvis and urine where these agents are concentrated, a loss of signal intensity can be observed due to T2 effects. The net result (positive or negative enhancement, and the degree of the effect) depends upon contrast dose, distribution, timing of the image acquisition, choice of pulse sequence, imaging field strength, and the native T1 and T2 values of the tissue of interest. With the recent interest in fast gradient echo techniques and echo-planar imaging, it is important to note that these sequences are quite sensitive to susceptibility effects. This can be turned to advantage in the use of gadolinium chelates as susceptibility agents (as in first pass studies) or in the application of iron oxide particles.

Another relatively recent innovation in pulse sequence design with applicability to body imaging is the use of fat suppression.[4] Fat has a short T1, in common with enhancing tissue (following gadolinium chelate administration). This situation can lead to a loss of lesion conspicuity following contrast administration, in regions with abundant fat. The wide distribution of fat in the body and its presence within tissue planes leads to substantial problems in image interpretation outside the central nervous system. Several different techniques have been developed to effectively suppress the signal from fat. Of these, the two most commonly employed are STIR (short tau inversion recovery) and the application of frequency selective saturation pulses. The latter can be applied in theory to any pulse sequence, although the sensitivity to field inhomogeneity has limited application. Frequency selective fat suppression is relatively easy to implement successfully in areas of the body with small cross sections, such as the neck. However, difficulties have been encountered in areas with large cross sections, such as the abdomen and pelvis. Advances continue to be made in this area, with encouraging results on current generation imaging systems. When effective fat saturation can be achieved, its use is strongly advocated for improved detection of contrast enhancement.

Head and Neck

Magnetic resonance is being increasingly used for examination of the extracranial head and neck.[5] The superior soft tissue contrast resolution of MR enables improved depiction, as compared to computed tomography, of lesion margins and differentiation of inflammatory change from space occupying lesions. Localization of lesions to specific tissue compartments is also superior due to the ability to directly acquire images in all three planes. An additional advantage of MR is the ability to identify vascular channels, adding specificity with lesions such as paragangliomas and hemangiomas.[6,7]

Enhancement of normal structures in the extracranial head and neck on MR following gadolinium chelate administration is similar to that seen on CT following iodinated contrast media. The mucosal surfaces demonstrate moderate contrast enhancement. The salivary, parathyroid, and thyroid glands show prominent enhancement. The remaining normal structures demonstrate no substantial contrast enhancement.

The fat in soft tissue and bone marrow is of high signal intensity on T1-weighted scans, as well as fast T2-weighted scans. The use of fat-saturation techniques to null the signal of fat markedly improves the detection of abnormal soft tissue lesions in the head and neck region. This is particularly true on scans following contrast administration, where — with the application of fat saturation — abnormal soft tissue enhancement is readily evident (figure 1).

The use of contrast media solves many diagnostic problems associated with unenhanced MR imaging in the head and neck. Contrast administration helps characterize lesions and assists in determining lesion margins. Contrast use also increases the sensitivity for detection of perineural tumor spread and metastatic lymphadenopathy. Inflammatory lesions involving the skull base and vital structures are also more likely to be correctly identified after the contrast injection.

In 1994, Hudgins reviewed the use of contrast enhancement, both on MR and CT, in head and neck imaging.[8] On MR (unlike CT), contrast administration is not needed to opacify blood vessels. Furthermore, good differentiation between lesions and normal tissue is often achieved on pre-contrast scans, with proper selection of imaging technique. Despite these advantages (of unenhanced MR as opposed to CT), intravenous (IV) contrast administration is routinely employed today in head and neck MR imaging, for the following reasons. Use of IV contrast improves the detection of perineural and intracranial spread of disease. Necrosis within lymph nodes, abscesses, or tumors is also best delineated on post-contrast studies. Most importantly, post-contrast scans often more accurately delineate the full extent of disease within surrounding soft tissue.

MR is the imaging modality of choice for the detection of lesions in the temporal bone and internal auditory canal (IAC). The most common tumor in this area is an acous-

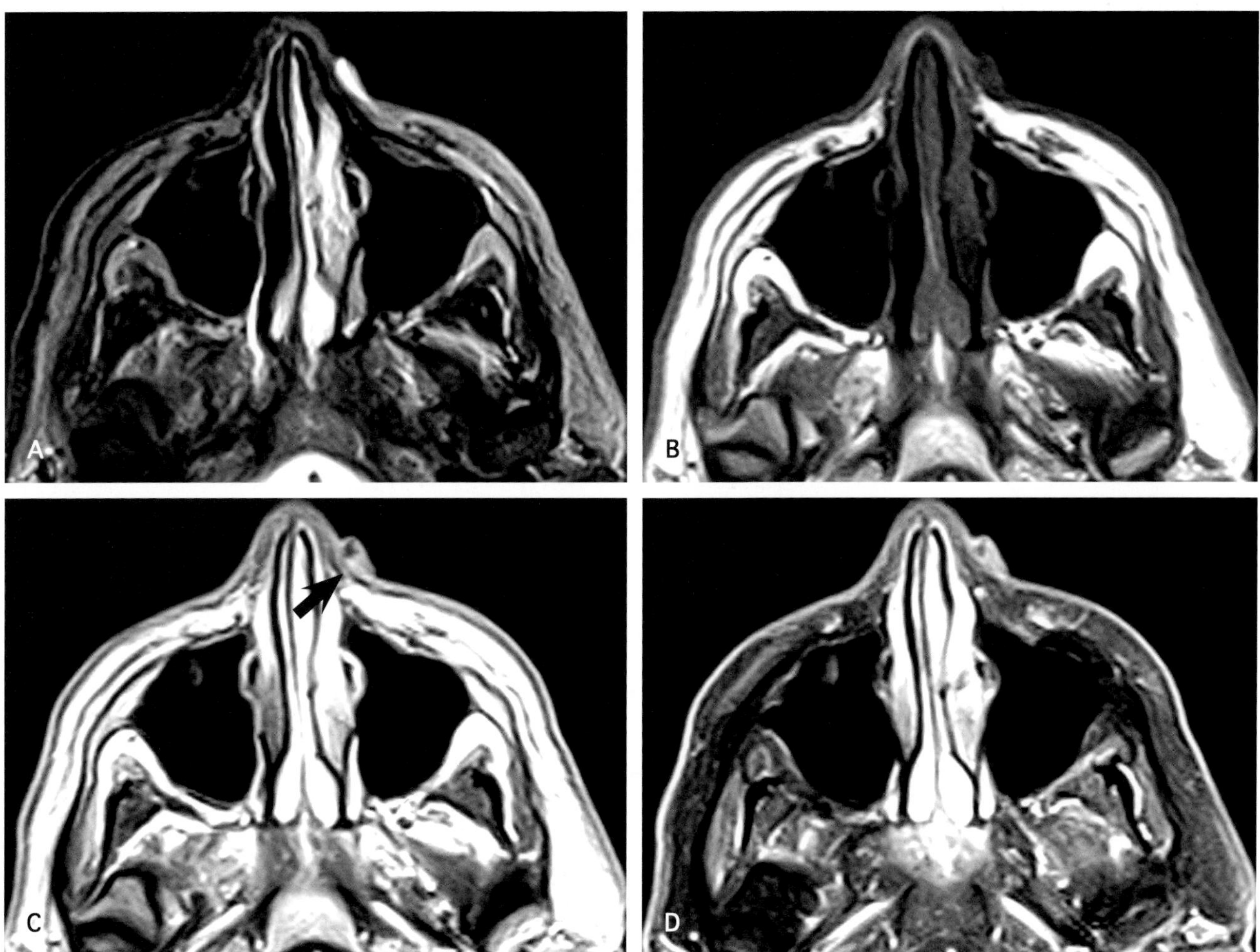

Figure 1. Basal cell carcinoma. On (A) the T2-weighted scan, a small, superficial, high signal intensity lesion is noted over the left nares. The lesion is of soft tissue signal intensity on (B) the pre-contrast T1-weighted scan. There is enhancement of the mass (arrow) on (C) the post-contrast T1-weighted scan. Differentiation between the lesion and surrounding soft tissue is poor, however, due to the high signal intensity of surrounding normal adipose tissue. (D) The post-contrast fat suppressed T1-weighted scan more clearly reveals the enhancement of the lesion and the lack of deep invasion.

tic nerve schwannoma. Differentiation from other lesions, including an arachnoid cyst (which may accompany a schwannoma), is readily accomplished on both pre- and post-contrast scans due to differences in signal intensity and contrast enhancement.[9,10]

In Bell's palsy, a viral neuritis, abnormal contrast enhancement of the facial nerve can be noted along its course from the internal auditory canal to the mastoid foramen. Most often seen is enhancement of the segment adjacent to the geniculate ganglion, on the basis of entrapment in the narrowest portion of the fallopian canal.[11,12]

Key to interpretation of images in the nasopharynx and skull base is the differences in tissue signal intensity on various pulse sequences. T1-weighted images best outline the muscular and fascial anatomy. T2-weighted images readily differentiate the mucosal surfaces from superficial lymphoid tissues in Waldeyer's ring. Contrast enhancement permits the differentiation of cysts from solid lesions. Cysts should not show substantial contrast enhancement. Occasionally, there may be enhancement of a thin cyst wall. Solid tumors display contrast enhancement, which may be either homogeneous or heterogeneous (figure 2). Metastatic lymph nodes, when necrotic, will display rim enhancement, adding to diagnostic specificity.[13,14] Tumor vascularity is also readily appreciated following contrast administration.

Chordomas typically enhance in a non-uniform pattern following gadolinium chelate administration.[15] Juvenile nasopharyngeal angiofibromas show marked contrast enhancement, greater than that of most primary malignant lesions in this area (figure 3).[16] These benign lesions, which

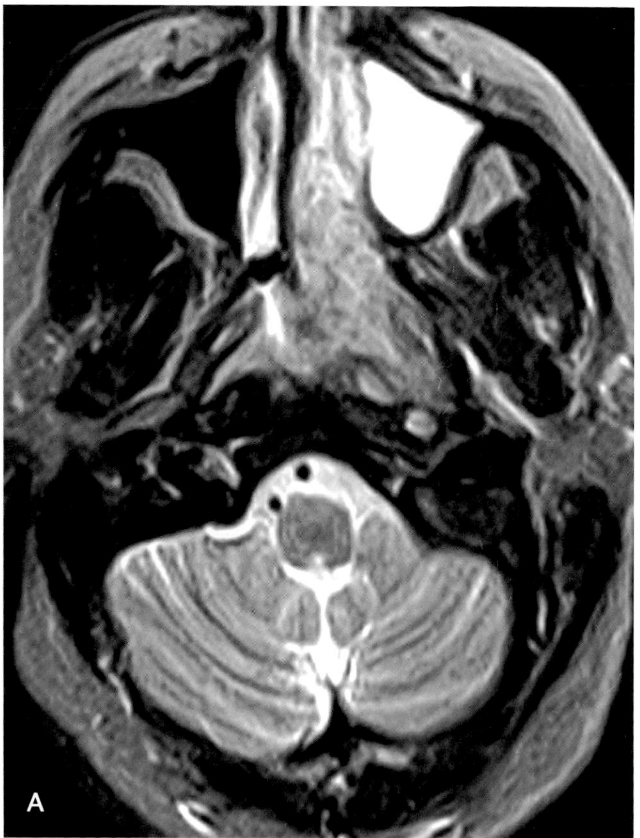

Figure 2. Squamous cell carcinoma of the nasopharynx. On (A) the T2-weighted scan, a large soft tissue mass with intermediate signal intensity is noted in the posterior nasopharynx. The lesion extends anteriorly into the left nasal cavity. Retained secretions, with high signal intensity, are noted in the left maxillary sinus. On (B) the pre-contrast T1-weighted scan, neoplastic tissue, retained secretions, and the normal turbinates are all intermediate signal intensity. (C) Following contrast administration, there is intense enhancement of the turbinates and the mucosal lining of the left maxillary sinus. Neoplastic tissue enhances, but to a lesser degree, permitting differentiation. *(From Runge VM, Brack MA, Garneau RA, Kirsch JE. Magnetic resonance imaging of the brain. Philadelphia, JB Lippincott, 1994).*

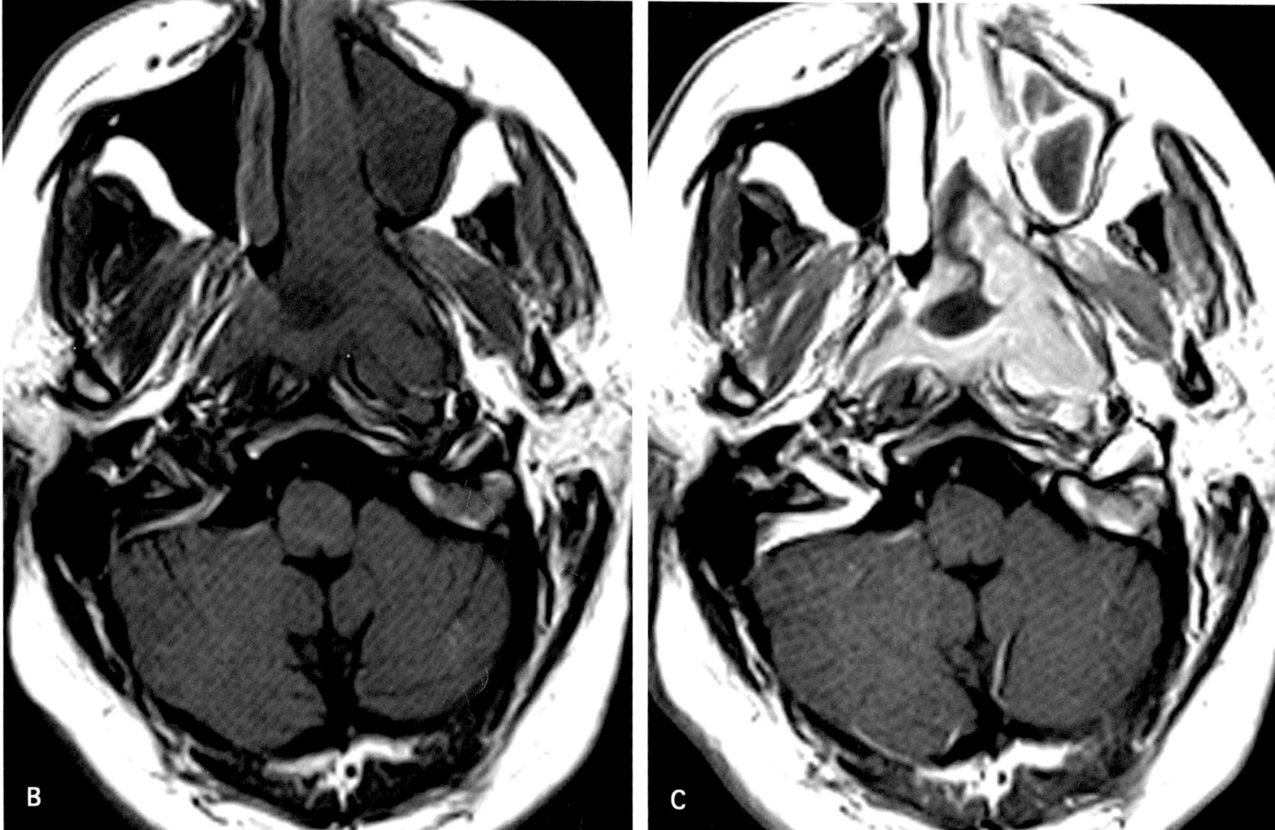

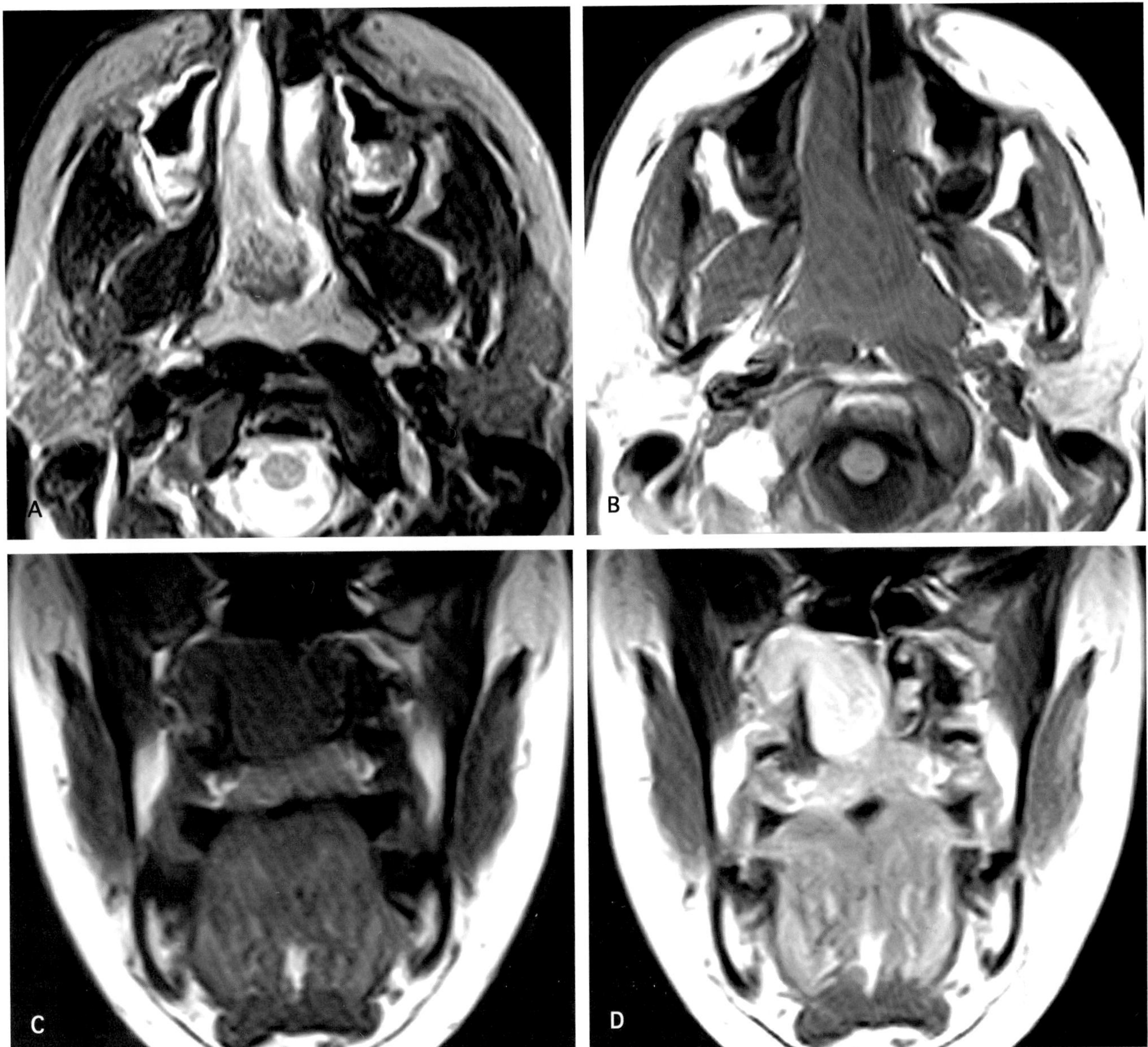

Figure 3. Juvenile angiofibroma. On (A) the T2-weighted scan, a large soft tissue mass with intermediate signal intensity fills the nasal passages and nasopharynx. Inflammatory changes are noted in the maxillary sinuses bilaterally. On pre-contrast (B) axial and (C) coronal T1-weighted scans, the mass is isointense with muscle. (D) Following contrast administration, there is intense lesion enhancement. Abnormal soft tissue expanding the right pterygopalatine fossa is well seen on the post-contrast scan. The borders of the lesion are also best delineated post-contrast. *(From Runge VM, Brack MA, Garneau RA, Kirsch JE. Magnetic resonance imaging of the brain. Philadelphia, JB Lippincott, 1994).*

are highly vascular, are characterized on pre-contrast scans by a salt and pepper like pattern, with low signal intensity vessels seen within a fibrous stroma.

Paragangliomas are an additional benign highly vascular tumor found in the head and neck. These occur in the middle ear (glomus tympanicum), jugular foramen (glomus jugulare), and carotid space (glomus vagale). MR is superior to CT for depiction of the vascularity of these tumors. Hypointense regions within these tumors on pre-contrast T1 and T2-weighted scans reflect flowing blood and vascular structures. Contrast enhanced MR shows prominent lesion enhancement. Paragangliomas demonstrate rapid contrast enhancement followed by gradual washout. This pattern assists in differential diagnosis from schwannomas, which enhance more slowly. Vascular malformations also demonstrate rapid enhancement, but can be distinguished from paragangliomas by means of MR or conventional angiography.[17,18]

In a study by Vogl, 167 patients with abnormalities of the skull base were examined by MR with and without fat saturation technique, and the diagnostic information thus obtained correlated with histopathological findings.[19] The number of lesions detected was not changed by the use of fat saturation. However, the visualization of soft tissue lesions was improved. On statistical analysis, post-contrast fat saturation scans proved superior for lesion delineation and visualization. The addition of contrast enhanced fat saturated scans specifically resulted in improved diagnosis of lesions at the skull base and the craniocervical junction.

In the soft tissues of the neck, the multiplanar capability of MR enables optimal localization of mass lesions within the cervical spaces. However, without the use of contrast media, differentiation of a mass from neighboring normal soft tissue may be difficult. Hemangiomas are the most common benign neck mass in a child, with the administration of contrast on MR providing marked lesion enhancement, aiding in differential diagnosis. MR also provides improved differentiation between recurrent tumor and postoperative fibrosis, as compared with CT.[20] Several months after surgery, fibrosis becomes intermediate in signal intensity on T2-weighted images, and thus difficult to distinguish from residual or recurrent tumor. In such cases, the use of contrast is helpful. Nodular irregular enhancement along the margins of the surgical bed is suggestive of tumor recurrence. However, biopsy may be necessary in many cases to provide absolute differentiation between fibrosis and recurrent tumor.

Perineural spread of malignant lesions is noted on imaging as a smooth thickening of cranial and spinal nerves. Concentric expansion of the foramina and fissures through which the nerves course may also be noted. Nerve infiltration by tumor is best identified on post-contrast scans.[21,22]

Lung

One of the advantages of MR over CT in the mediastinum and pulmonary hili is that a contrast agent is not necessary for the identification of blood vessels (and for differentiation of these from soft tissue). Depending upon the choice of imaging technique, flowing blood can be displayed as either high or low signal intensity. The latter is common, due to dephasing effects with conventional spin echo sequences. Thus normal blood vessels can be readily distinguished from soft tissue lesions.

Although spatial resolution on clinical MR studies is typically inferior to CT, soft tissue contrast is superior. The result is rough equivalence between CT and MR in many clinical body applications, not the least of which being the staging of bronchogenic carcinoma. Here both techniques contribute significant clinical information. Unfortunately, neither technique can discriminate at present between enlarged nodes containing tumor and those with only inflammatory change. It is in this differentiation that small iron oxide particles like AMI-227 may find clinical application. Glazer concluded that accurate staging of the pulmonary hili was not possible by MR or CT in patients with lung cancer.[23] Other groups, including the Radiologic Diagnostic Oncology Group, have concluded that both modalities display poor sensitivity and specificity for the detection of nodal metastases and chest wall involvement.[24,25]

Heart

MR can be used for the identification and quantification of myocardial infarction. The application of extracellular contrast agents, specifically the gadolinium chelates, has been explored with attention to improving diagnostic accuracy. T2-weighted scans provide a reasonable depiction of acute myocardial infarction. However, pitfalls include high signal intensity from slow flowing blood adjacent to the area of infarction and other motion related artifacts. On gated post-contrast spin echo scans, acute myocardial infarction demonstrates positive enhancement. The accumulation of contrast agent in damaged myocardium is felt to be secondary to reduced washout. In normal tissue, these agents are effectively cleared by 10 to 15 minutes post-injection. Contrast enhancement is seen during the first two weeks after acute infarction, but not in chronic myocardial infarction, after scar has formed.[26,27,28,29] De Roos[30] has described four patterns of enhancement in acute infarction: uniform diffuse, subendocardial, inhomogeneous (with dark areas in or adjacent to the area of enhancement), and doughnut like (with a non-enhancing core). The doughnut-like pattern is thought to be due to the lack of blood flow centrally. These patterns have been observed in both reperfused and nonreperfused infarcts.

Early post-contrast studies may be capable of differentiating reperfused from nonreperfused infarction after treatment with fibrinolysis. A reduction in apparent infarct size on MR has been demonstrated with successful reperfusion. Techniques for the estimation of myocardial infarct size, based on post-contrast scans, have been implemented by de Roos.[31] Echo-planar imaging and other subsecond scan techniques hold promise for improved assessment of myocardial perfusion when combined with bolus contrast administration.

Breast

Heywang has shown in extensive clinical studies that all breast carcinomas demonstrate substantial positive contrast

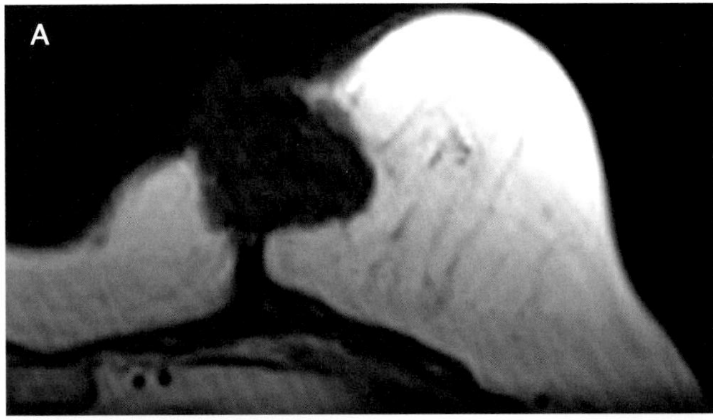

Figure 4. Ductal adenocarcinoma of the left breast. (A, B) Pre- and post-contrast T1-weighted axial scans, (C) the difference image between B and A, and (D, E) pre- and early dynamic post-contrast gradient echo (FLASH) T1-weighted axial scans are presented. A contrast dose of 0.3 mmol/kg gadoteridol was employed. A large relatively well defined mass is noted, which distorts the normal breast contour. There is associated skin thickening, best seen on the difference image. Best defined post-contrast is deep muscle invasion. The rapid, substantial, positive contrast enhancement of the mass within the first few minutes following contrast administration (E) is consistent with the tissue diagnosis, that of breast carcinoma.

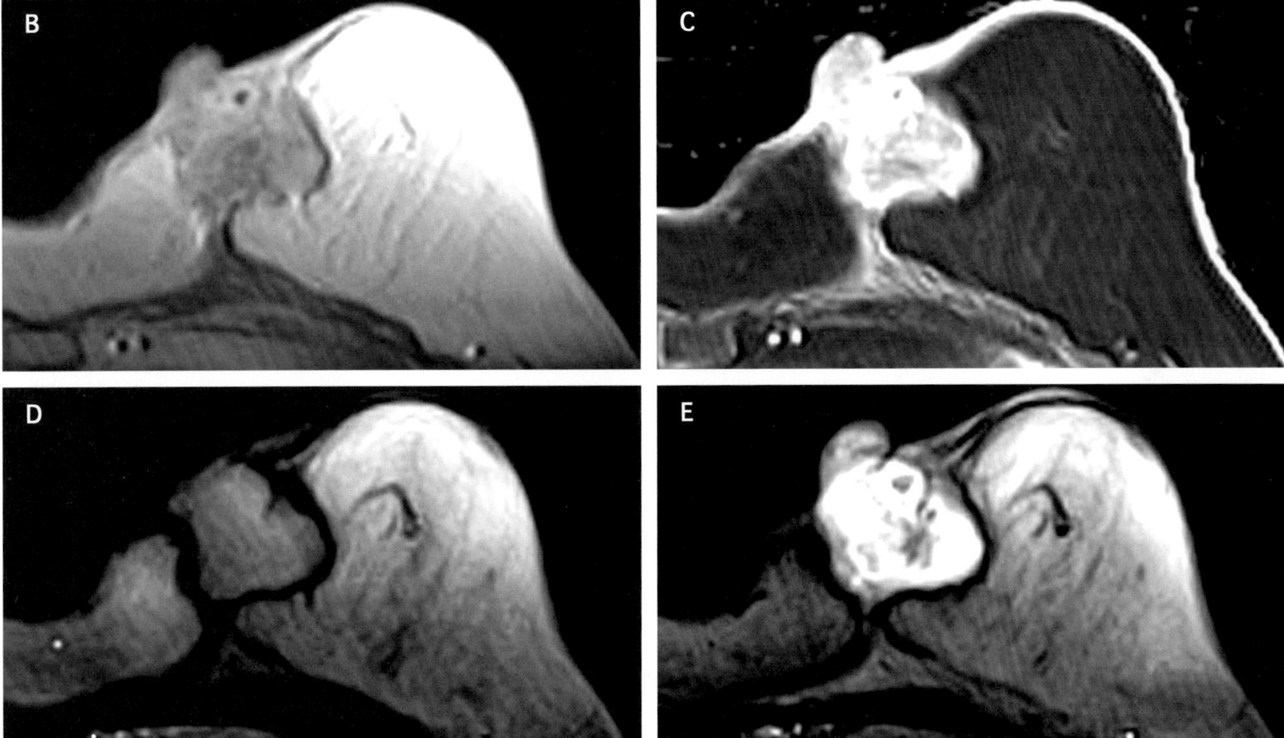

enhancement.[32,33] Focal enhancement can also occur in fibroadenomas, papillomas and proliferative dysplasia. Diffuse enhancement is most frequently seen in proliferative dysplasia or inflammatory change. This occurs, infrequently, in malignant disease. There is no significant enhancement in normal breasts, cysts, nonproliferative dysplasia and chronic scar tissue. Evaluation of the rate of enhancement on dynamic scans performed during the first few minutes following contrast administration shows a fast rise in signal enhancement in most carcinomas and a delayed rise in many benign lesions (figure 4). However, delayed enhancement cannot be used as a reliable criterion for excluding malignancy, since a small number of carcinomas display this pattern.

Heywang has proposed the following rules for interpretation of contrast enhanced MR studies of the breast. In cases with no significant enhancement, a malignancy larger in diameter than the slice thickness can be excluded. If focal contrast enhancement is present, biopsy is indicated to distinguish malignancy, benign tumors, and (rarely) focal proliferative dysplasia. Diffuse enhancement is nonspecific and also warrants biopsy if a focal abnormality is questioned.

The most clinically useful result of these studies is the high negative predictive value for the exclusion of malignancy when contrast enhancement is not present. Contrast enhanced MR is also valuable for the differentiation of irregular dysplasia and carcinoma, carcinoma and scar (provided at least six months have elapsed since surgery or 18 months since radiotherapy). Contrast enhanced MR is of further use in the evaluation of radiographically dense breasts when neoplastic involvement is suspected. The latter situation includes cases with a palpable abnormality, the search for a primary tumor, and patients in whom a limited excision is planned.

Liver and Spleen

Initial clinical trials with contrast agents in liver MR were limited to the use of Gd DTPA, an early extracellular agent, with mixed results. Unlike findings in the brain — where Gd DTPA rapidly found clinical acceptance, in the liver lesion detectability did not consistently improve post-contrast. Diminished lesion conspicuity was noted post-contrast in many instances. Differences in tissue relaxation characteristics, and the rapid extracellular distribution in the liver — without a structure comparable to the blood-brain barrier, were responsible for these disappointing findings and forced broad reassessment.

With liver metastases in particular, reduced lesion conspicuity was noted post-contrast in early clinical trials. This was due to distribution of the agent in the extracellular space, with the extracellular space relatively small in normal liver. In metastatic lesions, it is considerably larger. During the long imaging times of early clinical trials, Gd DTPA diffused into the lesions, which prior to contrast administration were hypointense (on T1-weighted studies). Thus post-contrast, the lesions became isointense to normal surrounding liver.[37] Early clinical trials did however hold some promise for improved lesion detection, with post-contrast studies revealing some lesions that were otherwise poorly demonstrated. Subsequently, the imaging techniques employed for contrast detection were reexamined and new agents developed, with rapid progress on both fronts achieved in recent years.

In terms of chemical design, MR contrast media share much in common with radiopharmaceuticals. Although the majority of clinical work to date has been performed with extracellular agents, including specifically Gd HP-DO3A and Gd DTPA, agents within two other major classes have been developed and are undergoing clinical evaluation. Metal chelates with substantial hepatobiliary uptake have been developed and tested (Gd BOPTA and Mn DPDP), with continuing research in this area. Preliminary results with hepatobiliary gadolinium chelates are favorable in regard to efficacy, although these agents remain in clinical trials. Two types of particulate agents have reached clinical trials, one with preferential uptake by the reticuloendothelial system (AMI-25), and the other a blood pool agent (AMI-227). Although particulate agents have also been designed which are targeted to cell receptors, these have not yet reached clinical trials.

MR imaging studies have revealed that the choice of pulse sequence is critical for visualization of a contrast agent in the liver, with marked differences depending upon agent class. T1-weighted techniques are employed for detection of gadolinium and manganese chelates, and T2-weighted techniques for detection of iron particles. The timing of image acquisition, quantity of pharmaceutical injected, and rate of injection are also important, in particular for routine clinical use at present — which is restricted to the gadolinium chelates with extracellular distribution.

The gadolinium chelates which are distributed in the extracellular space and excreted principally by the kidneys have been extensively evaluated in the liver with respect to improved lesion characterization and detection. In the past few years, attention has been paid in particular to rapid imaging following bolus administration and the use of doses higher than 0.1 mmol/kg. Extracellular MR agents are designed to have minimal binding to serum proteins, diffuse freely through the extracellular space, and undergo glomerular filtration.[34] This pattern of biodistribution is reflected in the name "extracellular" or "nonspecific" for this class of contrast agents. Analogous to iodinated low molecular weight contrast agents, extracellular MR agents show maximum liver to tumor contrast in the first few minutes after administration. However, unlike iodinated contrast agents, Gd DTPA and other agents in this class are not taken up significantly by hepatocytes.

Gd DTPA (gadopentetate dimeglumine or Magnevist) became the first MR contrast agent to be approved for clinical use in the United States in 1988, followed by Gd HP-DO3A (gadoteridol or ProHance) in 1992 and Gd DTPA-BMA (gadodiamide or Omniscan) in 1993. Gd DOTA (gadoterate meglumine or Dotarem) has received approval for clinical use in France, Switzerland, and Portugal. The recommended dose of Gd DTPA is 0.1 mmol/kg administered at a rate of 10 ml/min. (5 mmol/min.), although Hamm[35] have suggested that doubling the dose may improve liver lesion characterization and detection. Gd DTPA is well tolerated with adverse reactions occurring in only 1.0% - 2.6% of the population.[36] Patients with previous allergies have a higher incidence of adverse side effects.

As previously noted, the initial clinical experience with contrast enhancement in MR of the liver was disappointing.[37] As with CT, fast scanning is necessary to image the liver early in the vascular phase of contrast agent distribution, immediately following injection.[38,39] A delay in imaging the liver following contrast injection allows the contrast agent to redistribute from the vascular space of the liver into the interstitial space of tumors, reducing tumor to liver contrast. As a result, metastases are poorly seen on delayed Gd DTPA images, similar to the case with delayed iodine enhanced CT scans.

Modern rapid T1-weighted scanning techniques, including short TE fast low angle shot (FLASH), magnetization prepared rapid gradient echo (MP-RAGE) and inversion recovery echo-planar have largely overcome the limitations of older scan techniques.[40,41] In clinical practice today, the availability of these high quality fast scans makes possible routine acquisition of early dynamic scans following contrast administration. Acquisition of such scans provides improved visualization of most liver lesions (figure 5), which in the early dynamic time period following bolus contrast administration enhance substantially less than normal liver.[42] The conspicuity of hypervascular lesions is also increased using this approach. In the first few minutes following contrast administration, these demonstrate substantially greater enhancement than normal liver. The enhancement fades with time, with lesions typically isointense with liver by five to ten minutes following contrast administration.[43]

The choice between CT and MR as a screening technique for the liver is complex. Clinical studies have shown that the sensitivity of contrast-enhanced CT for detecting individual hepatic lesions is only 38%.[44] Although MR imaging has proven as effective as contrast enhanced CT of the liver, CT is superior for detecting most extrahepatic lesions in the abdomen.[45,46] Dynamic contrast enhanced MR, using T1-weighted sequences, has improved lesion detection[47] and offers today better image quality than non-breathhold scans.

Characterization of metastases on MR is accomplished primarily with T2-weighted sequences based on signal intensity, margin sharpness, and internal morphology.[48] After administration of a gadolinium chelate, the periphery of malignant tumors may show early increased enhancement. On delayed scans, some hypervascular metastases show diffusely increased enhancement, likely due to greater interstitial space as compared to normal hepatic parenchyma.[49]

The most common hepatic neoplasm is the cavernous hemangioma. Heavily T2-weighted sequences are the most reliable in distinguishing other lesions, and in particular other neoplasms, from a hemangioma.[50] In hemangiomas that are less than three centimeters in diameter, lesion enhancement is initiated by puddling in the periphery. This is followed by progressive centripetal filling and finally by homogeneous enhancement on delayed scans. Exceptions occur to this filling pattern. For example, large hemangiomas with central changes (thrombosis or scarring) will not enhance homogeneously on delayed scans.

Hamm studied the appearance of metastases and hemangiomas on MR, using both dynamic and delayed post-contrast scans.[43] Hemangiomas were characterized (as previously noted) by early peripheral contrast enhancement, with subsequent fill-in of the hypointense center. Metastases demonstrated variable enhancement. On delayed post-contrast scans, a number of the hemangiomas demonstrated very high homogeneous contrast enhancement. On these same scans, metastases were characterized by inhomogeneous and hyperintense to isointense enhancement.

The detection and characterization of cysts greater than one centimeter in diameter can easily be accomplished by ultrasound. The lesions that challenge ultrasound include those in obese patients, those that are less than one centimeter in diameter and lesions that lie close to the diaphragm.[51] Homogeneous high signal intensity on T2-weighted spin echo scans and the lack of enhancement on dynamic scans are characteristic findings for cysts.

Solid lesions like hepatocellular carcinoma (HCC), focal nodular hyperplasia (FNH), and liver adenoma have no specific features for characterization. Distinction of these lesions may rest on features such as arteriovenous shunting (HCC), and central feeding vessels, spoke wheel pattern, and central scar (FNH), but such findings are not specific.[52] The role of contrast enhancement under these circumstances is still evolving. Hepatocellular carcinomas may demonstrate either a hyper- or hypovascular pattern of enhancement following contrast administration. Like metastases, the enhancement is usually inhomogeneous. About half of all lesions have delayed enhancement in the area of the pseudocapsule. In distinction, hemangiomas typically have intense enhancement on delayed scans. Yoshida specifically examined the appearance of small hepatocellular carcinomas and hemangiomas on MR, comparing dynamic scans post-contrast with pre-contrast T1 and T2-weighted scans. Most hemangiomas (89%) were iso- or hypointense on pre-contrast T1-weighted scans and hyperintense on delayed post-contrast scans. By using pre- and post-contrast scans, along with T2 measurements, 30 of 32 lesions (94%) could be correctly differentiated.[53] In about half of the hepatocellular carcinomas studied, peak enhancement occurred by 10 seconds after contrast injection. In the hemangiomas, peak enhancement occurred more than two minutes after contrast injection in 72%.

Two ring chelates, Gd DOTA and Gd HP-DO3A, are in clinical use worldwide. Of these, only Gd HP-DO3A (gadoteridol or ProHance) is available in the United States. These two extracellular agents were developed after Gd DTPA and offer a possible safety advantage over linear chelates due to higher in vivo stability. Food and Drug Administration approval for Gd HP-DO3A is for doses of 0.1 to 0.3 mmol/kg, with that for Gd DTPA being just 0.1 mmol/kg. For linear chelates, such as Gd DTPA and Gd DTPA-BMA, the degree to which release of free gadolinium ion occurs is an issue due to lower in vivo stability.[54,55]

Patient studies with Gd HP-DO3A have evaluated the entire dose range of 0.1 to 0.3 mmol/kg in the liver.[56] In the author's experience, high dose has been more effective, with 5 of 7 patients in one trial demonstrating improved lesion detection at 0.3 mmol/kg, a result not seen at 0.1 mmol/kg.[57] Post-contrast scans at 0.1 mmol/kg using Gd HP-DO3A should be comparable to that using Gd DTPA, with the two agents sharing similar relaxation and distribution profiles. The reported frequency of adverse clinical reactions is similar, not a surprising result.[58] High dose has also been evaluated in animal models of liver disease. In an abscess model,

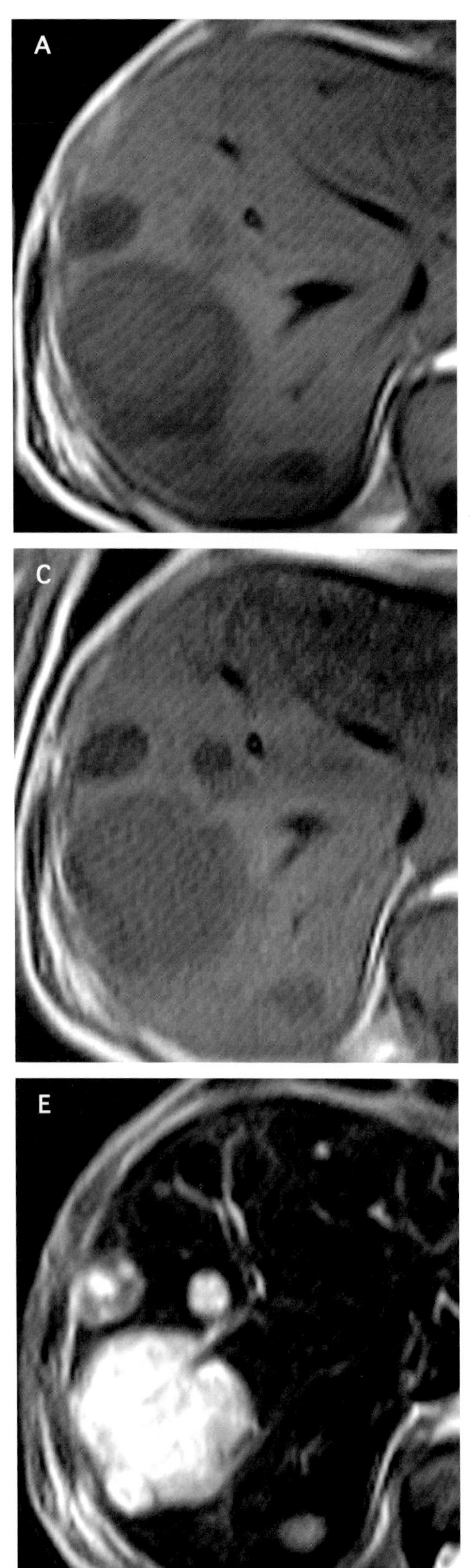

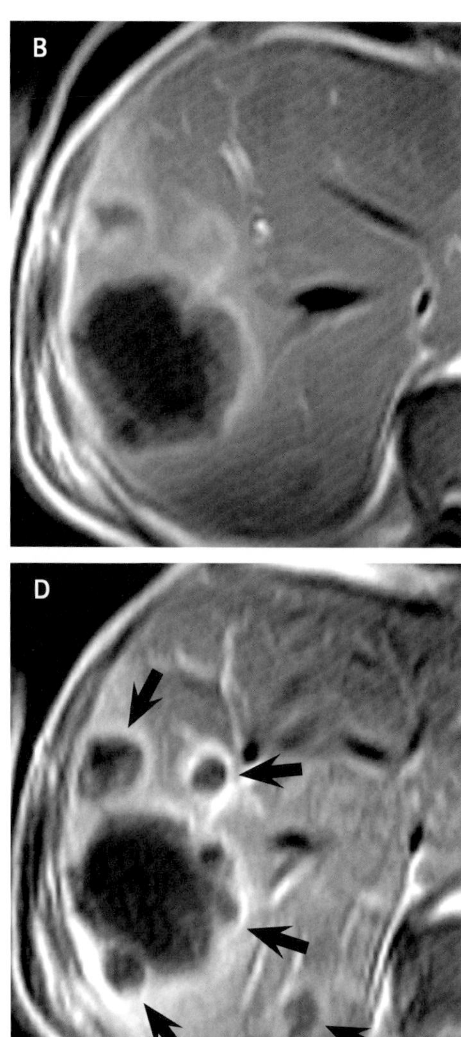

Figure 5. Metastases to the liver from lung carcinoma. (A, B) Pre- and post-contrast T1-weighted, (C, D) pre- and dynamic post-contrast breathhold T1-weighted, and (E) pre-contrast T2-weighted scans are presented. A contrast dose of 0.3 mmol/kg gadoteridol was employed. Respiratory artifacts degrade the non-breathhold T1-weighted scans. Motion during the long acquisition time, in addition to the delay following contrast administration, accounts for the poor visualization of several lesions (B) post-contrast. At least five metastatic lesions (arrows) are well seen on (D) the breathhold high dose post-contrast scan. Although the lesions can be identified on the T2-weighted scan, the contrast between the lesions and normal liver is lower than on the breathhold post-gadoteridol scan. The scan times differ as well by almost two orders of magnitude. *(From Runge VM, Kirsch JE, Wells JW, et al. Enhanced liver MR: contrast agents and imaging strategy. Critical Reviews in Diagnostic Imaging 1993;34:1-30).*

0.5 mmol/kg proved superior to both 0.25 and 0.1 mmol/kg for lesion detectability, as assessed by signal intensity measurements and film readers blinded to scan technique.[59] Recent results with a model of liver metastatic disease have been similar — favoring high dose, although in this experimentation 0.3 mmol/kg was compared with 0.1 mmol/kg.

Arterial portography with MR using extracellular gadolinium chelates has also been shown to be of value for improving liver lesion conspicuity.[60] In the spleen, dynamic scans following intravenous contrast injection provide greater lesion conspicuity than conventional Tl- and T2-weighted scans alone.[61]

As previously noted, an alternative approach to rapid imaging following gadolinium chelate injection is the use of magnetic iron oxide particles.[62,63,64] These preparations are injected intravenously and are taken up by the reticuloendothelial system. The iron particles have a large magnetic susceptibility effect, which leads to a substantial reduction in the T2 of tissues in which they accumulate. Severe hypotension was encountered in initial clinical trials, leading to reformulation and development of alternative agents. Gradient echo scans have increased sensitivity to the effects of iron particles, allowing a reduction in dose. Manganese DPDP has also been evaluated as a hepatobiliary agent, with improved tumor to liver contrast and visualization of focal lesions demonstrated in certain cases.[65] However, much greater enthusiasm has been voiced for future clinical application of hepatobiliary gadolinium chelates, such as Gd BOPTA, as opposed to particulate agents or manganese chelates.

Bowel

The need to opacity the bowel has been evident since the very first studies with abdominal MR. Numerous agents have been proposed, with many evaluated in volunteers and patients.[66] Both positive agents (which increase the signal intensity of the bowel contents) and negative agents (which decrease the signal intensity of the bowel contents) have been tested. Positive agents include oils[67] and fats, as well as paramagnetic metals such as iron salts (specifically Geritol) and gadolinium chelates.[68] Negative agents include gas or air, perfluorocarbons,[69] and magnetic iron oxide particles.[70,71,72] With both the gas preparations and the perfluorocarbons, the lack of mobile protons results in an absence of signal intensity. With magnetic iron oxide particles, the reduction in T2 is the cause of the loss of signal intensity of bowel contents. Although a perfluorocarbon preparation was made commercially available in the last few years, its use did not gain widespread acceptance due to side effects and poor bowel opacification.

Positive agents suffer from artifacts caused by bowel motion. The high signal intensity of the bowel contents, with peristalsis, causes ghosting across the image in the phase encoding direction. Such motion artifacts are either minimized or absent with the use of negative agents. The bowel wall itself, however, is often best visualized following administration of a positive agent. This is provided that peristalsis is minimized by the use of glucagon. Due to susceptibility effects, nearby tissues and lesions adjacent to the bowel may be poorly visualized following oral administration of iron oxide particles. Difficulty has also been encountered in obtaining simultaneous opacification of the small and large bowel. Reported side effects with gadopentetate dimeglumine (formulated specifically for oral use) and magnetic iron oxide particles are few.

Kidney

In renal imaging, contrast media can be used both to assess the functional status of the kidney (figure 6) and to improve the diagnosis of structural lesions (figure 7). The advent of fast scans, whether gradient echo or echo-planar in type, has permitted improved assessment of renal function following contrast administration.[73,74] Within ten to twenty seconds following bolus IV contrast administration (using a gadolinium chelate), enhancement of renal tissue is noted. Maximum enhancement is reached within a minute, followed by a slow gradual fall in signal intensity. The fall in signal intensity is principally due to excretion. The enhancement of the renal medulla is delayed by 10 to 20 seconds as compared to the cortex.

Gadolinium chelates are concentrated in the urine, due to reabsorption of water. As these contrast agents pass into the calyces, T2 shortening effects dominate (due to the high concentration of the agent), producing a loss in signal intensity. Thus low signal intensity within the calyces, renal pelves, and bladder is a common observation on T1-weighted scans following contrast administration. A layering effect can also be seen in the bladder on the basis of gravitational effects, with hyperintensity anteriorly (due to a lower concentration of the contrast agent) and hypointensity posteriorly (due to a higher concentration).

From dynamic scans, using region of interest analysis, the signal intensity of renal cortex and medulla can be plotted versus time. This analysis is of clinical use in the evaluation of renal function. In acute urinary obstruction, the enhancement of renal cortex is similar to that of normal patients. However, the enhancement of renal medulla is delayed and greater than normal. In chronic obstruction, cortical enhancement is less than normal, with medullary enhancement diminished or absent. Good correlation exists between enhanced MR and nuclear medicine studies.

On pre-contrast scans, renal masses may be isointense with surrounding normal tissue. In this situation, diagnosis

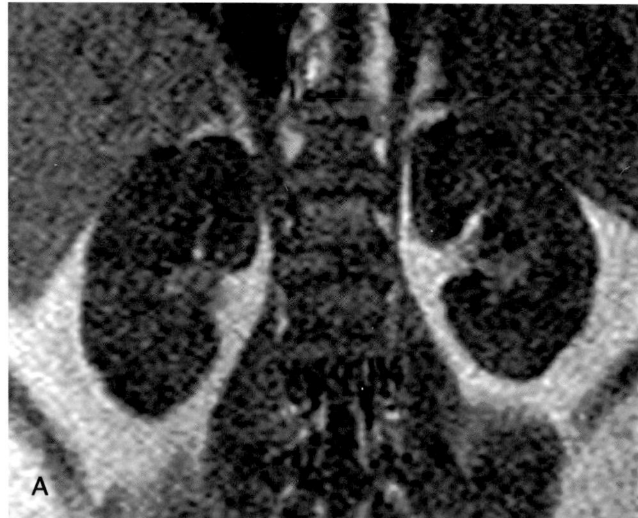

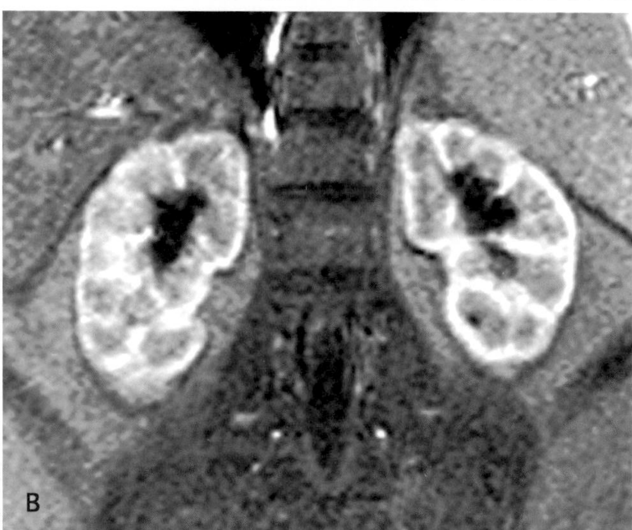

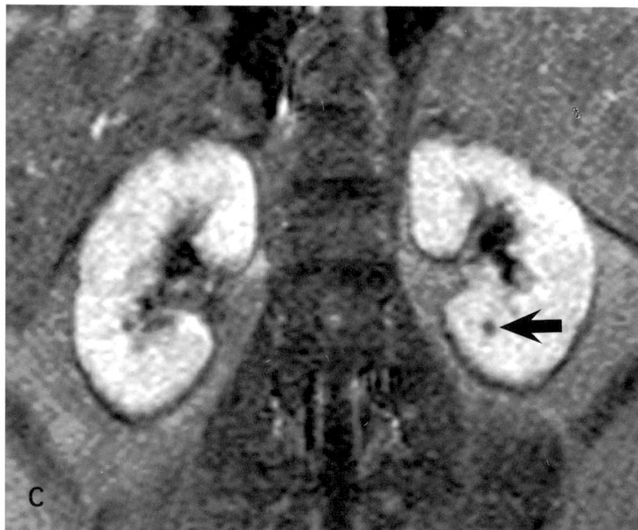

Figure 6. Dynamic renal imaging. Coronal (A) pre-contrast and (B, C) early dynamic post-contrast gradient echo breathhold scans are presented of the upper abdomen. (B) At one minute following bolus contrast injection, prominent enhancement of the renal cortex leads to improved corticomedullary differentiation. (C) By two minutes following contrast injection, sufficient enhancement of the medulla has occurred to render the cortex and medulla isointense. A small simple renal cyst (arrow) is well identified in the lower pole of the left kidney on the dynamic contrast enhanced scans.

can be made only by anatomic deformation or following contrast administration. With extracellular gadolinium chelates, few renal masses enhance on early scans. Thus, definition of lesions is typically improved post-contrast. Lesions appear hypointense relative to the normal surrounding renal parenchyma (which displays marked enhancement). The use of fat saturation techniques is also valuable in the evaluation of renal and extra-renal masses, in combination with contrast use.[75]

Adrenal Glands

Adrenal masses are relatively common, with most being benign adenomas. The adrenal glands are also a preferred site for blood borne metastatic disease, with MR reasonably successful in differential diagnosis.[76,77,78] In regard to contrast use, dynamic imaging improves lesion differentiation.[79] Enhancement of the normal adrenal gland is seen within the first minute following IV bolus contrast injection. Enhancement peaks by two to three minutes, followed by a gradual reduction in signal intensity due to washout of the agent. Adenomas demonstrate moderate enhancement, with malignant lesions displaying greater enhancement, followed by slower washout. With malignant lesions, enhancement can persist for ten to fifteen minutes. On T2-weighted images alone, the accuracy in differentiation of benign and malignant adrenal masses is about 70%. By using contrast enhanced MR in equivocal cases, the accuracy in differential diagnosis can be improved to about 90%.

Pelvis

Magnetic resonance is employed in many centers as a primary imaging modality for the staging of endometrial, cer-

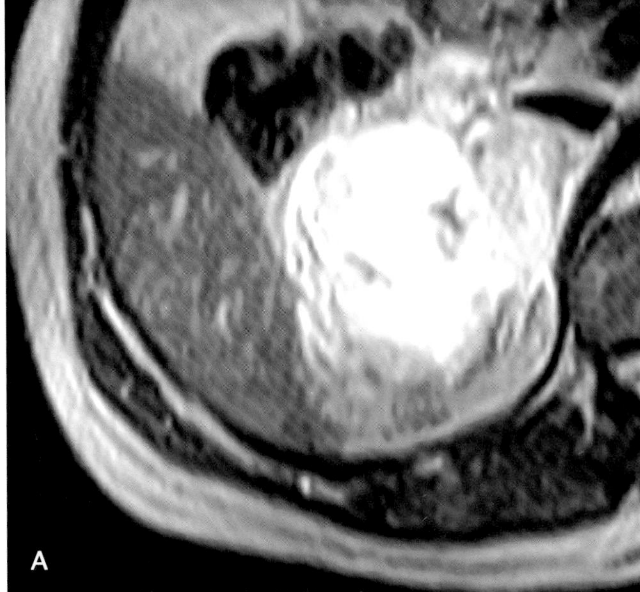

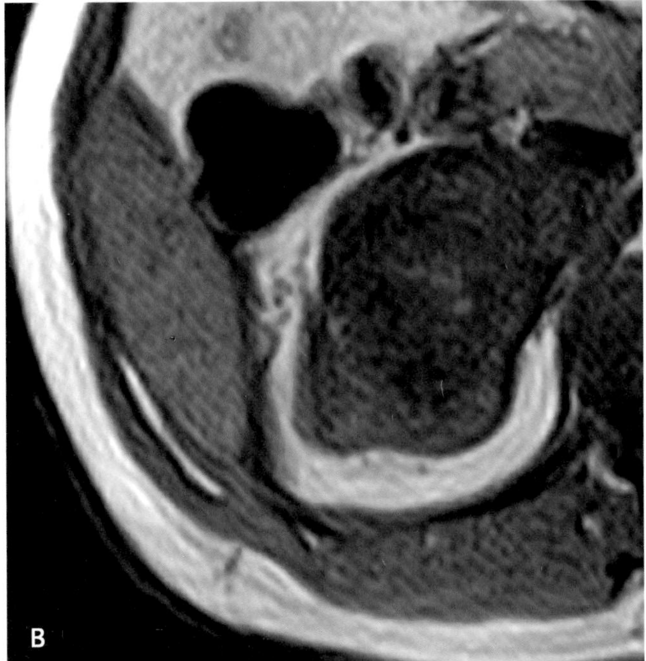

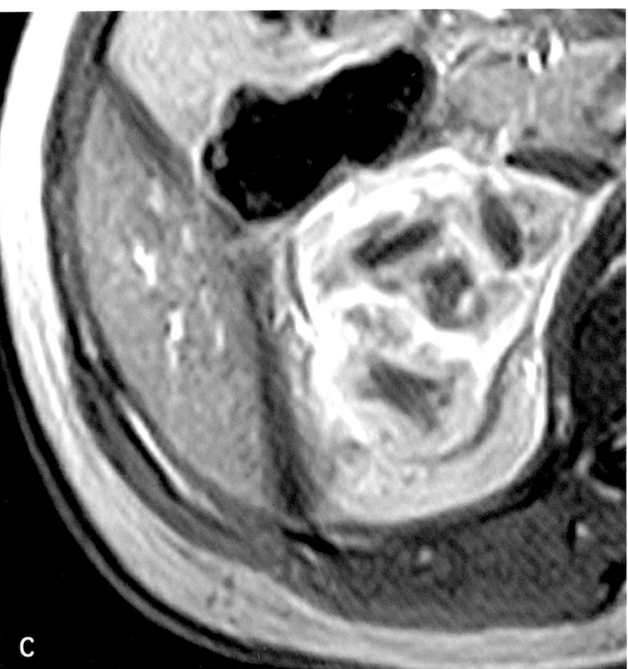

Figure 7. Renal cell carcinoma. On (A) the T2-weighted scan, a high signal intensity mass, measuring seven centimeters in diameter, is noted to occupy almost the entire superior pole of the right kidney. The lesion is slightly lower in signal intensity as compared to normal renal tissue, seen posteriorly, on (B) the pre-contrast T1-weighted scan. (C) Following contrast administration, the mass enhances in an inhomogeneous pattern. Several regions within the mass do not enhance, suggesting necrosis. Although dynamic scans were not acquired in this instance, contrast administration improves the demarcation of tumor from normal renal tissue.

vical, and vaginal carcinoma.[80] In this patient population, the administration of a gadolinium chelate improves tissue differentiation. Although T2-weighted scans can be used to demonstrate zonal anatomy, this is also well shown on post-contrast T1-weighted scans. The mucosa and endometrium enhance post-contrast. The junctional zone remains low signal intensity, due to the smaller extracellular space. The normal paracervical tissue and mucosal surface enhance, whereas cervical tissue remains low intensity. The mucosal surface of the vagina shows marked contrast enhancement. Normal ovarian tissue enhances, however cysts do not.

Leiomyomas demonstrates two patterns of enhancement. Nondegenerate lesions usually do not enhance, whereas degenerate or vascular lesions demonstrate varying degrees of enhancement.[81,82,83] Endometrial carcinoma demonstrates a similar degree of enhancement as compared to normal myometrium, but less than that of the endometrium. Contrast administration improves the distinction between viable tumor and necrotic tissue, as well as between tumor and residual secretions in the endometrial cavity. In regard to the assessment of tumor invasion, fat-saturation techniques may prove valuable in combination with contrast enhancement.

Staging of cervical carcinoma includes the assessment of parametrial, pelvic side wall, para-aortic lymph node, and uterine body involvement. On T2-weighted images, cervical cancer demonstrates abnormal high signal intensity that can be distinguished from the normal low signal intensity of the cervical stroma. Tl-weighted images provide good differentiation between pelvic tissues and cervical tumor. The use of intravenous contrast on MR has not been shown to improve diagnostic accuracy. Tumor heterogeneity is however better demonstrated following contrast administration.

In primary bladder tumors, contrast administration can improve the differentiation between the lesion and adjacent blood clot. However, on images without fat saturation, the ability to identify perivesical tumor extension, lymph node involvement, and bony metastases is reduced post-contrast.[84,85] The signal intensity from the bladder contents is variable post-contrast. Layering is frequently observed, with the signal intensity dependent upon concentration. Flow effects may be seen, especially involving the ureteric orifices.

Enhancement of most primary bladder tumors is heterogeneous. No relation to tumor histology has been noted. Intravesical clot does not enhance, a finding previously noted to be useful in differentiation from adjacent tumor. Recurrent and residual tumor typically show enhancement following contrast administration. However, enhancement can be seen in both normal and abnormal bladder walls. Enhancement of the mucosal lining can also occur following chemotherapy, radiation therapy, and instrumentation.

Musculoskeletal System

MR has become the preferred modality for the imaging evaluation of musculoskeletal tumors.[86] In specific clinical situations, contrast enhancement proves useful. In particular, contrast administration improves the differentiation of recurrent tumor from postoperative change. Value is also ascribed to the assessment of tumor vascularity and the identification of necrotic and cystic areas on post-contrast scans. This information can prove valuable in planning biopsy.

With musculoskeletal tumors, signal heterogeneity on pre- and post-contrast scans, as well as the presence of extensive edema, favor malignancy. Homogeneous enhancement is more common in benign lesions.

As in other areas of the body, contrast administration aids in the differentiation of viable from necrotic tumor (figure 8). Most malignant lesions exhibit a rapid increase in enhancement following bolus contrast injection. Benign tumors demonstrate slower uptake. Nerve sheath tumors have homogeneous enhancement, unless recurrent (figure 9).[87] This feature can aid differentiation from normal tissues and other pathologic processes. Differentiation between benign and malignant lesions on the basis of temporal enhancement is however difficult, since necrotic malignant lesions may also show slow uptake of contrast. Similar findings can be seen following radiation therapy.[88,89] In tumors that respond to therapy, enhancement is generally reduced. Contrast administration is of substantial value in identifying tumor recurrence.

Conclusion

From a practical perspective, intravenous contrast use in body MR is limited to the application of gadolinium chelates. Although magnetic iron oxide particles have been extensively evaluated in clinical trials, these have not yet achieved approval by the US Food and Drug Administration (FDA). Concerns also remain for the magnetic iron oxide particles regarding side effects and practical utility. In regard to oral contrast agents, although many are currently available, clinical use is still limited. The advent of fast imaging techniques and fat suppression has markedly improved the utility of body MR, aiding as well contrast application. The extracellular distribution of the gadolinium chelates places a premium on dynamic studies. Scans acquired in the early time period following contrast administration often add clinically significant information regarding diagnosis. Static post-contrast scans, as routinely acquired in the study of the central nervous system, are of lower utility in many instances.

In body applications, MR is noted for its high intrinsic tissue contrast. The application of intravenous contrast is often of most value in specific clinical problems. These include the identification of tumor necrosis, the differentiation between benign and malignant lesions, and the detection of recurrent tumor. Initial studies focused on tumor detection and differential diagnosis, with wider investigation and application in recent years.

Portions of this chapter are reprinted with permission from Runge VM, Pels Rijcken TH, Davidoff A, Wells JW, Stark DD. Contrast enhanced MR imaging of the liver. *J Magn Reson Imaging* 1994;4:281-289.

References

1. Hamm B, Laniado M, Saini S. Contrast enhanced magnetic resonance imaging of the abdomen and pelvis. Magn Reson Q 1990; 6:108-135.

2. Bloem JL, Reiser MF, Vanel D. Magnetic resonance contrast agents in the evaluation of the musculoskeletal system. Magn Reson Q 1990;6:136-163.

3. Saini S, Modic MT, Hamm B, Hahn PF. Advances in contrast enhanced MR imaging. AJR 1991;156:235-254.

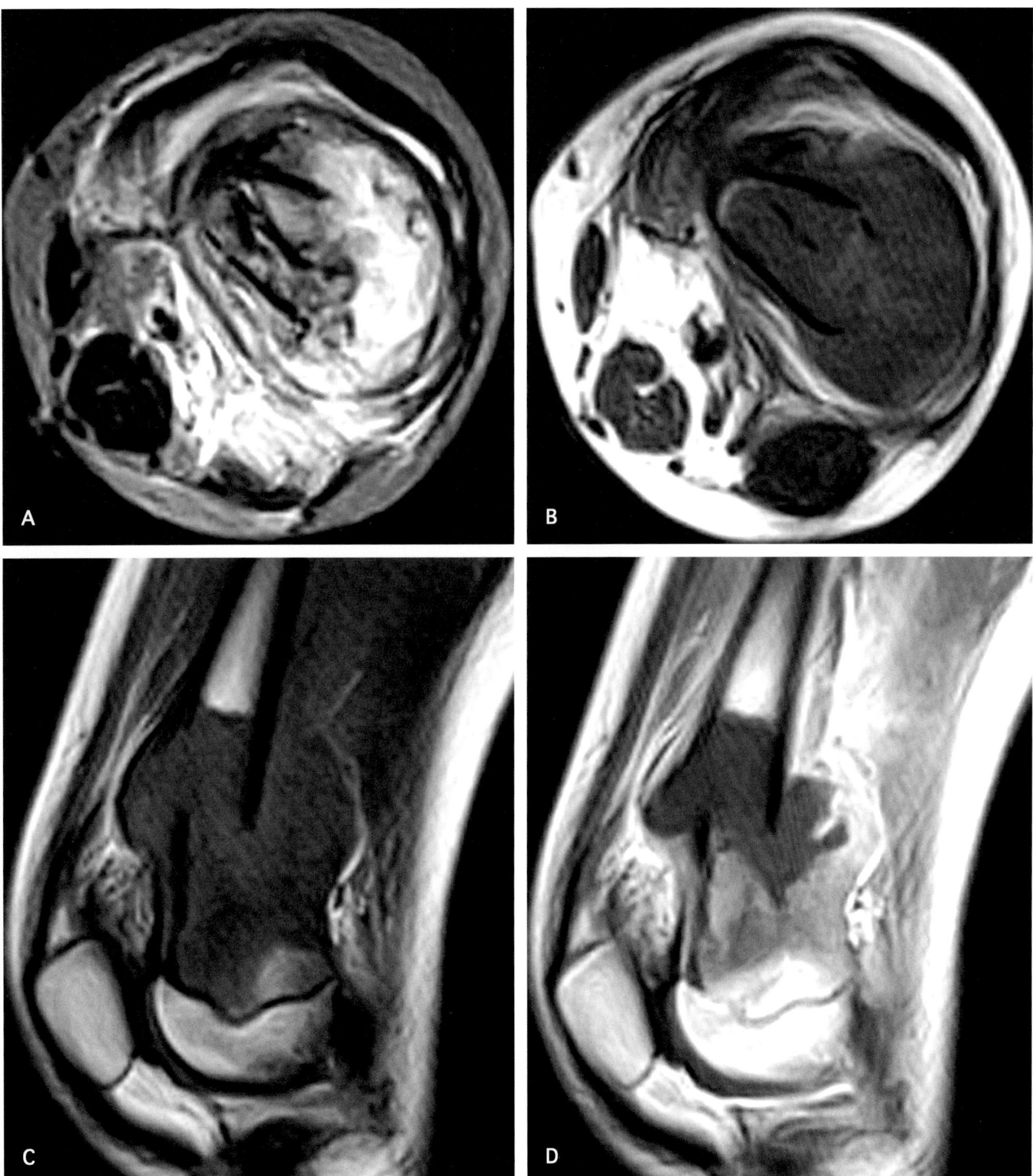

Figure 8. Osteosarcoma. On (A) the axial T2-weighted scan through the distal left femur, a high signal intensity mass involving the marrow space and extending into soft tissue is noted. High signal intensity in adjacent normal muscles is consistent with edema. The involvement of marrow, cortical breakthrough, and extension into adjacent tissue is better visualized on (B) the axial T1-weighted scan. (C) A sagittal pre-contrast T1-weighted scan reveals the mass to involve both the distal metaphysis and diaphysis. The epiphysis is not involved. A pathologic fracture is also identified. (D) Following contrast administration, much of the mass enhances, although the more proximal portion does not. Enhancement of adjacent musculature reflects edematous changes, as opposed to tumor infiltration. In selected cases, contrast enhanced MR can be used to direct biopsy, identifying a vascular, presumed viable portion of the tumor, and avoiding cystic or necrotic areas.

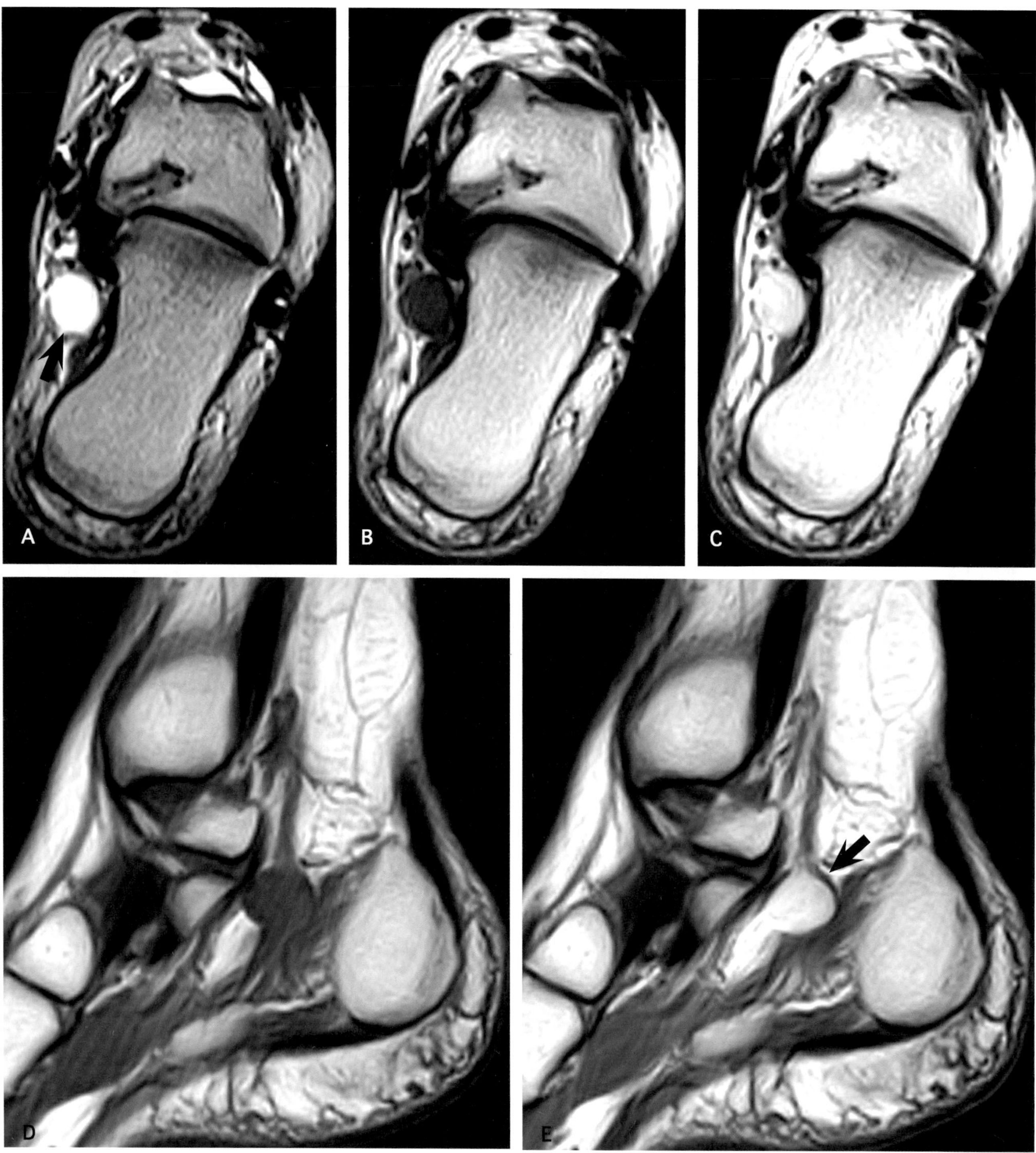

Figure 9. Schwannoma of the left tibial nerve. (A) Axial T2-weighted, (B, C) axial pre- and post-contrast T1-weighted, and (D, E) sagittal pre- and post-contrast T1-weighted scans are presented. A round, well-demarcated soft tissue lesion is noted medial to the calcaneus. The mass (arrow, A) demonstrates homogeneous high signal intensity on the T2-weighted scan and intermediate signal intensity, isointense with muscle, on the pre-contrast T1-weighted scan. Following contrast administration, there is moderate homogeneous enhancement of the mass. On the sagittal images, the lesion (arrow, E) is noted to be contiguous with the tibial nerve as it descends between the medial malleolus and heel.

4. Simon JH, Szumowski J. Chemical shift imaging with paramagnetic contrast enhancement for improved lesion depiction. Radiology 1989;171:539-543.
5. Hasso AN, Brown KD. Use of gadolinium chelates in MR imaging of lesions of the extracranial head and neck. J Magn Reson Imaging 1993 Jan-Feb;3(1):247-263.
6. Crawford SC, Harnsberger HR, Lufkin RB, Hanafee WN. The role of gadolinium-DTPA in the evaluation of extracranial head and neck mass lesions. Radiol Clin North Am 1989;27:219-242.
7. Hudgins PA, Gussack GS. MR imaging in the management of extracranial malignant tumors of the head and neck. AJR 1992; 159:161-169.
8. Hudgins PA. Contrast enhancement in head and neck imaging. Neuroimaging Clin N Am 1994 Feb;4(1):101-115.
9. Hasso AN. Infratentorial neoplasms, including the internal auditory canal and cerebellopontine angle regions. Top Magn Reson Imaging 1989:1:37-51.
10. Hasso AN, Smith DS. The cerebellopontine angle. Semin Ultrasound CT MR 1989;10:280-301.
11. Daniels DD, Czervionke LF, Millen SJ, et al. MR imaging of facial nerve enhancement in Bell's palsy or after temporal bone surgery. Radiology 1989;171:807-809.
12. Han MH, Jabour BA, Andrews JC, et al. Nonneoplastic enhancing lesions mimicking intracanalicular acoustic neuroma on gadolinium-enhanced MR images. Radiology 1991;179:795-796.
13. Dillon WP, Mills CM, Kjos B, et al. Magnetic resonance imaging of the nasopharynx. Radiology 1984;152:731-738.
14. Vogl T, Dresel S, Bilaniuk LT, et al. Tumors of the nasopharynx and adjacent areas: MR imaging with Gd-DTPA. AJR 1990; 154:585-592.
15. Laine FJ, Nadel L, Braun IF. CT and MR imaging of the central skull base. RadioGraphics 1990;10:797-821.
16. Ginsberg LE. Neoplastic disease affecting the central skull base: CT and MR Imaging. AJR 1992;159:581-589.
17. Olsen WL, Dillon WP, Kelly WM, et al. MR imaging of paragangliomas. AJR 1987;148:201-204.
18. Vogl T, Brüning R, Schedel H, et al. Paragangliomas of the jugular bulb and carotid body: MR imaging with short sequences and Gd-DTPA enhancement. AJR 1989;153:583-587.
19. Vogl TJ, Mack MG, Juergens M, Stark M, Deimling M, Knobber W, Grevers G, Felix R. Fat suppression in contrast-enhanced MRT of the base of the skull and of the head-neck area: its clinical value. Rofo 1994 May;160(5):417-424.
20. Pollei SR, Harnsberger HR. The radiologic evaluation of the parotid space. Semin Ultrasound CT MR 1990;11:486-503.
21. Laine FJ, Braun IF, Jensen ME, et al. Perineural tumor extension through the foramen ovale: evaluation with MR imaging. Radiology 1990;174:65-71.
22. Parker GD, Harnsberger HR. Clinical-radiologic issues in perineural tumor spread of malignant disease of the extracranial head and neck. RadioGraphics 1991;11:383-399.
23. Glazer GM, Gross BH, Aisen AM, et al. Imaging of the pulmonary hilum: a prospective study in patients with lung cancer. AJR 1985;145:245-248.
24. Grenier P, Dubray B, Corette MI, et al. Pre-operative thoracic staging of lung cancer. Diagn Intervent Radiol 1988;1:23-28.
25. Webb WR, Gatsonis C, Zerhouni EA, et al. CT and MR imaging in staging non-small cell bronchogenic carcinoma: report of the Radiologic Diagnostic Oncology Group. Radiology 1991;178:705-713.
26. Nishimura T, Kobayashi H, Okora Y, et al. General assessment of myocardial infarction by using gated MR imaging and gadopentetate dimeglumine. AJR 1989;153:715-720.
27. Eichstaedt HW, Felix R, Dougherty FC, et al. Magnetic resonance imaging (MRI) in different stages of myocardial infarction using the contrast agent gadolinium-DTPA. Clin Cardiol 1986; 9:527-535.
28. Postenia S, de Roos A, Doornbos J, et al. Acute myocardial infarction: detection and localisation by magnetic resonance imaging and thallium. J Med Imaging 1989;3:68-74.
29. De Roos A, van Roosin AC, van der Wall EE, et al. Reperfused and non-reperfused myocardial infarction: value of gadolinium DTPA enhanced MR imaging. Radiology 1989;172:717-720.
30. Van der Wall EE, van Dykman PRM, de Roos A, et al. Diagnostic significance of gadolinium-DTPA enhanced magnetic resonance imaging on thrombolytic treatment for acute myocardial infarction: its potential in assessing reperfusion. Br Heart J 1990,63:12-17.
31. De Roos A, Matheijssen NAA, Doornbos J, et al. Myocardial infarct size after reperfusion therapy: assessment with gadopentetate dimegiumine enhanced MR imaging. Radiology 1990;176:517-521.
32. Heywang SH, Hahn D, Schmidt H, et al. MR imaging of the breast using gadopentetate dimeglumine. J Comput Assist Tomogr 1986;10:199-204.
33. Heywang-Kobrunner SH. Contrast enhanced MRI of the breast. Munich: SH Karger, 1990.
34. Weinmann HJ, Brasch RC, Press WR, Wesbey GE. Characteristics of gadolinium DTPA complex: a potential NMR contrast agent. AJR 1984;142:619-624.
35. Hamm B, Wolf KJ, Felix R. Conventional and rapid MR imaging of the liver with Gd DTPA. Radiology 1987;164:313-320.
36. Neindorf HP, Haustein J, Cornelius I, et al. Safety of gadolinium DTPA: extended clinical experience. Magn Reson Med 1991; 22:222-228.
37. Carr DH, Brown J, Bydder GM, et al. Gadolinium DTPA as a contrast agent in MRI: initial clinical experience in 20 patients. AJR 1984;143:215-224.
38. Mano I, Yoshida H, Nakabayaski K, et al. Fast spin echo imaging with suspended respiration: gadolinium enhanced MR imaging of liver tumors. J Comput Assist Tomo 1987;11:73-80.
39. Mirowitz SA, Lee JKT, Brown JJ, et al. Rapid acquisition spin echo (RASE) MR imaging: a new technique for reduction of artifacts and acquisition time. Radiology 1990;175:131-135.
40. Chien D, Atkinson DJ, Edelman RR. Strategies to improve contrast in TurboFLASH imaging: reordered phase encoding and k-space segmentation. JMRI 1991;1:63-70.
41. Saini S, Stark DD, Rzedzian RR, et al. Forty-millisecond MR imaging of the abdomen at 2.0 T. Radiology 1989;173:111-116.
42. Hamm B, Wolf KJ, Felix R. Conventional and rapid MRI of the liver with gadolinium-DTPA. Radiology 1987;164:313-320.
43. Hamm B, Fisher E, Taupite M. Differential of hepatic hemangioma from hepatic metastases by using dynamic contrast enhanced MR imaging. J Comput Assist Tomogr 1990;14:205-216.
44. Freeny PC, Marks WM, Ryan JA, Bolen JW. Colorectal carcinoma evaluation with CT: preoperative staging and detection of post-operative recurrence. Radiology 1986;158:347-353.
45. Barakos J, Goldberg H, Brown JJ, et al. Comparison of com-

puted tomography and magnetic resonance imaging in the evaluation of focal hepatic lesions. Gastrointest Radiol 1990;15:93-101.
46. Chezmar JL, Rumancik WM, Megibow AJ, et al. Liver and abdominal screening in patients with cancer: CT versus MR imaging. Radiology 1988;168:43-47.
47. Edelman RR, Siegel JB, Singer A, et al. Dynamic MR imaging of the liver with Gd DTPA: initial clinical results. AJR 1989; 153:1213-1219.
48. Rummeny E, Saini S, Wittenberg J, et al. MR imaging of liver neoplasms. AJR 1989;152:493-499.
49. Ohtomo K, Itai Y, Yoshikawa K, et al. Hepatic tumors: dynamic MR imaging. Radiology 1987;163:27-31.
50. Stark DD, Felder RC, Wittenberg J, et al. Magnetic resonance imaging of cavernous hemangioma of the liver: tissue specific characterization. AJR 1985;145:213-220.
51. Brick SH, Hill MC, Lande IM. The mistaken or indeterminate CT: diagnosis of hepatic metastases: the value of sonography. AJR 1987;148:723-726.
52. Rummeny E, Weissleder R, Sironi S, et al. Central scars in primary liver tumors: MR features, specificity, and pathologic correlation. Radiology 1989;177:323-326.
53. Yoshida H, Itai Y, Ohtomo K, et al. Small hepatocellular carcinoma and hemangioma: differentiation with dynamic FLASH MR imaging with gadopentetate dimeglumine. Radiology 1989; 171:339-342.
54. Wedeking P, Kumar K, Tweedle MF. Dissociation of gadolinium chelates in mice: relationship to chemical characteristics. MRI 1992;10:641-648.
55. Tweedle MF. Physicochemical properties of gadoteridol and other magnetic resonance contrast agents. Invest Rad 1992;27:S2-6.
56. Seltzer SE, Hamm B. Evaluation of gadoteridol for MR imaging of the liver. Radiology 1993;189(P):202.
57. Runge VM, Kirsch JE, Wells JW, et al. Enhanced liver MR: contrast agents and imaging strategy. Critical Reviews in Diagnostic Imaging 1993;34:1-30.
58. Runge VM, Bradley WG, Brant-Zawadzki MN, et al. Clinical safety and efficacy of gadoteridol: a study in 411 patients with suspected intracranial and spinal disease. Radiology 1991;181:701-709.
59. Runge VM, Kirsch JE, Thomas GS. High dose applications of gadolinium chelates in magnetic resonance imaging. Magn Reson Med 1991;22:358-363.
60. Pavone P, Giuliani S, Cardone G, et al. Intraarterial portography with gadopentetate dimeglumine: improved liver-to-lesion contrast in MR imaging. Radiology 1991;179:693-697.
61. Mirowitz SA, Brown JJ, Lee JKT, Heiken JP. Dynamic gadolinium enhanced MRI of the spleen: normal enhancement patterns and evaluation of splenic lesions. Radiology 1991;179:681-686.
62. Stark DD, Weissleder R, Elizondo G, et al. Superparamagnetic iron oxide: clinical application as a contrast agent for MR imaging of the liver. Radiology 1988;168:297-301.
63. Weissleder R, Stark DD, Rummeny EJ, et al. Splenic lymphoma: ferrite enhanced MR imaging in rats. Radiology 1988;166:423-430.
64. Hahn PF, Stark DD, Saini S, et al. Clinical trials of a superparamagnetic iron oxide gastrointestinal agent. Radiology 1990;175:695-700.
65. Lim KO, Stark DD, Leese PT, et al. Hepatobiliary MR imaging: first human experience with Mn DPDP. Radiology 1991;178: 79-82.
66. Tart RP, Li KC, Storm BL, Rolfes RJ, Ang PG. Enteric MRI contrast agents: comparative study of five potential agents in humans. Magn Reson Imaging 1991;9(4):559-568.
67. Li KC, Ang PG, Tart RP, Storm BL, Rolfes R, Ho-Tai PC. Paramagnetic oil emulsions as oral magnetic resonance imaging contrast agents. Magn Reson Imaging 1990;8(5):589-598.
68. Laniado M, Kornmesser W, Hamm B, et al. MR imaging of the gastrointestinal tract: value of Gd DTPA. AJR 1988;150:817-821.
69. Mattrey RF, Hajeck PC, Gylys-Morin VM, et al. Perfluorochemicals as gastrointestinal agents for MR imaging. AJR 1987;148:1259-1263.
70. Hahn PF, Stark DD, Saini S, et al. Ferrite particles for bowel contrast in MR imaging: design issues and feasibility studies. Radiology 1987;164:37-40.
71. Lönnemark M, Hemmingsson A, Carlsten J, et al. Superparamagnetic particles as an MRI contrast agent for the gastrointestinal tract. Acta Radiol 1988;29:599-602.
72. Lönnemark M, Hemmingsson A, Ericsson A, et al. The effect of oral superparamagnetic particles in plain and viscous aqueous suspensions. Acta Radiol 1990;29:303-307.
73. Choyke PL, Frank JA, Girton ME, et al. Dynamic gadolinium DTPA enhanced MRI of the kidneys: a physiologic correlation. Radiology 1989;170:713-720.
74. Patel SK, Stock CM, Turner DA. Magnetic resonance imaging in staging of renal cell carcinoma. Radiographics 1987;7:703-728.
75. Semelka RC, Hricak H, Stevens SK, et al. Combined gadolinium-enhanced and fat-saturation MR imaging of renal masses. Radiology 1991;178:803-809.
76. Reinig JW, Doppman JL, Dwyer AJ, et al. Adrenal masses differentiated by MR. Radiology 1986;158:81-84.
77. Chang A, Glazer HS, Lee JKT, et al. Adrenal gland: MR imaging. Radiology 1987;163:123-128.
78. Falke THM, te Strake L, Shaff MI, et al. MR imaging of the adrenals: correlation with computed tomography. J Comput Assist Tomogr 1986;10:242-253.
79. Krestin GP, Steinbrich W, Friedmann G. Adrenal masses: evaluation with fast dynamic gradient echo MR imaging and gadopentetate dimeglumine enhanced dynamic studies. Radiology 1989;171:675-680.
80. Hricak H. Magnetic resonance of the female pelvis: review. AJR 1986;146:1115-1122.
81. Hricak H, Hamm B, Semelka R, et al. Carcinoma of the uterus: use of gadopentetate dimeglumine in MR imaging. Radiology 1991;181:95-106.
82. Mawhinney RR, Powell MC, Worthington BS, et al. Magnetic resonance imaging of benign ovarian masses. Br J Radiol 1988;61:179-186.
83. Chang YCF, Hricak H, Thurnher S, Lacey CG. Vagina: evaluation with MR imaging. Part II. Neoplasms. Radiology 1988;160:431-435.
84. Johnson RJ, Carrington BM, Jenkins JPR, et al. Accuracy in staging carcinoma of the bladder by magnetic resonance imaging. Clin Radiol 1990;41:258-263.
85. Neuerburg JM, Bohndorf K, Sohn M, et al. Urinary bladder neoplasms: evaluation with contrast enhanced MR imaging. Radiology 1989;172:739-743.
86. Kransdorf MJ. The use of gadolinium in the MR evaluation of musculoskeletal tumors. Top Magn Reson Imaging 1996;8(1):15-23.

87. Loke TK, Ma HT, Ward SC, et al. MRI of intraspinal nerve sheath tumours presenting with sciatica. Australas Radiol 1995 Aug;39(3):228-232.
88. Erlemann R, Reiser MF, Peters PE, et al. Musculoskeletal neoplasms: static and dynamic gadopentetate dimeglumine MR imaging. Radiology 1989;171:767-773.
89. Erlemann R, Sciuk J, Bosse A, et al. Response of osteosarcoma and Ewing sarcoma to preoperative chemotherapy: assessment with dynamic and static MR imaging and skeletal scintigraphy. Radiology 1990;175:791-796.

Chapter 6

Safety, New Applications, and New Agents

Val M. Runge, M.D. and John W. Wells, R.T.

Introduction

In just over a decade, magnetic resonance (MR) has become the imaging modality of choice for the study of central nervous system disease. Concurrent development of contrast media, now in widespread use, has aided the rapid expansion of this field and increased clinical efficacy. Magnetic resonance imaging offers high spatial resolution and soft tissue contrast, with a sensitivity to contrast media greater than that of x-ray computed tomography (CT). First pass brain studies now make possible the assessment of regional cerebral blood volume, with high spatial and temporal resolution. New hardware developments, together with advances in contrast media design, continue to drive expansion of contrast media applications, building upon the large base of current clinical use. This chapter discusses safety data concerning the gadolinium chelates in current clinical use, new agents and directions for future development, and new clinical applications.

Design Requirements

Investigation by industry in the field of MR pharmaceuticals began in 1982. Research led to the synthesis and initial evaluation of Gd DTPA. This agent became the first compound to be approved for human use, with clinical application now of this and other related agents world-wide.

Prior to 1982, the relaxation effects of the paramagnetic metals, which include gadolinium, were well known. However, the toxicity of these metals in their ionic form appeared to prevent use in humans. In order to design a safe agent, it was proposed that the metal ion be tightly bound by a chelate, permitting the metal to exhibit its paramagnetic effect yet limiting toxicity by achieving rapid and total renal excretion.[1] The gadolinium ion emerged as the most favorable choice in regard to paramagnetic effect, and specifically enhancement of T1 relaxation.[2]

The clinical safety of a gadolinium chelate is to a large extent dependent upon its stability in vivo. Key factors include thermodynamics, solubility, selectivity, and kinetics. Gadolinium, administered as the free metal ion, is not suitable as a contrast agent due to its toxicity and biodistribution.[3]

Gadolinium Chelates

Indications for contrast media use in the head and spine have been well established through experience in clinical trials world-wide.[4,5,6] Administration of a gadolinium chelate can substantially improve lesion identification and characterization. With conventional spin echo techniques, contrast enhancement occurs on the basis of either blood-brain (or blood-cord) barrier disruption or lesion vascularity, the latter with extraaxial lesions. In this setting, it is the T1 effect of the agent upon surrounding water protons, producing "positive" enhancement, which is observed. At the dose most commonly used in clinical practice today, 0.1 mmol/kg, lesion enhancement on MR with a gadolinium chelate is equivalent to slightly superior to that observed on CT with iodinated agents. However, unlike CT, abnormal contrast enhancement is not obscured by adjacent bone or calcification. On MR, small intra- and extraaxial lesions (for example metastases and meningiomas) can appear isointense on precontrast images, with only the administration of a gadolinium chelate providing lesion recognition. Following therapeutic measures, recurrent disease can also be difficult to diagnose without contrast administration, given the background of associated treatment related tissue change. With perfusion studies, the contrast agent bolus itself is tracked during first pass through the brain. In this instance, it is the T2 and susceptibility effects of the agent, producing "negative" enhancement, which are observed.

In neoplastic disease, MR contrast administration improves visualization of both intra- and extraaxial lesions. Only in the case of metastases confined to the vertebral body is lesion visualization generally not improved, and in this instance may actually decrease. Small metastatic lesions within the central nervous system may not elicit sufficient edema to be recognized on unenhanced scans, mandating contrast administration for detection. Contrast use commonly improves lesion definition, permitting better evaluation of lesion margins and invasion of adjacent structures. Prior to surgery, contrast enhanced scans are valuable for planning lesion resection and defining areas for biopsy. Following surgery, contrast enhanced scans find utility for definition of recurrent tumor.

In infection, MR contrast administration finds utility primarily for lesion characterization and assessment of lesion activity. Acute disease can be differentiated from chronic change, such as gliosis, and disease progression or regression followed. Enhanced MR is particularly superior to enhanced CT for the depiction of meningeal disease. This is primarily due to the lack of beam hardening artifacts, which obscure visualization of tissue adjacent to bone. Active meningeal disease, whether inflammatory or neoplastic in nature, is well visualized with prominent enhancement. This is in distinction to the appearance of the normal falx and meninges, which on MR (unlike CT) do not demonstrate substantial enhancement.

In ischemia, MR contrast administration provides for temporal dating and assists in lesion characterization. Intravascular enhancement is observed in the first week following infarction, with parenchymal enhancement seen thereafter and up to eight weeks. These patterns of enhancement also assist in differential diagnosis. Not all infarcts can be diagnosed as such by their involvement of a characteristic arterial distribution, with intravascular or gyriform enhancement in this instance providing important information for differential diagnosis.

In the spine,[7] the indications for contrast use are quite broad, as in the head. Contrast enhancement is used routinely in the post-operative back, for the differentiation of scar from recurrent or residual disk material.[8] In the first twenty minutes following contrast injection, scar tissue will demonstrate enhancement, due to its vascular nature, while disk material will not. On unenhanced scans, this differentiation may not be possible. Contrast administration also markedly improves the detection of leptomeningeal metastases. Identification of tumor enhancement can aid in the differentiation of a tumor syrinx from a congenital or post-traumatic syrinx.[9] For intrinsic cord lesions, contrast administration also improves differential diagnosis.

In the head and neck, post-contrast images can provide important additional diagnostic information.[10] In a clinical trial using 0.1 mmol/kg Gd HP-DO3A in 122 patient studies, the additional information provided by contrast administration was judged by two blinded readers to likely have contributed to a change in diagnosis in 16%.[11] The additional information available post-contrast consisted principally of improved lesion visualization and definition of lesion margins.

Growing experience with gadolinium chelates has led to extensive discussion of the utility of high dose. This specifically refers to the injection of 0.3 mmol/kg, as compared to 0.1 mmol/kg. The latter dose is that most commonly employed in clinical practice. Whether given as a single dose, or as a supplemental injection, high dose has been shown to improve lesion enhancement over a broad range of pathology. In studying patients with possible metastatic disease to the brain, high dose contrast administration improves lesion detection and is strongly recommended. High dose also allows for the exclusion of abnormalities questioned on the basis of the standard dose post-contrast exam. Furthermore, first pass perfusion studies are improved, if the injection time is kept short, with the use of high dose.[12,13]

Cost concerns have limited high dose trials and clinical acceptance. The use of low dose, less than 0.1 mmol/kg, was advocated by numerous practitioners in the late 1980s and early 1990s, principally for financial reasons. This practice has fortunately been discontinued, with clinical experience demonstrating such scans to be nondiagnostic in many instances. Low contrast doses, such as 0.05 mmol/kg, have been shown to provide inferior tumor-brain contrast, and inadequate lesion delineation.[14]

As requirements for high dose have become more apparent, further research has been pursued to develop new agents with improved tolerance. Increased emphasis has been placed on physicochemical properties, including osmolality, viscosity and stability of the metal chelate in vivo. Agents with lower osmolality and viscosity can be administered faster and generally at higher doses, important features for first pass perfusion studies. Other avenues of research include development of compounds with higher relaxivity. Both approaches seek to lower the toxicity of the agent for a given effective dose. One step in development has paralleled the history of the iodinated agents. Nonionic (neutral) compounds, such as gadoteridol, have been perfected following the initial development of gadopentetate dimeglumine, an ionic (charged) compound.[15]

Gadolinium chelates were developed due to the high relaxivity of the gadolinium ion and relative low toxicity of the complex. With the agents in clinical use in the US, excretion is by glomerular filtration. The clinical safety of these agents is principally dependent upon the stability of the chelate in vivo. Key factors determining safety include thermodynamics, solubility, selectivity, and kinetics.[16,17,18] There

Table 1. Physicochemical properties of the gadolinium chelates

Trade Name	Chemical formula	T1 relaxivity	log K_{eq}	$k(obs')s^{-1}$	Osmolality (Osmol/kg)	Viscosity (cP)
ProHance	Gd HP-DO3A	3.7	23.8	6.3×10^{-5}	0.63	1.3
Magnevist	Gd DTPA	3.8	22.1	1.2×10^{-3}	1.96	2.9
Omniscan	Gd DTPA-BMA	3.8	16.9	$> 2 \times 10^{-2}$	0.65	1.4

must be a high affinity of the chelate for the metal ion, which is reflected by the thermodynamic binding constant of the complex. If the agent is not sufficiently soluble, precipitation of the gadolinium ion can occur, with potential toxicity. The chelate must have high selectivity for the gadolinium ion itself. This requirement is so that metal exchange with endogenous ions, such as zinc and copper, does not occur. And last, but not least, the compound must exhibit slow kinetics in regard to release of the gadolinium ion. This makes possible near complete excretion of the complex in the setting of normal renal function. One way to assess kinetics is by the rate of dissociation of the complex in acid solution. Table 1 presents a comparison of the three agents available in the US on the basis of these and other chemical characteristics. High thermodynamic stability, slow kinetics of dissociation (small $k(obs')s^{-1}$), low osmolality and low viscosity are favorable features.

To date, two basic types of chelates have been developed — linear and macrocyclic. Linear chelates include Gd DTPA and Gd DTPA-BMA. In the US, only one macrocyclic chelate is available, Gd HP-DO3A. In Europe, a second macrocyclic compound, Gd DOTA, is also in use. Both macrocycles exhibit higher thermodynamic and kinetic stability[19,20] leading to lower long term heavy metal (Gd^{3+}) deposition. In any chelate preparation, the addition of a small amount of excess of ligand will also diminish the potential for metal ion substitution.[21]

As a group, the gadolinium chelates have a good overall safety profile in regard to acute toxicity. The majority of adverse events encountered are mild and transient. However, the existence of severe anaphylactoid reactions, although rare, has been documented. Radiologists should be aware of potential complications, with adequate preparation for treatment of a major untoward event.[22]

Gd DTPA

Gadopentetate dimeglumine (Gd DTPA or Magnevist, Berlex Laboratories) was the first extracellular gadolinium chelate to be developed for clinical use (figure 1). It was approved for use in the U.S. by the Food and Drug Administration in 1988.[23] Currently, this approval includes use in adults and pediatrics (greater than 2 years of age), at a single dose of 0.1 mmol/kg. The pharmaceutical preparation contains 0.2% of the excess ligand. There is extensive experience with this agent, as well as with Gd DTPA-BMA and Gd HP-DO3A in the head, neck, and spine.[24,25,26] As with any such agent, caution should be exercised in renally impaired patients. The safety of the agent is dependent to a large extent upon its rapid excretion. Gd DTPA, like Gd DTPA-BMA and Gd HP-DO3A, is cleared by dialysis. Debate continues however on the rate and degree to which the agents are cleared.

Concern has also been raised with regard to the use of Gd DTPA in patients with hemolytic anemia, due to early observations of a transient elevation in serum iron and bilirubin following injection. These laboratory abnormalities are presumably due to the release from the chelate of a small amount of gadolinium ion, which then causes blood hemolysis. In a large early clinical study, 11% of men (34 of 308) had abnormal serum iron levels and 2.9% (11 of 379) had abnormal bilirubin levels at 24 hours following administration of Gd DTPA. In healthy volunteers, when 0.25 mmol/kg Gd DTPA was administered, an elevation in serum iron and total bilirubin could be observed by 3 hours, with a peak in levels between 6 and 12 hours, and return to baseline by 24 hours.[27] The implication of these findings in clinical application is unclear.

The effect of Gd DTPA, as with all the gadolinium chelates, upon the fetus is unknown. Injection during pregnancy is not recommended, except in extenuating clinical circumstances and with informed consent. The agent is known to cross the placenta.[28] Gd DTPA is also excreted in breast milk.[29] It is recommended that breast feeding of infants be discontinued for several days following the injection of contrast in the mother.

As with the other gadolinium chelates with extracellular distribution and renal excretion, there is a 3 to 5% rate of adverse reactions observed following IV administration. The majority are mild, including principally nausea and hives.[30] Caution should be exercised with bolus administration, particularly given the close confines of most MR units. In a large clinical trial of 4,260 patients, with bolus injection of Gd DTPA, emesis was reported in 12.[31] Anaphylactoid like reactions are rare, but have been reported.[32] Administration of the agent in the presence of a physician, or with a physician readily available, is recommended. Also important is proper instruction of personnel and ready availability of equipment for treatment of possible untoward events.

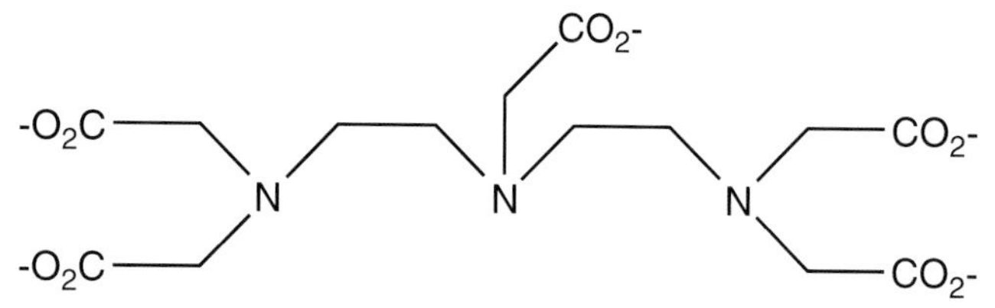

Figure 1. The chemical structure for DTPA (diethylenetriamine-pentaacetic acid), the chelate in gadopentetate dimeglumine (Magnevist).

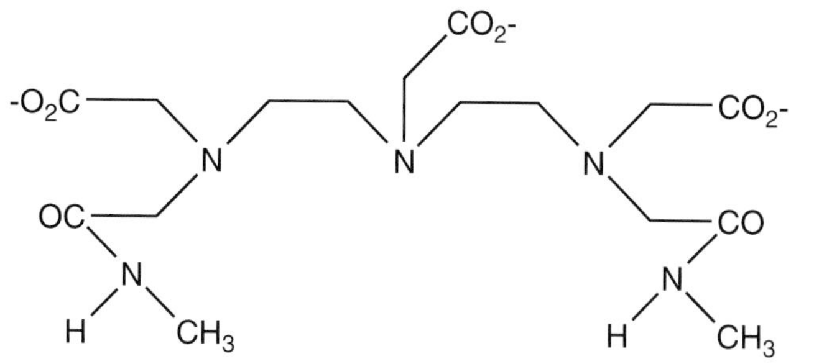

Figure 2. The chemical structure for DTPA-BMA (diethylene-triaminepentaacetic acid bis-methylamide), the chelate in gadodiamide (Omniscan).

Gd DTPA-BMA

Gadodiamide (Gd DTPA-BMA or Omniscan, Sanofi-Winthrop) is a neutral linear chelate which was approved for clinical use in the U.S. in 1993 (figure 2). The ligand, DTPA-BMA, is a derivative of DTPA. Neutrality is achieved by replacement of two anionic donors ($-CO_2^-$) with methylamide (BMA = bis-methylamide). This leads to a substantial decrease in the thermodynamic stability constant for the complex, with log K_{therm} for Gd DTPA-BMA being 16.9 and that for Gd DTPA being 22.5. The pharmaceutical preparation contains 5% of the excess ligand as calcium DTPA-BMA. Questions have been raised concerning acute toxicologic studies in animals and overall product tolerance.[33] A statistically significant change in serum iron has also been reported following administration of Gd DTPA-BMA, as with Gd DTPA.[34]

Transmetallation was investigated in a recent clinical study.[35] Patients were randomized into three groups, comparing Gd DTPA, Gd DTPA-BMA, and Gd HP-DO3A, all at a dose of 0.1 mmol/kg. Patients receiving Gd DTPA-BMA experienced a significant drop in serum zinc following contrast injection. This result was not seen with either Gd DTPA or Gd HP-DO3A. Urine zinc was 26-fold higher in patients receiving Gd DTPA-BMA, as compared to Gd HP-DO3A. These results imply greater gadolinium release in vivo with Gd DTPA-BMA.

No differences in lesion enhancement, at a dose of 0.1 mmol/kg, have been described as compared to Gd DTPA or Gd HP-DO3A. The conclusion from phase II-III trials in 439 patients was that Gd DTPA-BMA is an effective MR contrast agent for imaging of the head and spine.[36] In a study of 73 patients at a dose of 0.1 mmol/kg, abnormalities in serum iron were described in 6 (8%). No abnormalities in total bilirubin were reported.[37] However, post-contrast blood samples were obtained only between 24 and 36 hours following injection. This avoided the early post-contrast time period, during which peak changes due to blood hemolysis would be anticipated. The most common adverse reactions reported are headache, dizziness, and nausea.

Gd HP-DO3A

Gadoteridol (Gd HP-DO3A or ProHance®, Bracco Diagnostics) is a neutral (nonionic) ring chelate which was approved for clinical use in the U.S. in 1992 for a dose range of 0.1 to 0.3 mmol/kg (figure 3). The pharmaceutical preparation contains 0.1% of the excess ligand as calteridol calcium. Due in part to the ring (or macrocyclic) nature of the chelate, Gd HP-DO3A is more stable in vitro and in vivo than either Gd DTPA or Gd DTPA-BMA (figure 4). Gd HP-DO3A is thus relatively inert to metal ion substitution. With regard to potential long term toxicity, on the basis of heavy metal deposition, this agent should be superior.

The effects of contrast media extravasation in soft tissue have been studied in animals.[38] Gd HP-DO3A proved significantly less toxic than Gd DTPA, which caused moderate necrosis, hemorrhage, and edema. The changes noted with Gd DTPA were similar to that seen with a conventional radiographic contrast agent, meglumine diatrizoate.

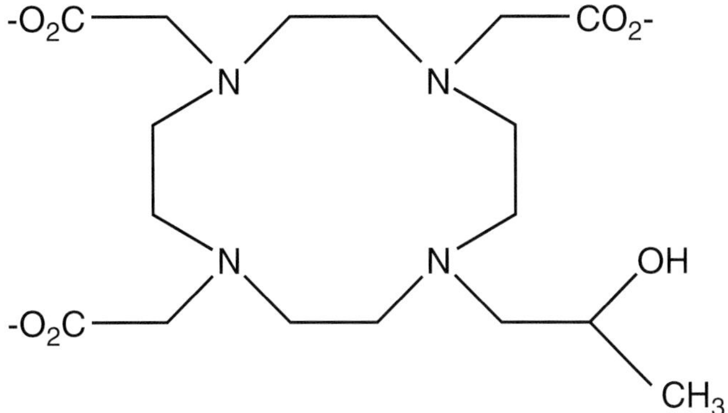

Figure 3. The chemical structure for HP-DO3A (1,4,7-tris(carboxymethyl)-10-2'-hydroxypropyl-1,4,7,10-tetraazacyclododecane), the chelate in gadoteridol (ProHance®). Formulated as the gadolinium (Gd^{3+}) chelate, ProHance® is a nonionic agent (neutral in solution, carrying a net charge of zero).

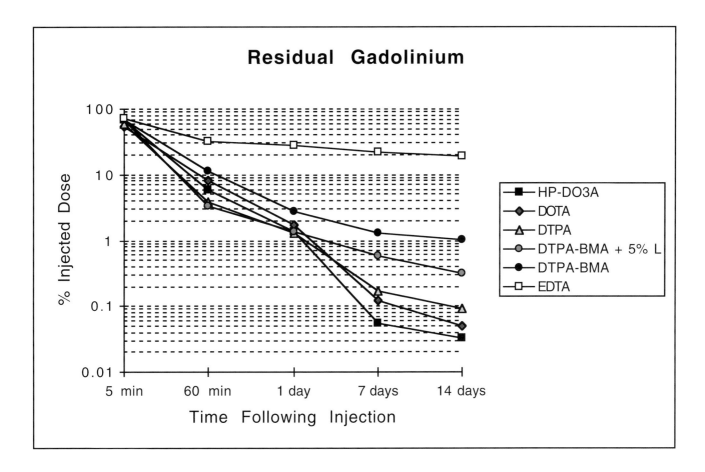

Figure 4. Whole body residual gadolinium (Gd) following intravenous administration of radiolabeled chelates. Gd EDTA dissociates rapidly in vivo and is poorly tolerated. The stability of each chelate, and the degree to which in vivo dissociation occurs, is reflected by the residual Gd at each time point. More stable chelates, with less release of Gd in vivo, leave less free metal ion. Of the agents approved for clinical use, Gd DTPA-BMA shows the greatest residual Gd. Addition of excess ligand (+ 5% L) improves excretion. Free gadolinium is deposited in liver and bone marrow, with the potential for chronic heavy metal toxicity. *(From Tweedle MF. Physicochemical properties of gadoteridol and other magnetic resonance contrast agents. Investigative Radiology 1992;27:S2-6).*

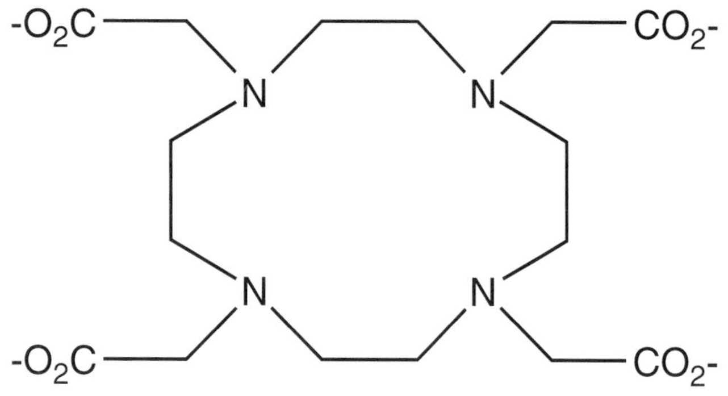

Figure 5. The chemical structure for DOTA (1,4,7,10-tetraazacyclododecane-N,N',N,N'-tetraacetic acid), the chelate in gadoterate meglumine (Dotarem).

Gd HP-DO3A, as noted earlier, is approved for high dose use (0.3 mmol/kg). Clinical trials with high dose have focused on the investigation of intracranial metastatic disease. Lesion enhancement is consistently improved at high dose, with a mean increase of 107% at 0.3 versus 0.1 mmol/kg demonstrated in one study.[39] In a study of 27 patients with clinically suspected brain metastases, 46 new lesions were noted in 19 patients with a dose of 0.3 as compared to 0.1 mmol/kg.[40] A marked improvement in lesion conspicuity was also found. In the phase III multicenter U.S. trial, 49 patients were studied with evidence of at least one metastatic lesion on MR.[41] On film review, both unblinded and blinded reviewers noted a marked improvement in diagnostic confidence and lesion detection at high dose. The increase in number of lesions detected was 51% (unblinded) and 32% (blinded), respectively. Two patients with normal scans at 0.1 mmol/kg demonstrated a single metastatic lesion at 0.3 mmol/kg. A study of cost-effectiveness revealed lower overall cost of patient management, despite the higher cost of contrast administration.[42] Craniotomies and aggressive courses of radiation therapy were avoided in five patients due to detection of additional lesions at high dose.

Other Compounds

Although not approved for clinical use in the U.S., gadoterate meglumine (Gd DOTA or Dotarem, Laboratoire Guerbet, figure 5) is currently used in some European and South American countries. Like Gd HP-DO3A, Gd DOTA is a ring chelate, with greater in vitro and in vivo stability than linear chelates. A randomized clinical trial comparing Gd DOTA and Gd DTPA in 300 patients found no difference in efficacy, with a similar frequency of adverse events.[43]

Gadobutrol (Gd DO3A-butrol, Schering AG) is a nonionic, cyclic paramagnetic metal ion chelate which has been studied in phase II clinical trials in Germany.[44] Post-contrast MR exams were obtained in 20 patients with metastatic disease, comparing doses of 0.1 and 0.3 mmol/kg Gd DO3A-butrol to 0.1 mmol/kg Gd DTPA. High dose Gd DO3A-butrol provided a statistically significant improvement in lesion enhancement, compared to the standard dose of either agent. 36 additional metastatic lesions were noted in 6 patients at high dose.

Gadoversetamide (Gd DTPA bis-methoxyethyl amide or Optimark, Mallinckrodt Medical), a linear chelate, was evaluated in 1994 in normal volunteers at doses of 0.1 to 0.7 mmol/kg. Serum iron increased transiently following injection in a dose dependent fashion.[45]

Although initially evaluated as a hepatobiliary contrast agent,[46] gadobenate dimeglumine (Gd BOPTA, Bracco Diagnostics) has recently received attention for CNS use. Investigation has focused on the use of Gd BOPTA in brain neoplasia and first pass cerebral blood volume studies.[47]

Special Applications

High Dose

High dose contrast administration with an agent such as Gd HP-DO3A has been shown to provide improved lesion detection, greater diagnostic confidence, and improved assessment of tissue perfusion, the latter with first pass studies. The original choice of contrast dose (0.1 mmol/kg for Gd DTPA, first used in 1984) was determined by safety concerns and not based on efficacy. Subsequent animal and clinical trials suggest efficacy for higher doses in a broad range of indications. The multicenter U.S. trial comparing 0.1 and 0.3 mmol/kg Gd HP-DO3A for the detection of brain metastases demonstrated an improvement of 32% in number of lesions detected at high dose (figure 6). In this trial, patients received an initial injection of 0.1 mmol/kg, followed by a supplemental injection of 0.2 mmol/kg (for a total dose of 0.3 mmol/kg) 30 minutes later. A subsequent multicenter U.S. trial compared doses of 0.1 and 0.3 given at different settings, separated by more than 1 day and less than 7 days. Results were similar, with the conclusion being that high dose is efficacious regardless of whether given as a split injection or as a single dose.[48] Metastatic lesions show consistently greater enhancement at high dose, leading to improved confidence in diagnosis of lesions questioned on the basis of

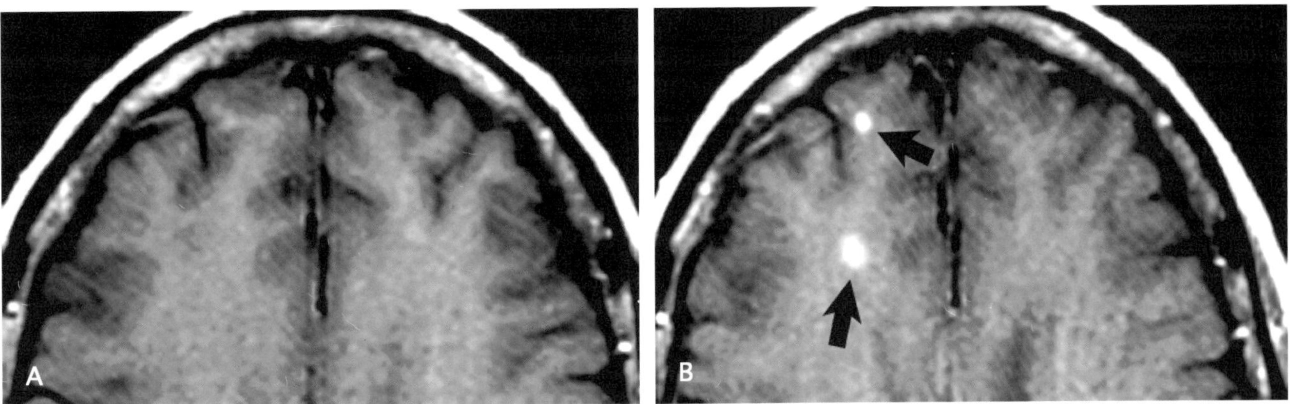

Figure 6. Detection of brain metastases only following high dose contrast administration (0.3 mmol/kg gadoteridol). (A) The T1-weighted scan following administration of 0.1 mmol/kg, standard dose, is normal. Identification of two metastatic lesions (arrows), from primary lung carcinoma in this instance, is possible only on (B) the high dose (0.3 mmol/kg) post-contrast T1-weighted scan. A recent multi-institutional study demonstrated a 32% increase in the number of metastatic lesions detected when a dose of 0.3 mmol/kg was used in comparison to a dose of 0.1 mmol/kg.

the standard dose exam (figure 7), as well as increased lesion detection. High dose makes possible the detection of additional lesions by raising the level of enhancement above the threshold necessary for visualization (figure 8).

There is limited experience with the application of high dose in brain neoplasia other than metastatic disease. In a phase II clinical trial involving 14 patients with intracranial neoplastic disease, higher contrast doses (0.2 and 0.3 mmol/kg) consistently improved lesion enhancement.[49] A subsequent study, which combined phase II and III results in 40 patients with intracranial neoplastic disease, concluded that "improved enhancement, detection, and delineation" of CNS neoplasms resulted from injection of higher contrast doses. It was further suggested that findings at high dose have the potential to be clinically significant and justify the higher cost.[50]

In gliomas of the brain, the administration of high contrast dose can lead to recognition of tumor outside the bounds defined by T2-weighted scans (figure 9). In a study of 23 patients with pathologically proven gliomas, twelve "demonstrated enhancement on T1-weighted images extending beyond the zone of apparent signal abnormality demonstrated on T2-weighted images." [51] This was not seen in any of the six patients receiving a contrast dose of 0.05 mmol/kg, in only one of five at 0.1 mmol/kg, in four of five at 0.2 mmol/kg, and in all seven at 0.3 mmol/kg. Thus improved definition of neoplastic extent is possible at high contrast dose in these infiltrative tumors, by recognition of subtle blood-brain barrier disruption.

In early subacute cerebral infarction, the degree of blood-brain barrier disruption may not be sufficient to produce abnormal contrast enhancement at standard contrast dose.[13] In an experimental animal study, administration of 0.3 mmol/kg (as opposed to 0.1 mmol/kg) produced a statistically significant increase in enhancement — more than double. In six early subacute infarcts, abnormal contrast enhancement was noted in only three animals at 0.1 mmol/kg, yet in all at 0.3 mmol/kg (figure 10). This phenomenon has also been observed in clinical studies (figure 11). Administration of high dose enables recognition of characteristic parenchymal enhancement, providing information for lesion dating and differential diagnosis.

In brain infection, administration of high contrast dose also produces greater lesion enhancement (figures 12 - 15). For early lesions, or in the immunocompromised patient, the use of high dose permits identification of blood-brain barrier disruption, which might otherwise not be identified, confirming lesion activity. This finding can be critical clinically, changing the assessment of the lesion from chronic to active.

Initial studies comparing 0.1 and 0.3 mmol/kg in the head and neck and in the spine suggest utility for high dose in both areas. In tumors of the head and neck, both the percent lesion enhancement and the visual assessment rating were improved at 0.3 mmol/kg.[52] Better lesion detection and delineation, as well as greater diagnostic confidence, were reported at 0.3 mmol/kg in 14 patients with suspected spinal cord lesions. The final diagnosis was altered in 39% after the high dose exam.[53]

Magnetization Transfer

Magnetization transfer (MT) techniques have recently been employed in MR imaging to influence tissue contrast. In this approach, off resonance pulses are used to saturate protons in macromolecules. The addition of MT pulses to standard imaging sequences can improve the visualization of contrast enhancement in the brain, with this observation specifically demonstrated in cerebral infarction.[54] However, in a comparison of high and standard dose, with and without MT,

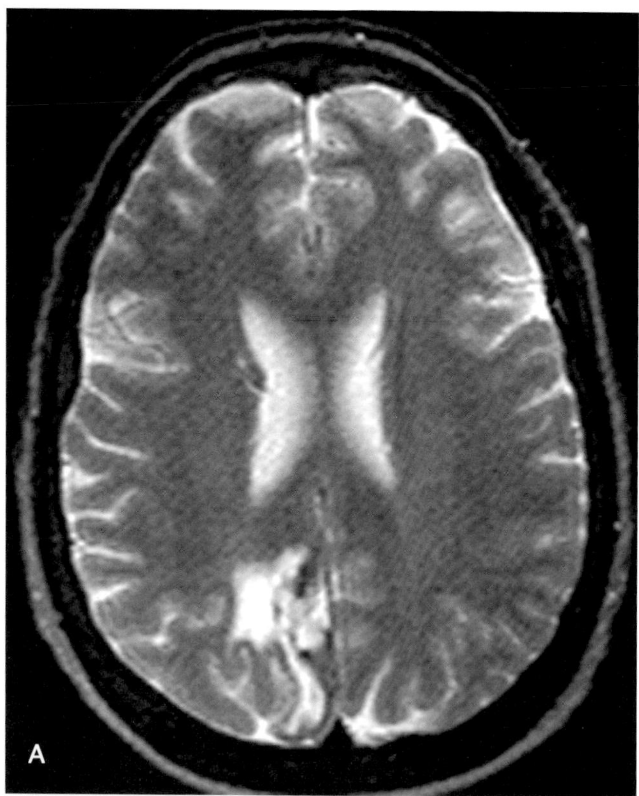

Figure 7. Improved visualization of brain metastases with high contrast dose (0.3 mmol/kg gadoteridol). High dose not only provides for the identification of additional lesions, but also improves reader confidence regarding identification of other metastases. The (A) pre-contrast T2-weighted scan and (B) standard dose post-contrast T1-weighted scan were interpreted prospectively as consistent with a single brain metastasis (with minimal contrast enhancement) along the lateral ventricular wall. The changes in the occipital lobe are due to prior surgical resection. (C) The high dose post-contrast T1-weighted scan, however, increases markedly the certainty of identification of this enhancing brain metastasis (arrow). *(From Runge VM, Wells JW, Nelson KL, Linville PM. MR imaging detection of cerebral metastases with a single injection of high-dose gadoteridol. Journal of Magnetic Resonance Imaging 1994;4(5):669-673).*

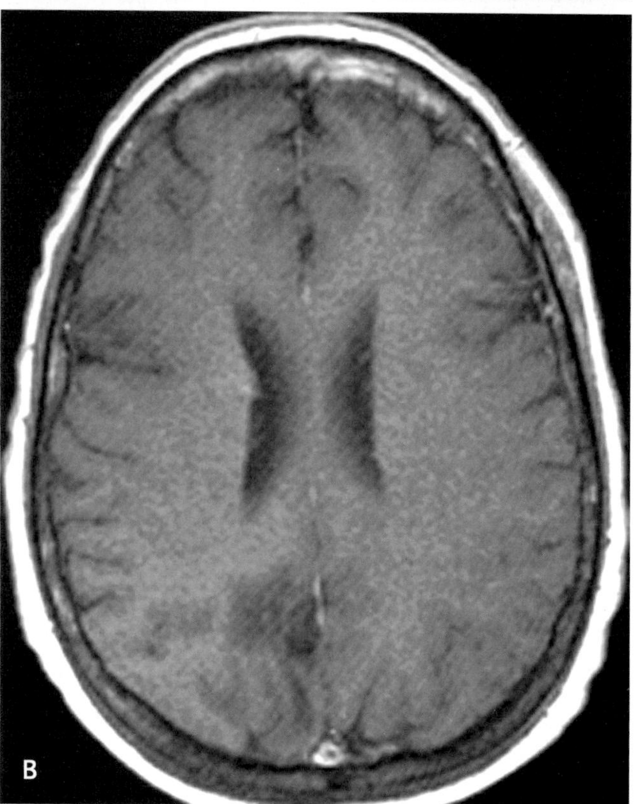

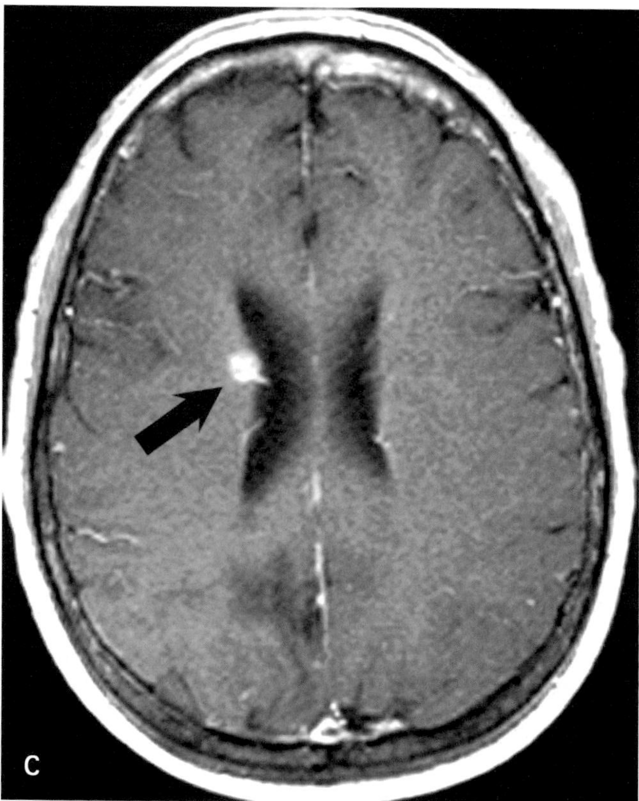

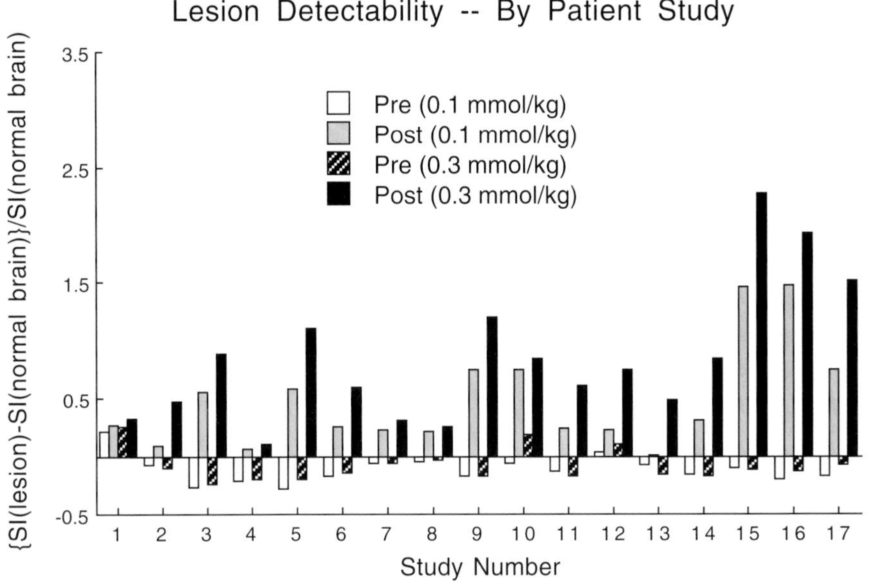

Figure 8. Improved detectability of brain metastases at high dose as quantitated by region of interest measurements. Lesion detectability was assessed by signal intensity analysis in 17 patients studied at both standard (0.1 mmol/kg) and high (0.3 mmol/kg) contrast dose (using gadoteridol). In patients in whom more than one metastasis was noted, measurements were averaged for all lesions. In each instance, lesion enhancement improved following a dose of 0.3 mmol/kg, as compared to a dose of 0.1 mmol/kg. This increase leads to improved lesion detection on film interpretation. No paradoxical decrease in lesion signal intensity was noted at high dose, a theoretical consideration due to the T2 effects of the contrast agent. *(From Runge VM, Wells JW, Nelson KL, Linville PM. MR imaging detection of cerebral metastases with a single injection of high-dose gadoteridol. Journal of Magnetic Resonance Imaging 1994;4(5):669-673).*

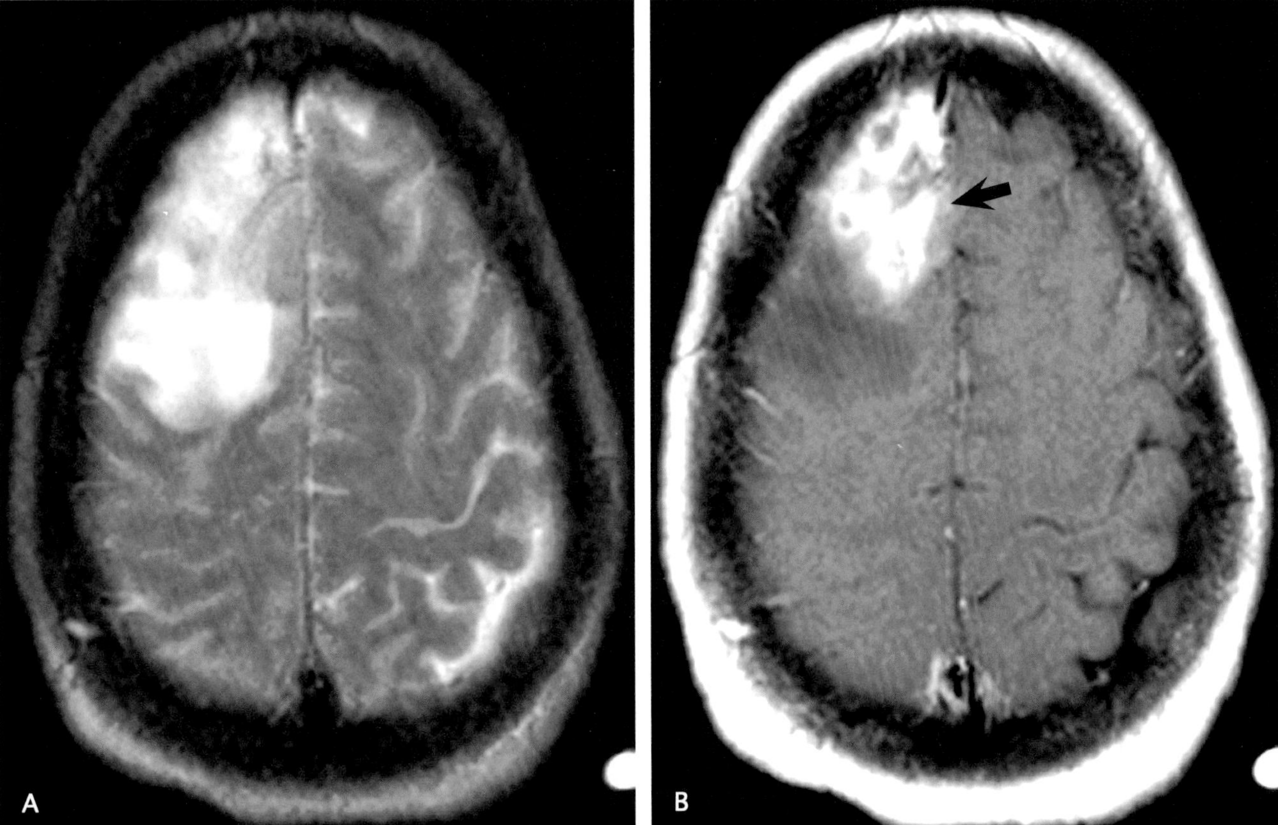

Figure 9. At high contrast dose, lesion extension beyond the border shown on T2-weighted scans is consistently noted in high grade astrocytomas. (A) T2-weighted and (B) high dose post-contrast (0.3 mmol/kg gadoteridol) T1-weighted scans are presented from a 62 year old female with a glioblastoma. Enhancement of the lesion medially (arrow) extends beyond the zone of high signal abnormality on the T2-weighted scan, providing a better estimate of gross tumor involvement.

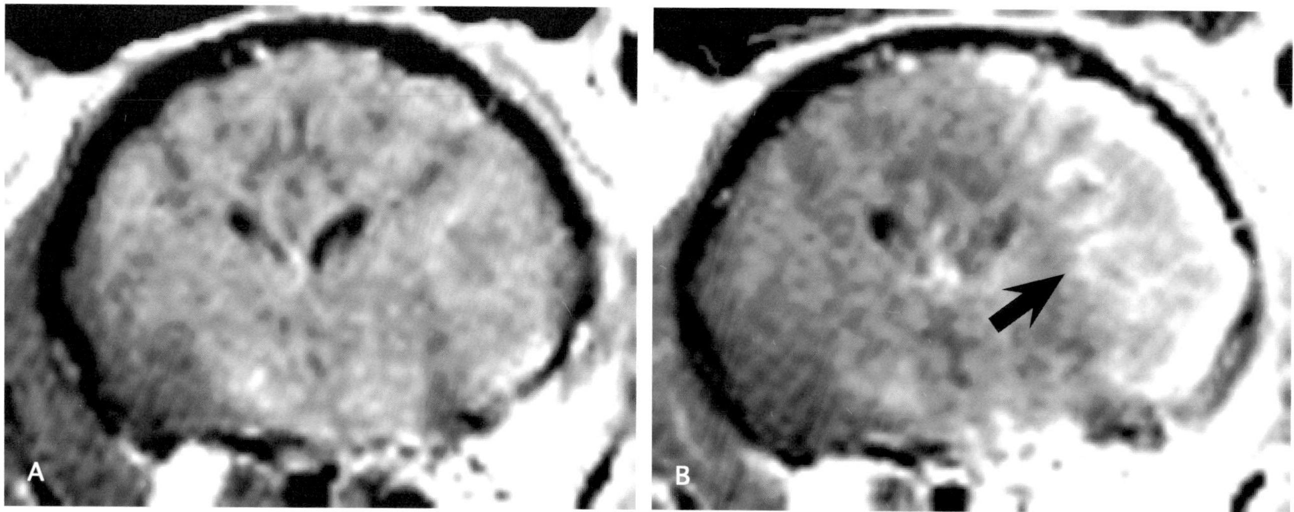

Figure 10. Improved detection of blood-brain barrier disruption in acute brain infarction following high dose contrast administration (using gadoteridol). In early infarction, the degree of disruption of the blood-brain barrier may be insufficient to visualize abnormal contrast enhancement at (A) standard dose (0.1 mmol/kg). In such a setting, (B) administration of high dose (0.3 mmol/kg) can provide for identification of abnormal parenchymal enhancement (arrow). The left hemispheric infarct in this experimental animal was created by surgical occlusion of the middle cerebral artery, followed by reperfusion. *(From Runge VM, Kirsch JE, Wells JW, Dunworth JN, Woolfolk CE. Visualization of blood-brain barrier disruption on MR images of cats with acute cerebral infarction: value of administering a high dose of contrast material. American Journal of Roentgenology 1994;162:431-435).*

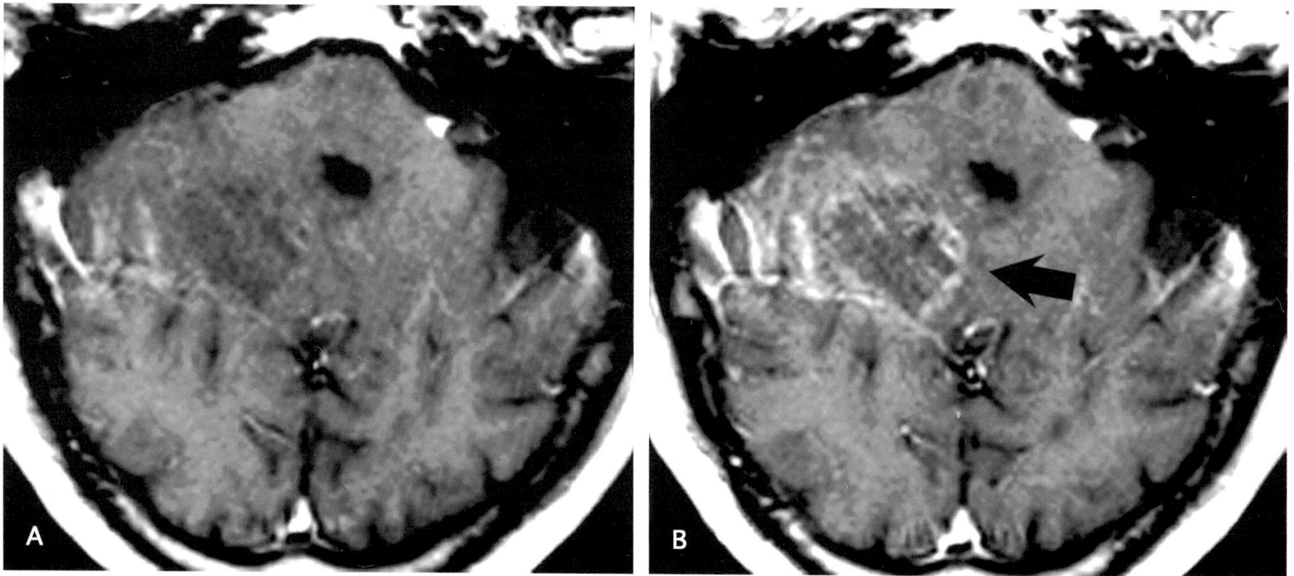

Figure 11. Visualization of blood-brain barrier disruption in an acute superior cerebellar artery infarct at 0.3 mmol/kg gadoteridol, with absence of enhancement at 0.1 mmol/kg. As noted in figure 10, blood-brain barrier disruption in early infarction may be of insufficient degree to manifest abnormal contrast enhancement (A) at standard dose. In such instances, administration of (B) high dose can reveal abnormal enhancement (arrow). This confirms the acute nature of the lesion, with the patient in this instance an elderly man studied one day following clinical presentation.

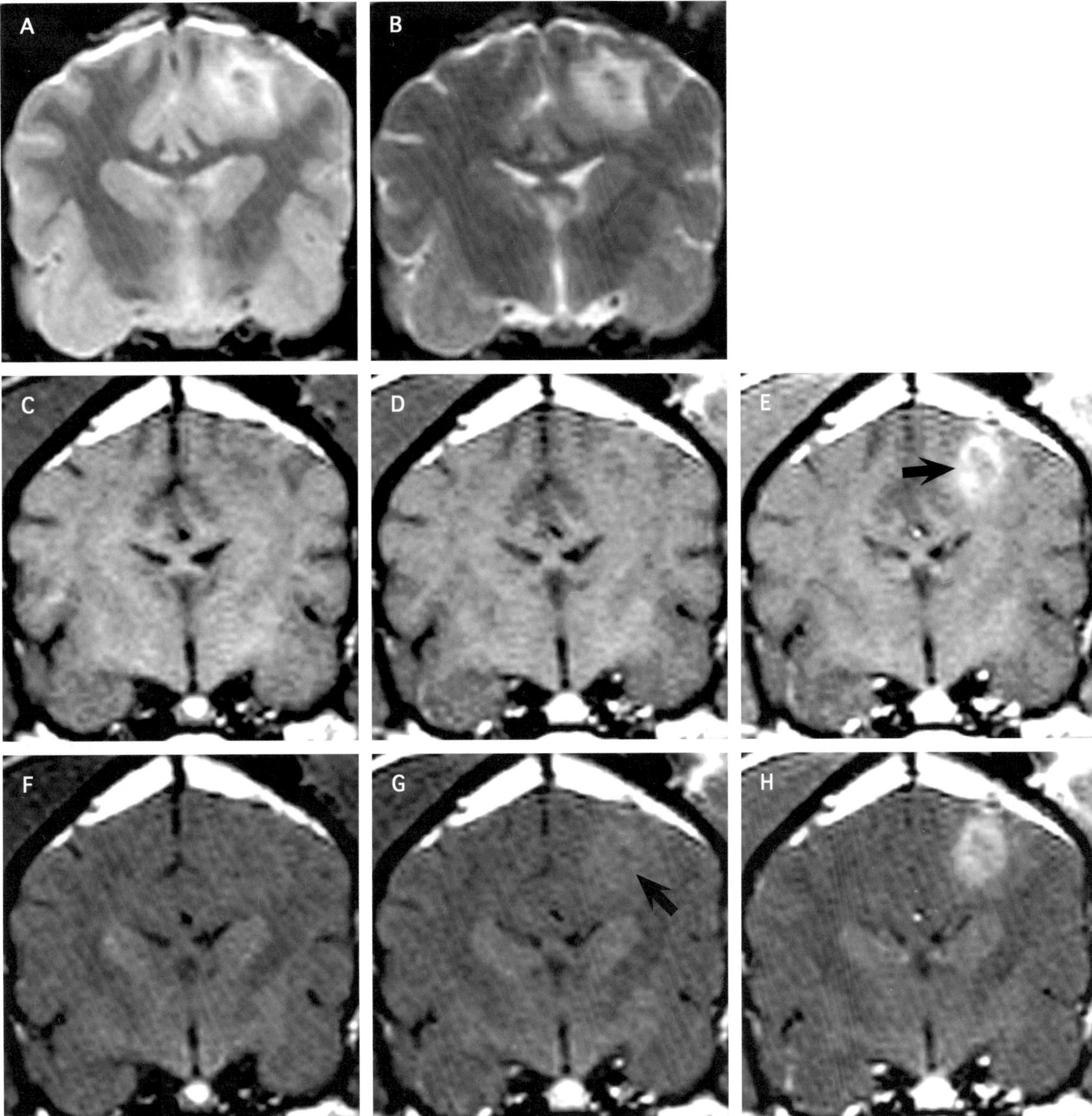

Figure 12. Improved identification of contrast enhancement in an early brain abscess by the use of high dose. Only a marginal additional increase is provided by the use of magnetization transfer (MT). Coronal T2- and T1-weighted scans are presented in a canine model one day after injection of a bacterial suspension. (A) First and (B) second echoes from the T2-weighted scan reveal vasogenic edema surrounding the lesion. The T1-weighted images are from (C, F) prior to and following, respectively, (D, G) 0.1 mmol/kg and (E, H) 0.3 mmol/kg contrast injection (gadoteridol). (C, D, E) Scans using conventional spin echo technique are compared to (F, G, H) scans using magnetization transfer. (C, F) Pre-contrast, the lesion is of slightly lower signal intensity than surrounding brain. The normal brain parenchyma is globally of lower signal intensity on (F) as compared with (C), consistent with the application of magnetization transfer. At standard contrast dose (D, G), there is minimal lesion enhancement. This is slightly better demonstrated (arrow, G) on the scan with MT. At high dose (E, H), there is prominent ring enhancement, which is equally striking on both scans. Lesion enhancement (arrow, E) on the (E) high dose scan without MT is substantially greater than that on (G) the standard dose scan with MT. *(From Runge VM, Wells JW, Kirsch JE. Magnetization transfer and high dose contrast in early brain infection on MR. Investigative Radiology 1995;30:135-143).*

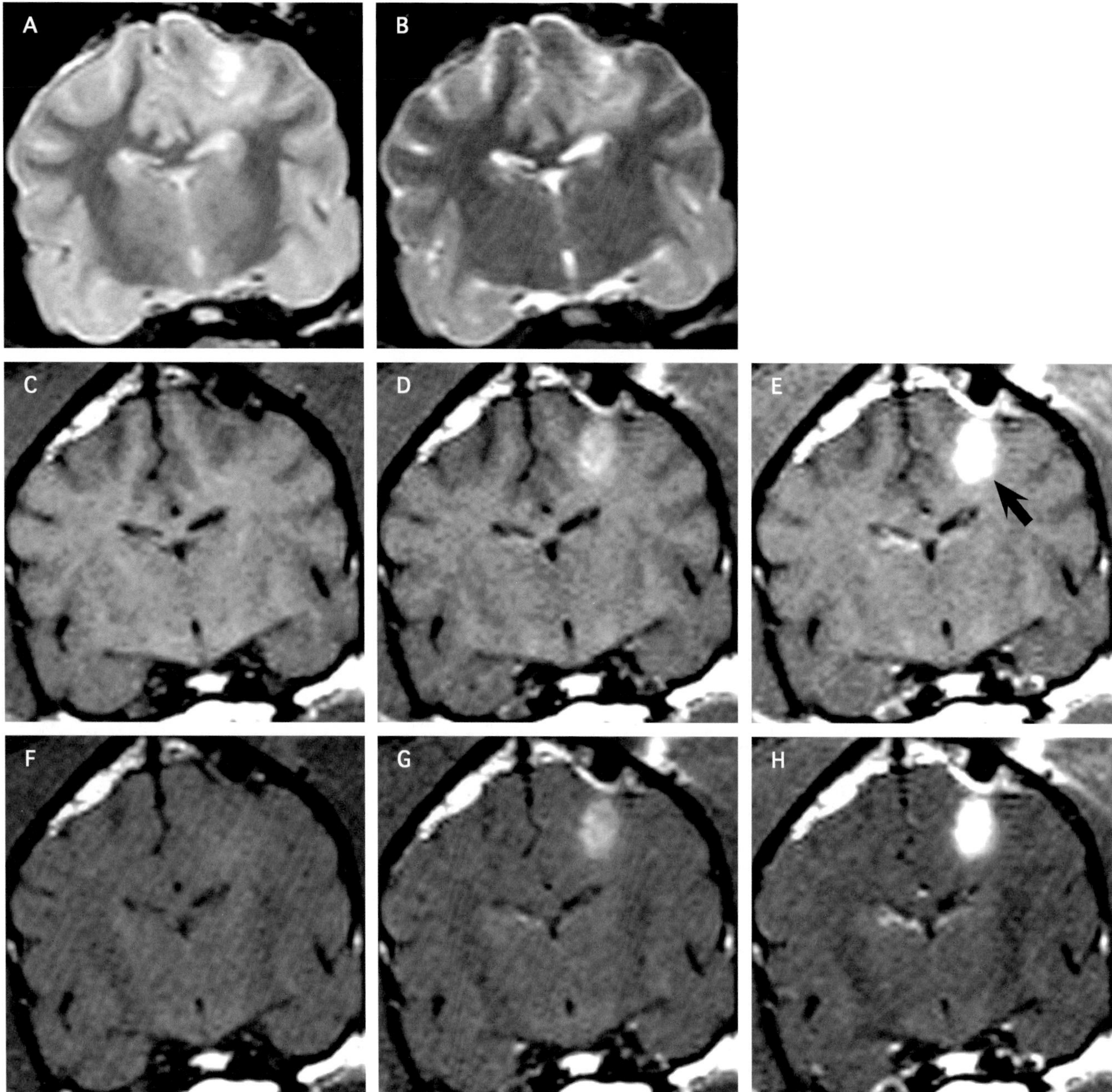

Figure 13. Improved identification of lesion activity (contrast enhancement) in a mature brain abscess, late cerebritis stage, by the use of high contrast dose (with gadoteridol). These results are in an animal model studied at five days following implantation of the bacterial nidus. Pre-contrast (A, B) T2- and (C, F — without and with MT) T1-weighted scans are compared to post-contrast T1-weighted scans using (D, G — without and with MT) a dose of 0.1 mmol/kg and (E, H — without and with MT) a dose of 0.3 mmol/kg. The degree of lesion enhancement was rated as mild by a reader blinded to imaging technique on both scans (D, G) at standard dose. (E, H) At high dose, lesion enhancement was rated as intense for both scans, without and with MT. There is little difference in the degree of lesion enhancement (arrow) on the high dose scans (E) without and (H) with MT. *(From Runge VM, Wells JW, Kirsch JE. Magnetization transfer and high dose contrast in early brain infection on MR. Investigative Radiology 1995;30:135-143).*

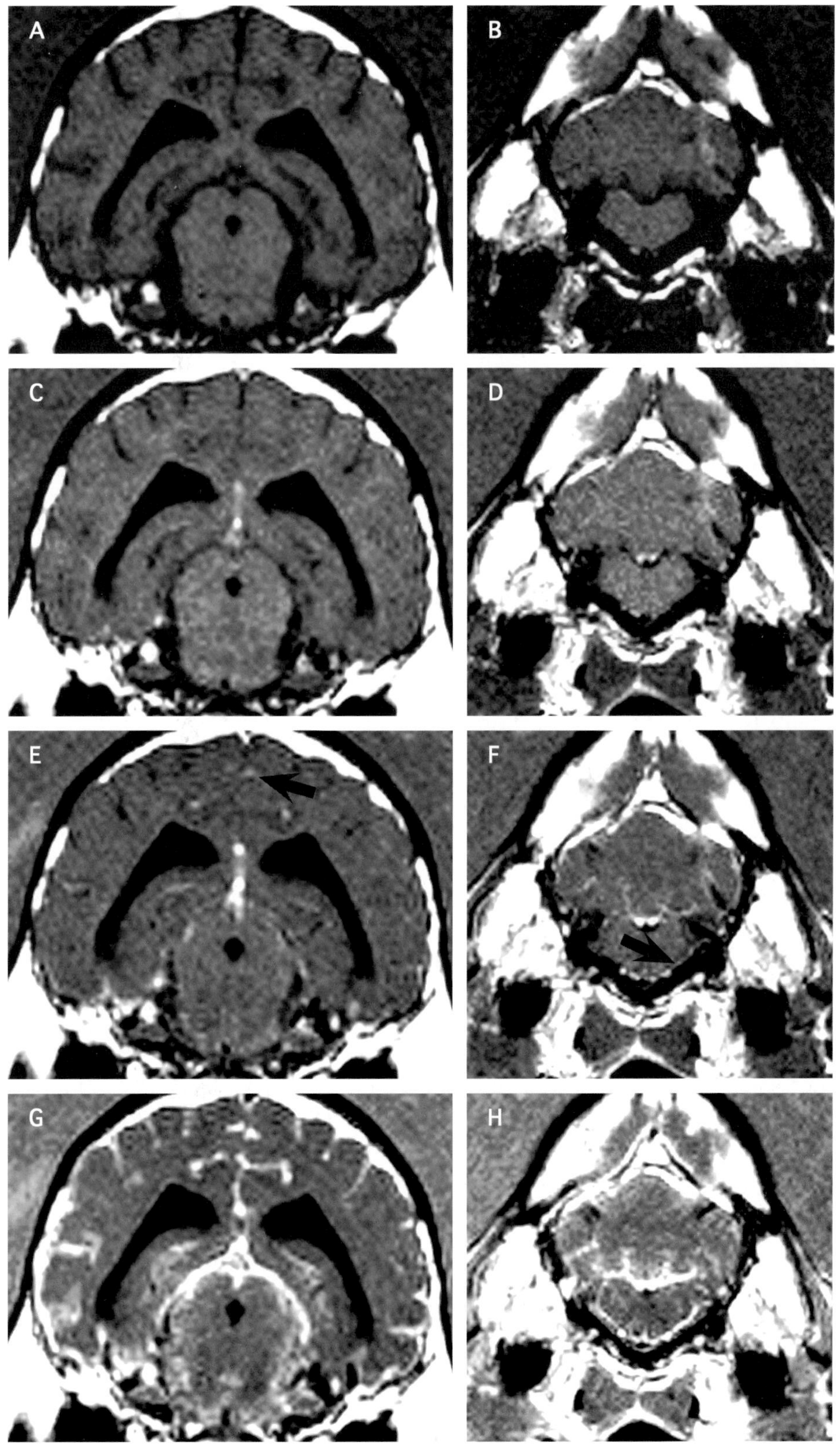

Figure 14. Early bacterial meningitis, detected only following high dose contrast administration. The scans illustrated are T1-weighted spin echo technique without the application of magnetization transfer. (A, B) are prior to contrast injection, with the remaining images immediately following contrast doses of (C, D) 0.1, (E, F) 0.3, and (G, H) 0.8 mmol/kg gadoteridol. Scans at both the level of the lateral ventricles (A, C, E, G) and the medulla (B, D, F, H) are shown. On prospective film interpretation, with the reader blinded to contrast administration and dose, no abnormality was noted pre-contrast. This included T2-weighted scans (not shown). In addition, no abnormality was identified on post-contrast scans using a dose of 0.1 mmol/kg. At 0.3 mmol/kg, mild abnormal meningeal enhancement (arrows) was identified both above and below the tentorium (the latter principally surrounding the brainstem). Using a dose of 0.8 mmol/kg, meningeal enhancement was diffuse and intense. *(From Runge VM, Wells JW, Williams NM, Lee C, Timoney JF, Young AB. Detectability of early brain meningitis on MR. Investigative Radiology 1995;30(8):484-495).*

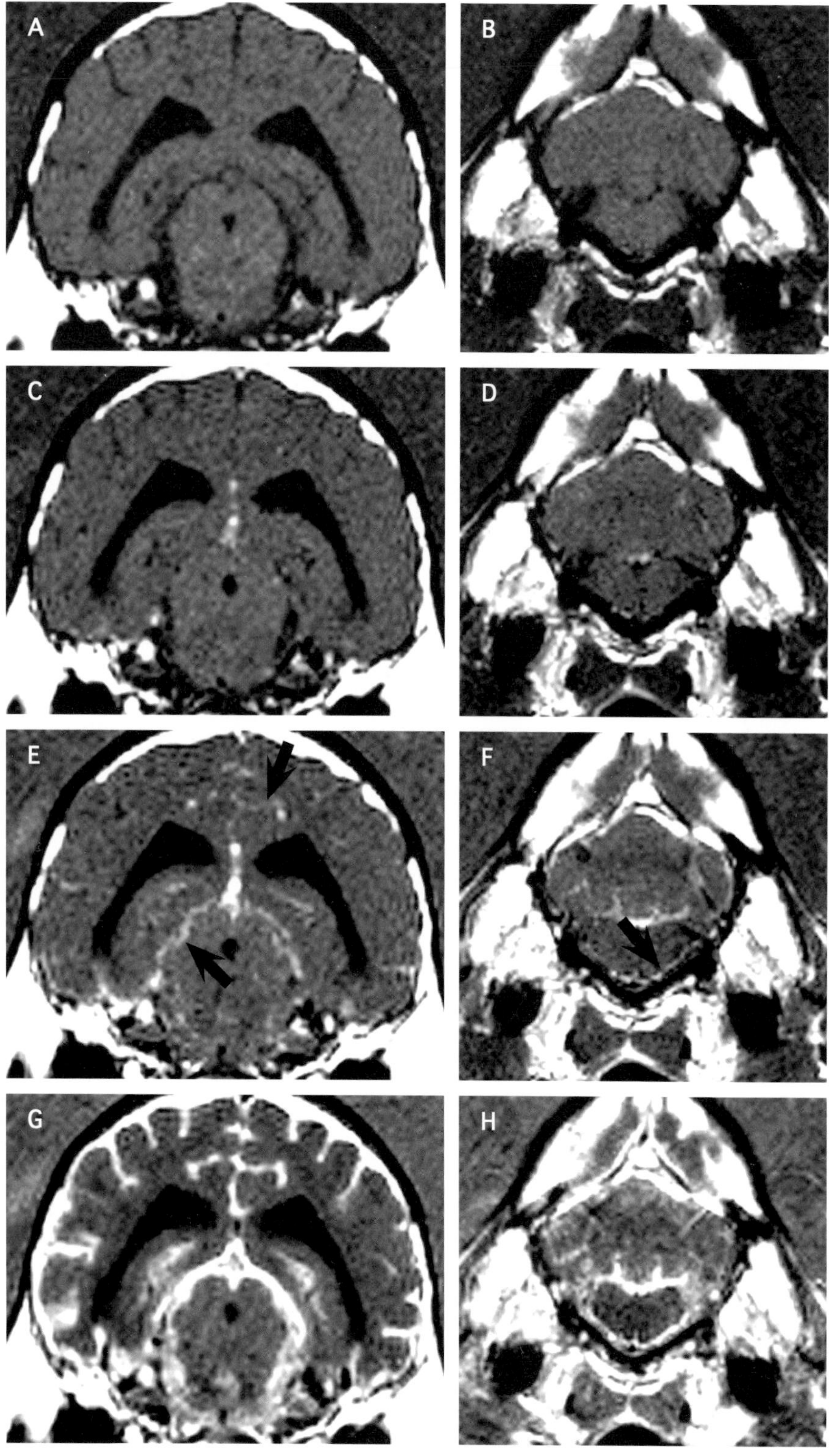

Figure 15. Early bacterial meningitis, improved visualization on post-contrast scans using magnetization transfer (MT). Images are from the same experimental animal as depicted in figure 14. The timing of scans pre- and post-contrast, and anatomic level, are also the same. All scans are T1-weighted spin echo technique with MT. (A, B) are prior to contrast injection, and the remaining images immediately following contrast doses of (C, D) 0.1, (E, F) 0.3, and (G, H) 0.8 mmol/kg gadoteridol. At 0.3 mmol/kg, moderate abnormal meningeal enhancement (arrows) was identified prospectively in the supratentorial space and surrounding the brainstem. Without MT (figure 14), the enhancement was graded as only mild in degree. With a contrast dose of 0.8 mmol/kg, meningeal enhancement was diffuse and intense both with and without the application of MT. *(From Runge VM, Wells JW, Williams NM, Lee C, Timoney JF, Young AB. Detectability of early brain meningitis on MR. Investigative Radiology 1995;30(8):484-495).*

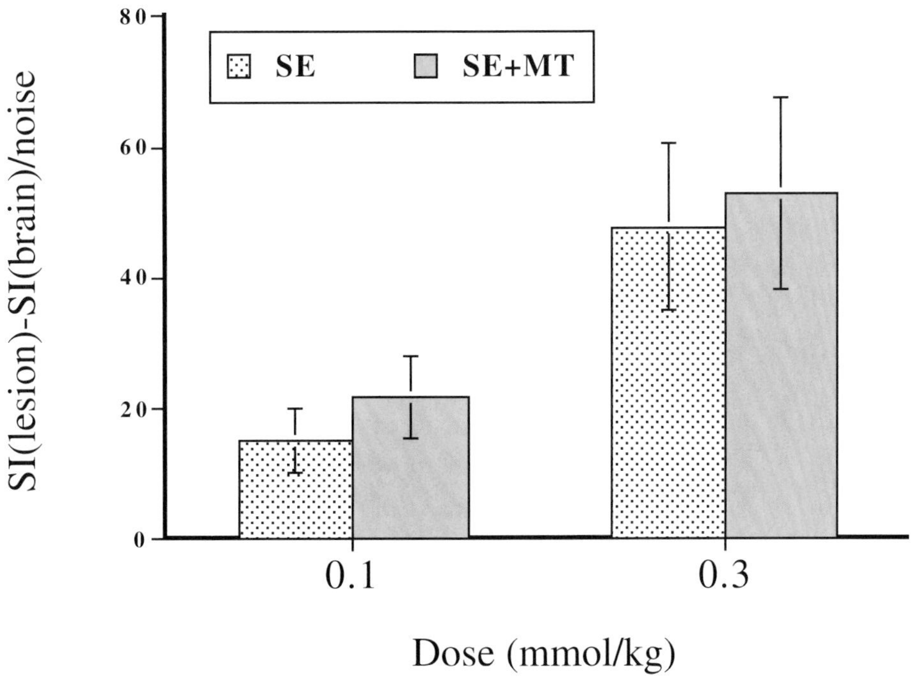

Figure 16. Comparison of lesion enhancement relative to contrast dose, with and without magnetization transfer (MT), from statistical image analysis. Results are from a brain abscess model. The effects of contrast dose dominate over that of scan technique, specifically the application of MT. SI stands for signal intensity, SE for spin echo T1-weighted technique without the application of MT, and SE+MT for spin echo T1-weighted technique with the application of MT. The mean plus or minus one standard deviation is plotted. Results with MT were marginally superior to that without MT, on statistical analysis, with contrast dose held constant. Results at high dose (0.3 mmol/kg) were substantially superior to that at standard dose (0.1 mmol/kg). The improvement in detection of lesion enhancement with MT alone was 44% at a dose of 0.1 mmol/kg and 11% at a dose of 0.3 mmol/kg. Comparing images using the same scan technique, the improvement with high dose (0.3 vs. 0.1 mmol/kg) was 214% (scans without MT) and 142% (scans with MT). *(From Runge VM, Wells JW, Kirsch JE. Magnetization transfer and high dose contrast in early brain infection on MR. Investigative Radiology 1995;30:135-143).*

high dose with or without MT ranked superior to all other imaging approaches (figure 16). The degree of lesion enhancement achieved with MT and standard contrast dose does not approach that achieved with high contrast dose, regardless of the application or not of MT.

MR Angiography

In specific instances, contrast enhanced MR angiography (MRA) can provide important additional diagnostic information (figures 17 and 18).[55] Advantages of post-contrast MRA include improved depiction of both fast and slow flow, less dependence on vessel orientation, and effective imaging of larger volumes. Disadvantages include display of both arteries and veins and increased background signal due to soft tissue enhancement.

First Pass Studies

First pass studies can be acquired on either conventional 1.5 T MR systems or newer echo-planar units. By observing with rapid dynamic imaging the bolus of the contrast agent as it passes through the brain, an assessment of cerebral blood volume and thus brain perfusion can be made. These studies typically depend upon observation of the T2* effect of the contrast agent. Dose has been evaluated in three studies.[12,56,57] The conclusion of each investigation has been that there is a dose dependent effect (figure 19), with improved sensitivity and efficacy at higher doses (up to 0.5 mmol/kg). This type of MR study has found clinical application in the evaluation of brain ischemia (figures 20 and 21) and brain neoplasia.

Both Gd HP-DO3A and Gd DO3A-butrol can be formulated at a concentration of 1.0 molar, twice that currently

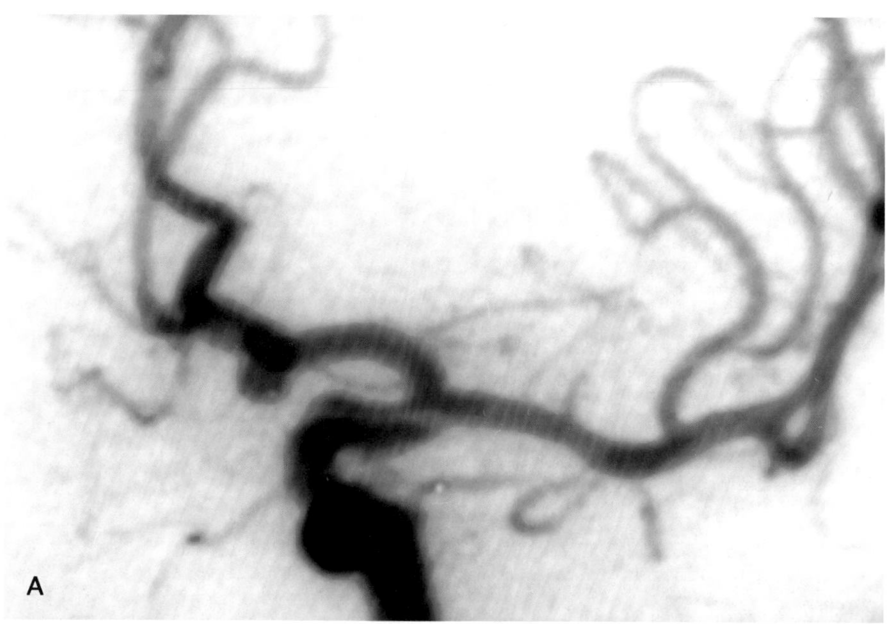

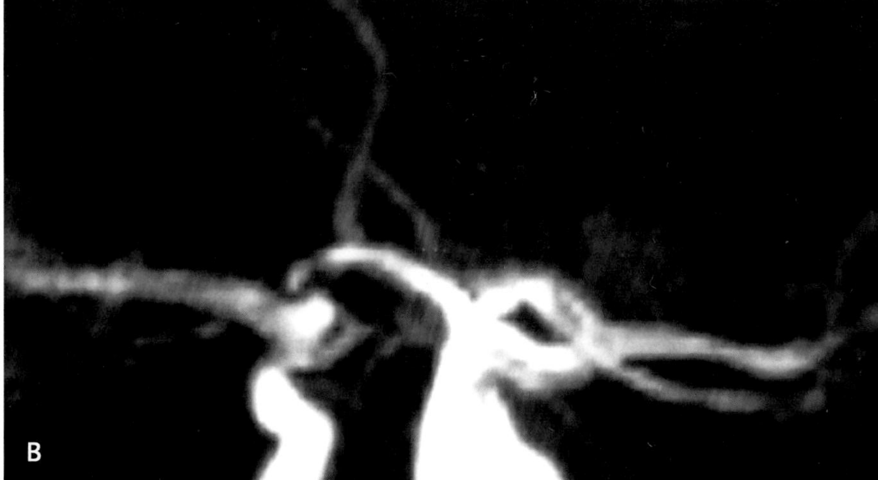

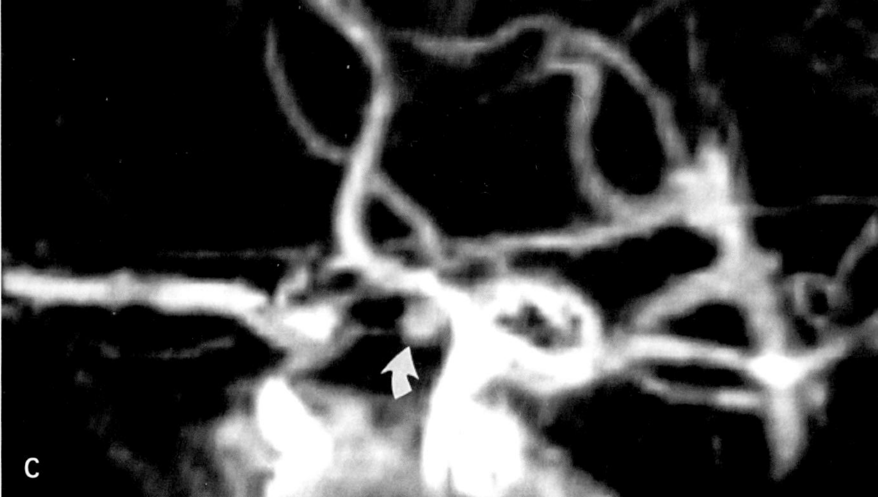

Figure 17. Left anterior communicating artery aneurysm, with improved visualization on post-contrast 3D time-of-flight MR angiography (MRA). (A) The aneurysm is well visualized on a right posterior oblique view from a conventional iodinated contrast angiogram. (B, C) Oblique coronal maximum intensity projections (MIP) are shown from the (B) pre- and (C) post-contrast MRA studies. The aneurysm is poorly visualized on the pre-contrast study. There is excellent opacification and visualization of this anterior communicating artery aneurysm (arrow, C) on the post-contrast (0.3 mmol/kg gadoteridol) MR angiogram. Large aneurysms will also, on occasion, be better depicted on post-contrast 3D time-of-flight MR angiography. The latter finding is due to the enhancement of slowly flowing blood. *(From Runge VM, Kirsch JE, Lee C. Contrast-enhanced MR angiography. Journal of Magnetic Resonance Imaging 1993;3: 233-239).*

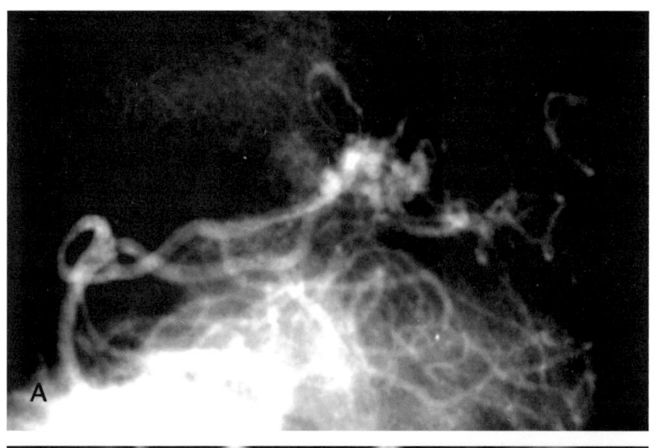

Figure 18. Right thalamic arteriovenous malformation (AVM), with improved visualization on post-contrast MRA. (A) The lateral projection from a x-ray angiogram depicts the nidus and feeding vessels. Using the angiogram, part of the AVM could be identified on routine axial T2- and T1-weighted scans, both pre- and post-contrast (images not shown). The lesion was seen on the basis of flow voids pre-contrast and due to partial enhancement post-contrast. Craniocaudal MIP projections from the (B) pre- and (C) post-contrast (0.3 mmol/kg gadoteridol) MRA studies are shown. On the pre-contrast MRA, the lesion cannot be seen. However, the nidus (arrow) is well identified on the post-contrast MR angiogram. Enlarged abnormal draining veins can also be seen on the post-contrast study, although these must be differentiated from enhancement of the adjacent choroid plexus. *(From reference 55).*

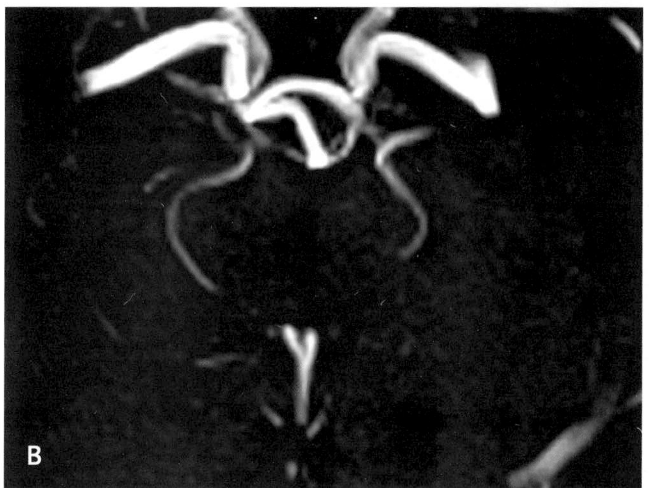

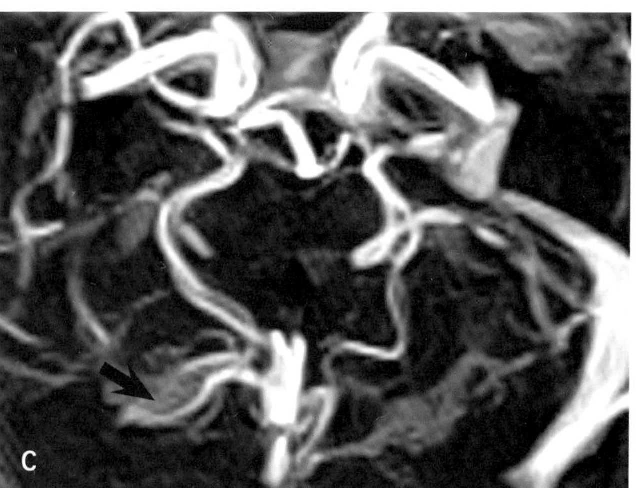

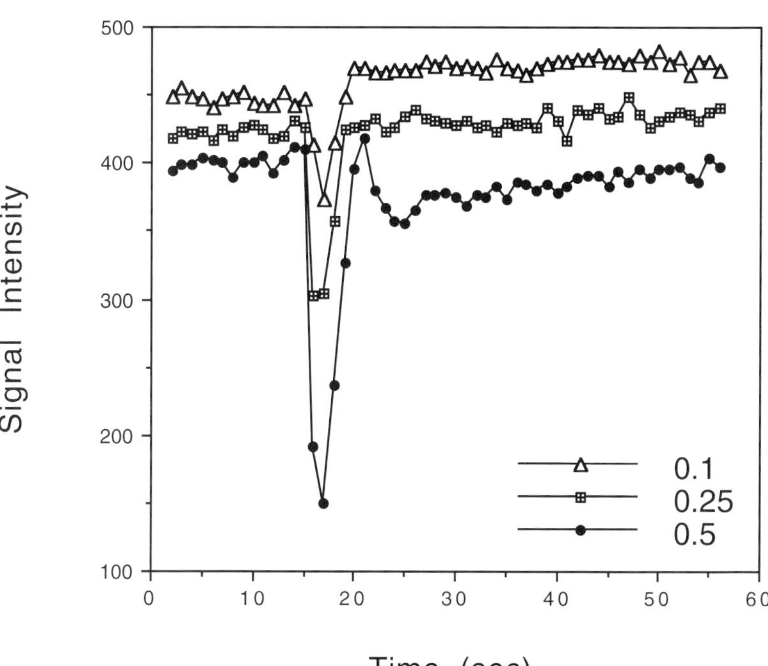

Figure 19. The first pass effect in brain, as observed on MR following bolus gadolinium chelate administration, is dose dependent. On SSFP and echo-planar imaging, the presence of contrast within capillaries during the first pass of an agent like gadoteridol (illustrated here) through the brain causes a reduction in signal intensity, due to T2 and susceptibility effects. A proportionally greater response, and thus more negative signal intensity change, is seen with higher contrast doses. Curves from normal brain are illustrated comparing doses of 0.1, 0.25, and 0.5 mmol/kg. *(From Runge VM, Kirsch JE, Wells JW, Woolfolk CE. Assessment of cerebral perfusion by first-pass, dynamic, contrast-enhanced, steady-state free-precession MR imaging: an animal study. American Journal of Roentgenology 1993;160:593-600).*

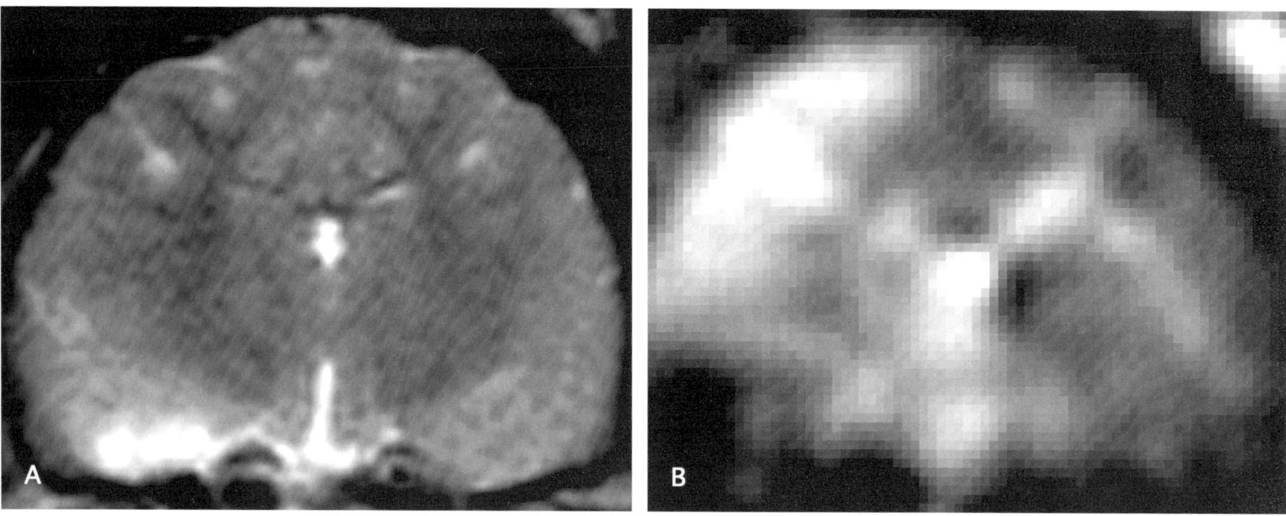

Figure 20. Information regarding regional cerebral blood volume is provided by first pass studies, permitting detection of early ischemic injury. In acute infarction, as illustrated in a cat model one hour following middle cerebral artery occlusion, there may not be sufficient vasogenic edema to permit lesion detection on (A) the T2-weighted scan. (B) At the peak of the first pass through the brain, the normal left hemisphere demonstrates a marked reduction in signal intensity due to presence of the contrast agent. However, the right hemisphere remains hyperintense, demarcating the region of ischemic insult. A dose of 0.3 mmol/kg gadoteridol (Gd HP-DO3A), injected at a rate of 9 cc/sec, was utilized in this instance.

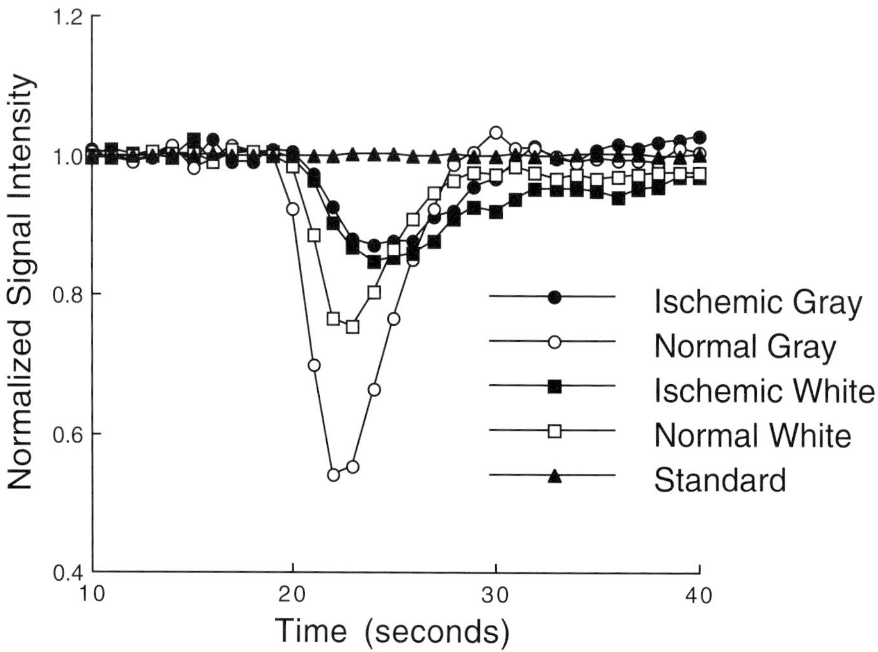

Figure 21. First pass MR studies can differentiate ischemic and normal gray and white matter in the brain. The change in signal intensity is graphed during transit of the contrast agent bolus, in this case gadoteridol. Results are from an experimental group of five animals, sixty minutes following occlusion of the middle cerebral artery. The curves for normal and ischemic gray and white matter are distinct from one another. The reduction in area under the curve for ischemic as compared to normal tissue reflects the reduction in regional cerebral blood volume. *(From Runge VM, Kirsch JE, Wells JW, Dunworth JN, Hilaire L, Woolfolk CE. Repeat cerebral blood volume assessment with first-pass MR imaging. Journal of Magnetic Resonance Imaging 1994;4:457-461).*

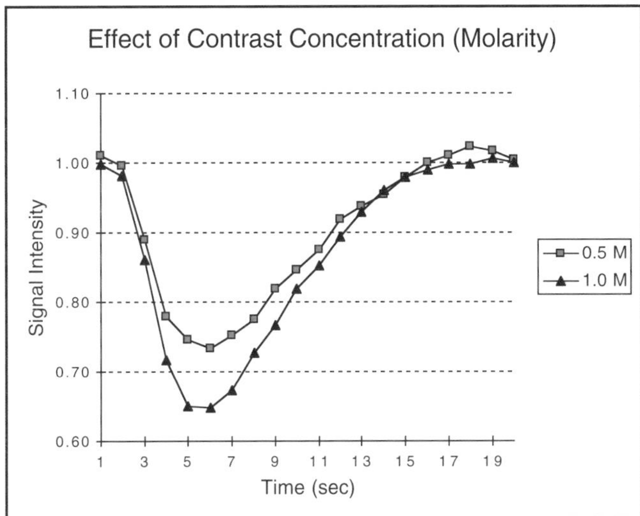

Figure 22. Higher concentration contrast formulations improve first pass regional cerebral blood volume studies. The results presented compare the 0.5 molar and 1.0 molar formulations of gadoteridol (Gd HP-DO3A). Contrast dose was held constant. Nonionic agents such as gadoteridol can be formulated at higher concentrations than currently used clinically (0.5 molar), with advantages in first pass perfusion studies due to delivery of a more compact bolus. The region of interest measurements presented here are from normal white matter. The higher concentration formulation produces a greater signal intensity decrease. A larger observed change leads to improved sensitivity and accuracy in the assessment of regional cerebral blood volume.

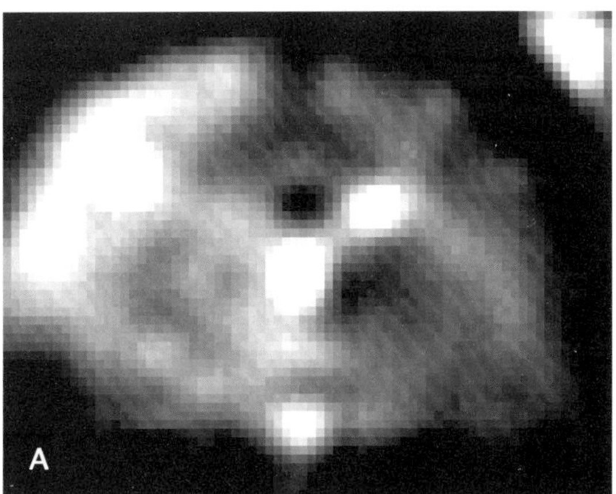

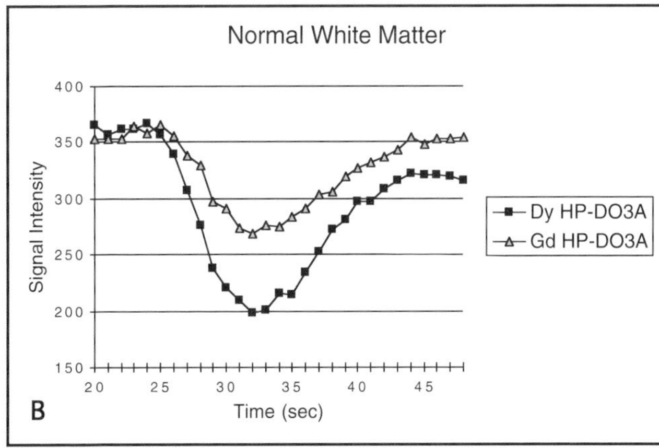

Figure 23. At 1.5 T, the use of a dysprosium chelate can lead to a further improvement in first pass brain perfusion studies. (A) At the peak of the first pass through the brain, following bolus injection of Dy HP-DO3A, the signal intensity of the normal left hemisphere is markedly reduced. The ischemic right hemisphere appears hyperintense in comparison, reflecting lower perfusion. In comparing this result to that with Gd HP-DO3A (figure 20), with dose and imaging parameters held constant, the effect of dysprosium is seen to be greater than that of gadolinium. This is quantitated in (B), which compares for the same animal the signal intensity curves during first pass in normal white matter for Dy HP-DO3A and Gd HP-DO3A.

used clinically for all extracellular gadolinium chelates (0.5 molar). Use of higher concentration formations in first pass studies has been shown to improve the reliability of regional cerebral blood volume measurements (figure 22). The smaller volume of contrast agent produces a sharper bolus.[58,59]

Dysprosium Chelates

The dysprosium (Dy) chelates represent a different avenue of contrast media development for MR. The compounds tested to date are analogs of the extracellular gadolinium chelates, with substitution of the dysprosium ion for the gadolinium ion. Dysprosium has a higher magnetic susceptibility than gadolinium, offering advantages in application on first pass MR studies. In this use, these compounds act as "negative" contrast agents, creating in vivo a small localized magnetic field gradient which causes a decrease in signal intensity in the perfused tissue on MR. Images are acquired on a rapid dynamic time frame immediately following bolus intravenous injection. Both Dy HP-DO3A and Dy DTPA-BMA[60,61] have been evaluated in animal studies, with limited clinical trials. The ability to assess brain and myocardial perfusion has been demonstrated.

For first pass brain studies, it is principally the T2* effect of the contrast media which is observed during bolus transit. Both gadolinium and dysprosium chelates have been used successfully in this application, at least in experimental investigation. In regard to dysprosium chelates, reports exist to date only with formulations of Dy HP-DO3A (figure 23)

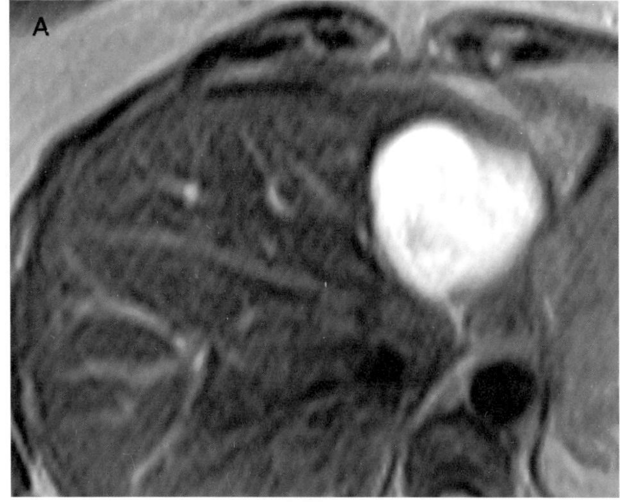

Figure 24. Liver hemangioma, illustrating improved lesion characterization following contrast administration. Pre-contrast (A) T2- and (B) T1-weighted scans are presented, together with (C) the post-contrast T1-weighted scan. The contrast dose was 0.1 mmol/kg, using a gadolinium chelate with extracellular distribution. A thick peripheral rim of intense enhancement is noted on (C) the post-contrast scan. This appearance is characteristic for a large hemangioma, as imaged on a non-dynamic post-contrast study. Dynamic imaging, viewing the temporal change in lesion enhancement within the first 15 minutes following contrast administration, offers further information in regard to differential diagnosis.

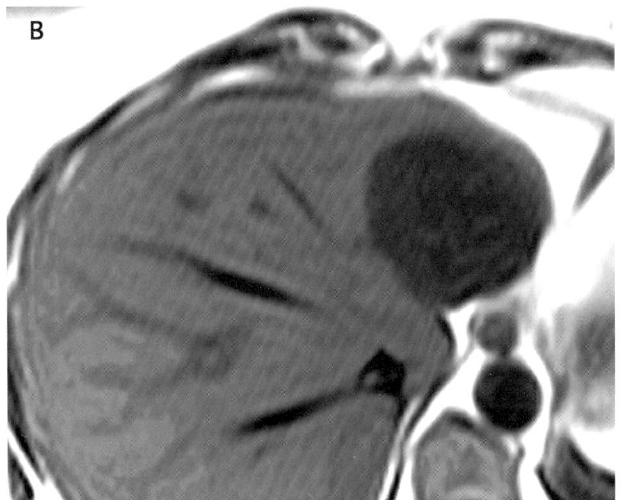

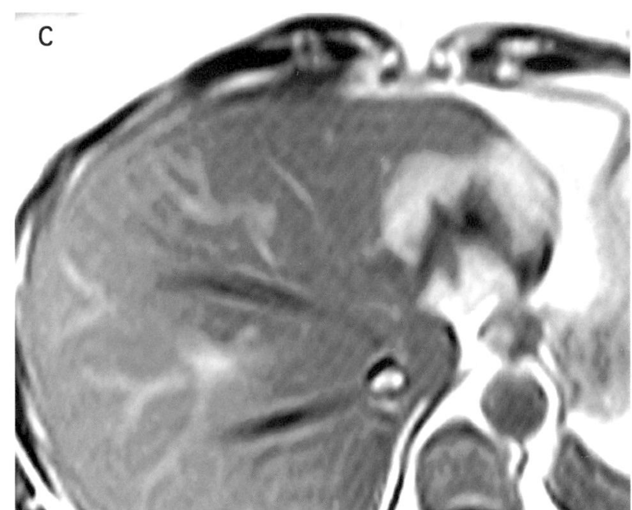

and Dy DTPA-BMA.[62,63] Improved results, specifically a greater magnitude of signal intensity change during first pass, are seen with dysprosium chelates as compared to the corresponding gadolinium chelates at high magnetic fields (1.5 to 2.0 T). This result is expected due to the higher T2 relaxivity and susceptibility effect of the dysprosium ion.

Liver Agents

In the development of liver contrast media, three major approaches have been explored.[64,65] The first is the targeting of water-soluble contrast media to hepatocytes, with examples being Gd BOPTA and Gd EOB-DTPA. These agents are taken up by hepatocytes and excreted into the bile, like bilirubin, by the organic anion transport mechanism. Unlike biliary iodinated contrast media, the high sensitivity of MR, combined with the increase in relaxivity inside hepatocytes, make such paramagnetic chelates very effective for improved liver lesion detection. Mn DPDP can be considered a variant of this class, with dechelation unfortunately demonstrated and enhancement properties in part dependent upon the presence of free metal ion (in this case manganese). The second approach is the targeting of agents (principally superparamagnetic iron oxide) to Kupffer cells in the liver. Problems have been encountered in development, due to limited knowledge regarding pharmacokinetics, difficulty in manufacturing, and cardiovascular tolerance. The third approach involves the application of macromolecular contrast media. The intent is to take advantage of differences in vessel permeability, vessel density, and lymphatics between normal and tumorous tissue. Research using this approach is still in its infancy.

In current clinical practice, liver imaging with contrast media is restricted to use of the gadolinium chelates with extracellular distribution. T1-weighted techniques are employed for detection of contrast enhancement (figure 24). Acquisition of dynamic post-contrast images, using a dose of 0.1 mmol/kg, improves lesion conspicuity and provides supplemental information regarding differential diagnosis (figure 25). The use of high dose (0.3 mmol/kg), combined

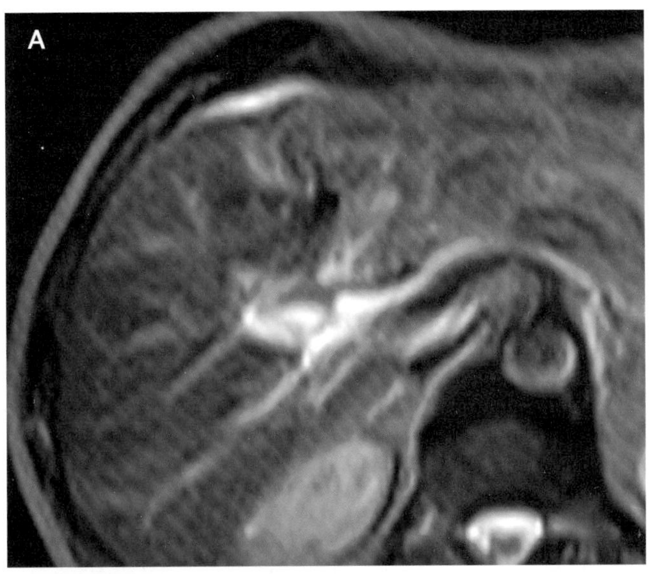

Figure 25. Residual Klatskin tumor, improved lesion identification on dynamic as opposed to non-dynamic post-contrast scans. (A) Pre-contrast T2, (B) pre- and (C) post-contrast T1, and (D) pre- and (E) dynamic post-contrast breathhold T1 scans are illustrated. The contrast agent is gadoteridol (Gd HP-DO3A), used at a dose of 0.1 mmol/kg dose. Residual tumor enhances to isointensity with respect to the normal liver on non-dynamic images. There is improved lesion conspicuity (arrow) on the dynamic breathhold post-contrast image. In the early dynamic time frame, most liver lesions enhance less than the normal parenchyma, and thus appear hypointense.

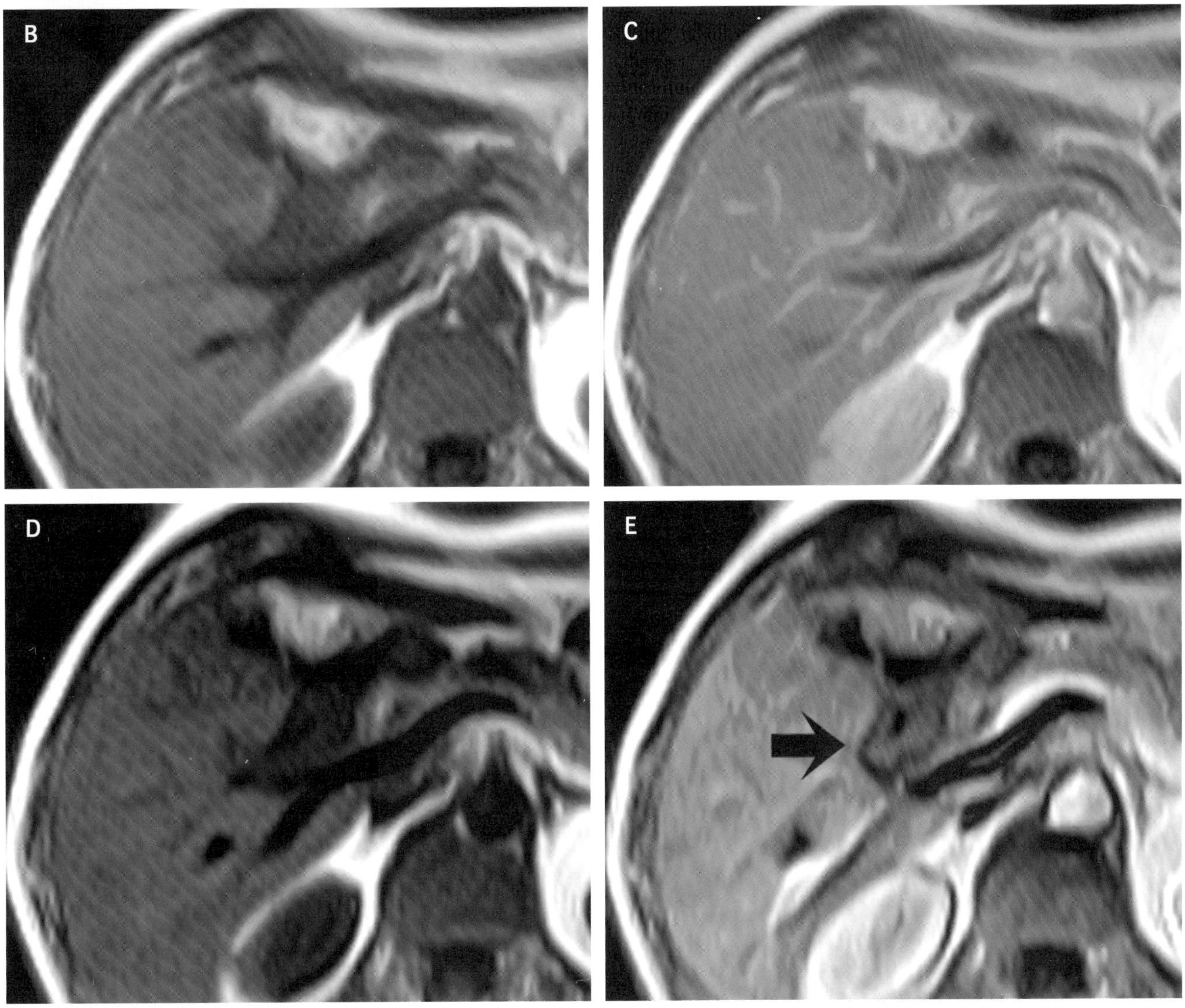

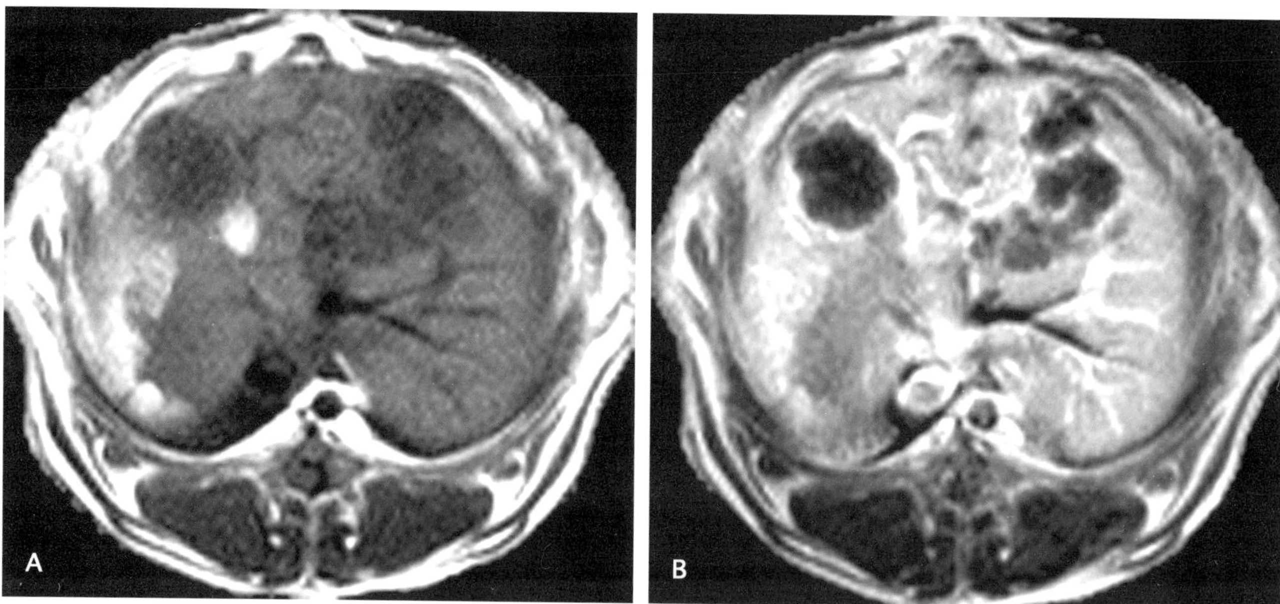

Figure 26. Contrast dose and lesion detectability in liver MR. Breathhold T1-weighted post-contrast scans are illustrated using two doses, (A) 0.1 and (B) 0.3 mmol/kg, in an animal model of liver metastatic disease. The agent is gadoteridol (Gd HP-DO3A). The metastases appear hypointense on both studies relative to the normal enhancing liver. Lesion conspicuity is highest on (B) the dynamic high dose (0.3 mmol/kg) post-contrast scan. Both scans were obtained in the first one to two minutes following intravenous contrast injection, the time period during which lesion visibility is typically greatest. *(From Runge VM, Pels Rijcken TH, Davidoff A, Wells JW, Stark DD. Contrast-enhanced MR imaging of the liver. Journal of Magnetic Resonance Imaging 1994;4:281-289).*

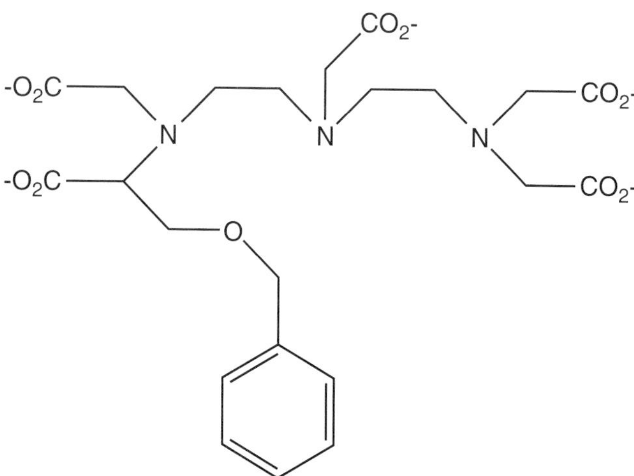

Figure 27. The chemical structure for BOPTA (4-carboxy-5,8,11-tris(carboxymethyl)-1-phenyl-2-oxa-5,8,11-triazatridecan-13-oic acid), the chelate in gadobenate dimeglumine.

with early dynamic imaging, can further improve lesion detectability (figure 26).

Two gadolinium based hepatobiliary agents (Gd BOPTA and Gd EOB-DTPA, figures 27 and 28) have received attention in Europe, with clinical trials currently in progress in the United States with Gd BOPTA. Other gadolinium containing agents are in pre-clinical development (figures 29 - 31). Attempts are also in progress to design agents with enhanced relaxivity by manipulation of electron relaxation times.[66]

Gd BOPTA

Preclinical studies with Gd BOPTA (MultiHance™, Bracco Diagnostics) demonstrated the agent to have low toxicity and to exhibit hepatobiliary uptake (figures 32 and 33).[67] The osmolality and viscosity of the agent in solutions at a clinically useful concentration are within acceptable physiologic range. Pharmacokinetic data reveals Gd BOPTA to have selectivity for the hepatobiliary system. Serious cardiovascular effects are absent, predicting safe clinical use. Toxicity

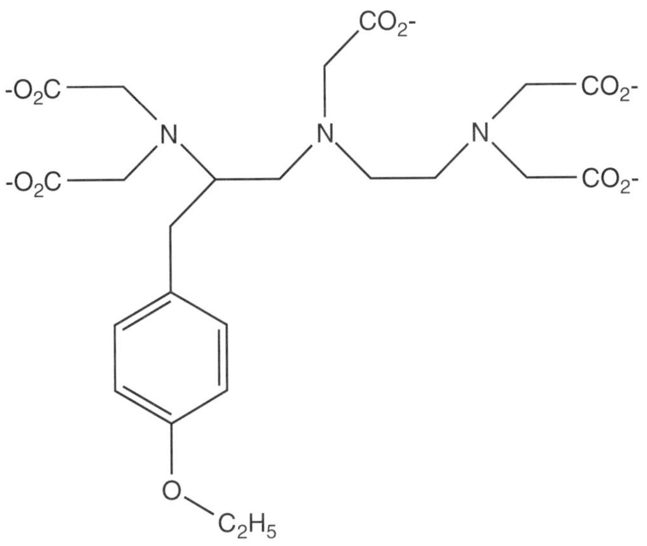

-O_2C CO_2- CO_2- N N N -O_2C CO_2- O C_2H_5

Figure 28. The chemical structure for EOB-DTPA, the chelate in gadolinium ethoxybenzyl diethylenetriaminepentaacetic acid.

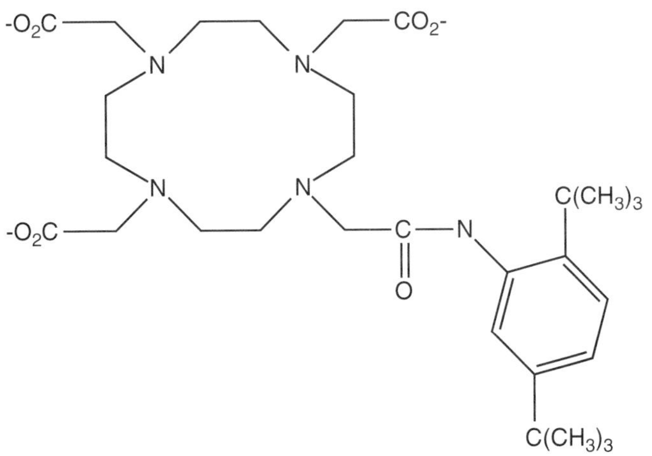

-O_2C N N CO_2- N N -O_2C C N O $C(CH_3)_3$ $C(CH_3)_3$

Figure 29. The chemical structure for 2,5-BPA-DO3A. When formulated as the gadolinium (Gd^{3+}) chelate, Gd 2,5-BPA-DO3A is a neutral or nonionic compound, carrying a net charge of zero. There is both hepatobiliary and renal excretion of this agent.

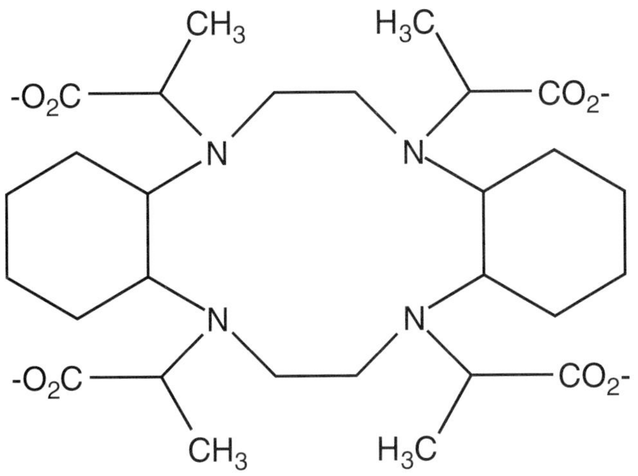

CH_3 H_3C -O_2C CO_2- N N N N -O_2C CO_2- CH_3 H_3C

Figure 30. The chemical structure for Cy_2-DOTMA. This macrocyclic chelate, formulated with the gadolinium ion, exhibits high hepatobiliary excretion. The basic structure of this molecule differs substantially from the hepatobiliary gadolinium chelates currently in clinical trials, Gd BOPTA and Gd EOB-DTPA.

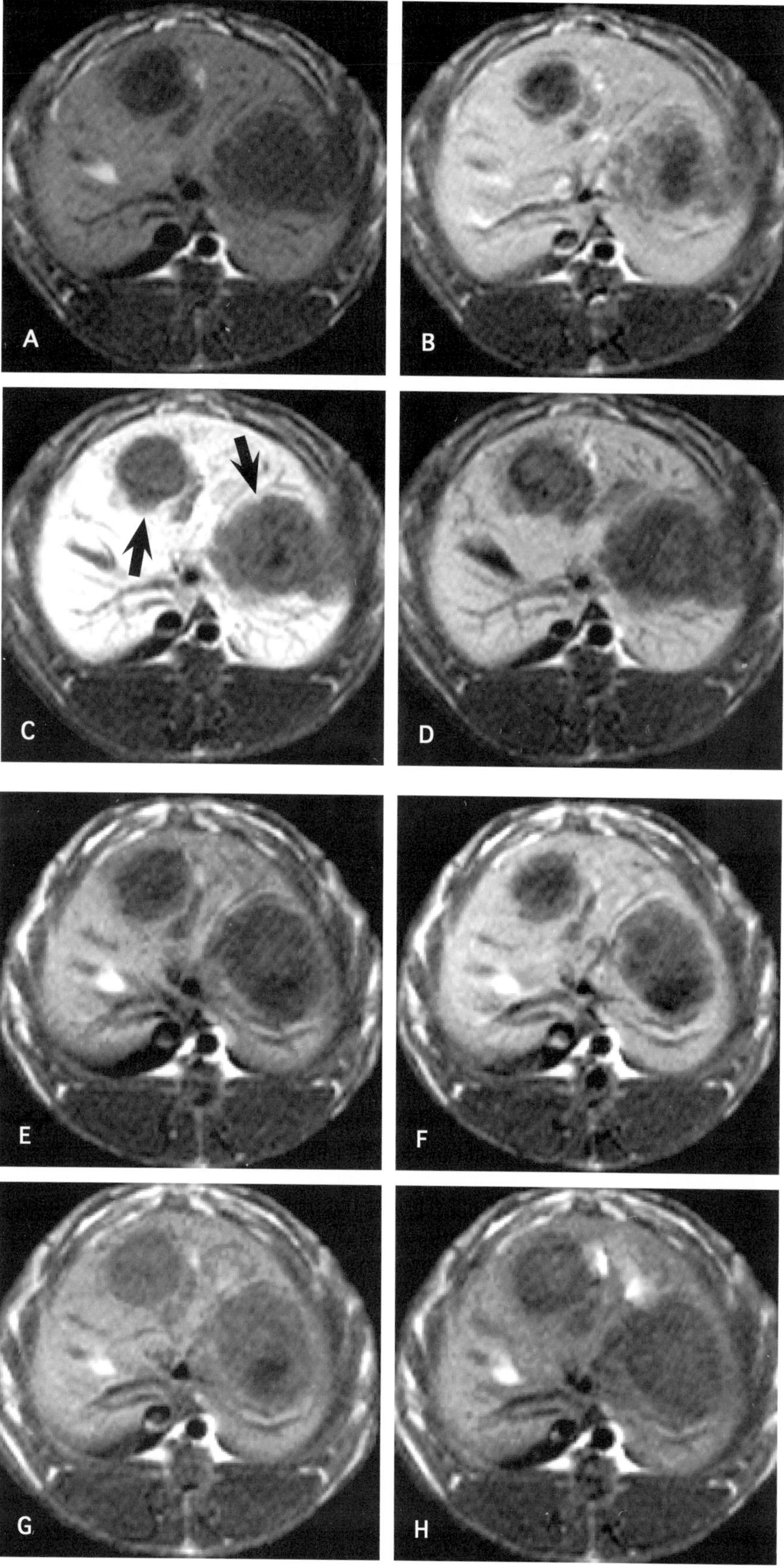

Figure 31. Improved visualization of liver metastases in an animal model following intravenous administration of 0.1 mmol/kg Gd 2,5-BPA-DO3A. Breathhold T1-weighted spin echo scans are illustrated (A) prior to and at (B) 1 minute, (C) 60 minutes, and (D) 180 minutes following contrast injection. Two large, low signal intensity, metastatic lesions (arrows) are best visualized on (C) the scan at 60 minutes following Gd 2,5-BPA-DO3A injection. Enhancement of normal liver parenchyma is greatest at this time, with little increase from baseline in the signal intensity of the metastatic lesions. For comparison, scans (E) prior to and at (F) 1 minute, (G) 60 minutes, and (H) 180 minutes following 0.1 mmol/kg Gd HP-DO3A injection are also illustrated. Although the metastatic lesions can be identified on these scans, the improvement in lesion visibility is substantially less (and occurs in the early dynamic time frame) with the extracellular chelate (Gd HP-DO3A). *(From Runge VM, Wells JW, Williams NM. Evaluation of gadolinium 2,5-BPA-DO3A, a new macrocyclic hepatobiliary chelate, in normal liver and metastatic disease on high field magnetic resonance imaging. Investigative Radiology 1996;31(1):11-16).*

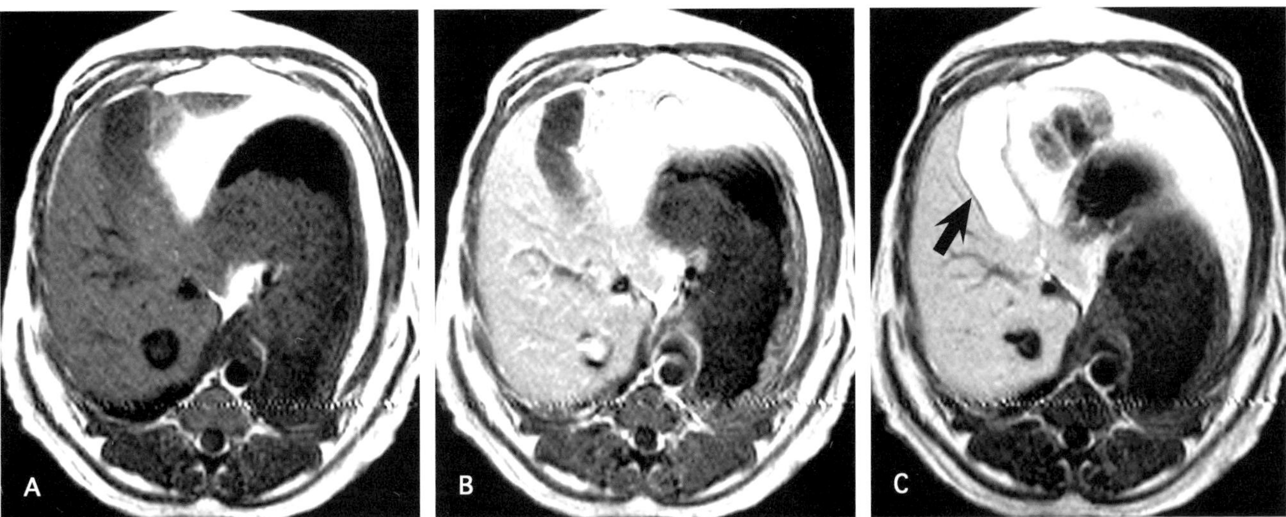

Figure 32. Enhancement of normal liver in the rhesus monkey following intravenous injection of 0.1 mmol/kg Gd BOPTA. Breathhold T1-weighted scans were acquired (A) prior to and at (B) two and (C) sixty minutes following contrast injection. Moderate enhancement of normal liver parenchyma is observed at two minutes, with a further increase by sixty minutes. Excretion of contrast into the gall bladder (arrow) is also noted on the sixty minutes post-contrast exam.

data show good systemic and neural tolerance. And last, but not least, animal imaging demonstrates hepatobiliary specificity, with prolonged enhancement of normal liver and high, persistent tumor-liver contrast.

Gd BOPTA has been evaluated in rats in models of both focal liver disease and acute myocardial ischemia.[68] Liver tumors were established by direct implantation and blood-borne dissemination. Acute myocardial ischemia was induced by occlusion of the lower anterior descending coronary artery. In the liver (using a dose of 0.25 mmol/kg), a large (370%), persistent (more than two hours) increase in tumor-liver contrast-to-noise ratio was observed. In the heart, Gd BOPTA administration produced enhancement of normal myocardium and differentiation from ischemic myocardium (on the basis of contrast-to-noise ratio) both greater and more persistent than following Gd DTPA administration. In an earlier liver study,[69] Gd BOPTA was also compared to Gd DTPA in the liver, evaluating doses of 0.25, 0.5, and 1.0 mmol/kg. Greater and longer lasting parenchymal enhancement was noted with Gd BOPTA, with the difference more evident at lower doses.

In phase I clinical studies in Germany, Gd BOPTA was evaluated at four doses — 0.005, 0.05, 0.1, and 0.2 mmol/kg.[46] Normal liver enhanced by 149% on gradient echo scans and 90% on spin echo scans 60 minutes after injection. Contrast enhancement of the liver remained virtually constant for 2 hours. Reported side effects included nausea, warmth at the injection site, and transient pruritus.

A preliminary report of phase II clinical trials with Gd BOPTA discussed results in 360 patients.[70] Within this population, 149 patients were evaluated for focal liver lesions, 127 for intracranial lesions, and 84 for acute myocardial infarction. The administered dose ranged from 0.05 to 0.2 mmol/kg. In liver imaging, liver-lesion contrast was maximal 60 to 120 minutes after injection. In the imaging of intracranial lesions, post-contrast studies provided better diagnostic information than pre-contrast studies in 95% of the studied population. In acute myocardial infarction, better localization and delineation of infarcted tissue was also obtained following Gd BOPTA administration in 95% of cases. In both brain and heart imaging, best lesion detectability occurred within the first 30 minutes following contrast administration. The safety and tolerability profile appears similar to other gadolinium chelates, with vomiting or nausea occurring in 1.6%. This was the most common adverse event reported, excluding altered sensation at the injection site and headache. The latter is likely related to the MR scan itself, and not the contrast injection.

One possible difficulty for hepatobiliary gadolinium chelates could be lesion detection in the presence of diffuse liver disease. To evaluate this concern, Gd BOPTA was studied in a liver tumor model with and without accompanying diffuse fatty liver disease.[71] Post-contrast scans were compared with conventional scans and chemical shift imaging. Fatty liver disease increased lesion conspicuity on unenhanced T1-weighted scans and decreased lesion conspicuity on unenhanced T2-weighted scans. Gd BOPTA was effective in both fatty and non-fatty liver for detection of liver tumors, and outperformed both chemical shift imaging and conventional pre-contrast MR scans.

An additional challenge to hepatobiliary agents is their performance across a range of tumor types. This was evalu-

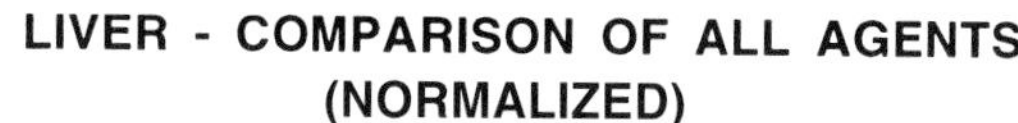

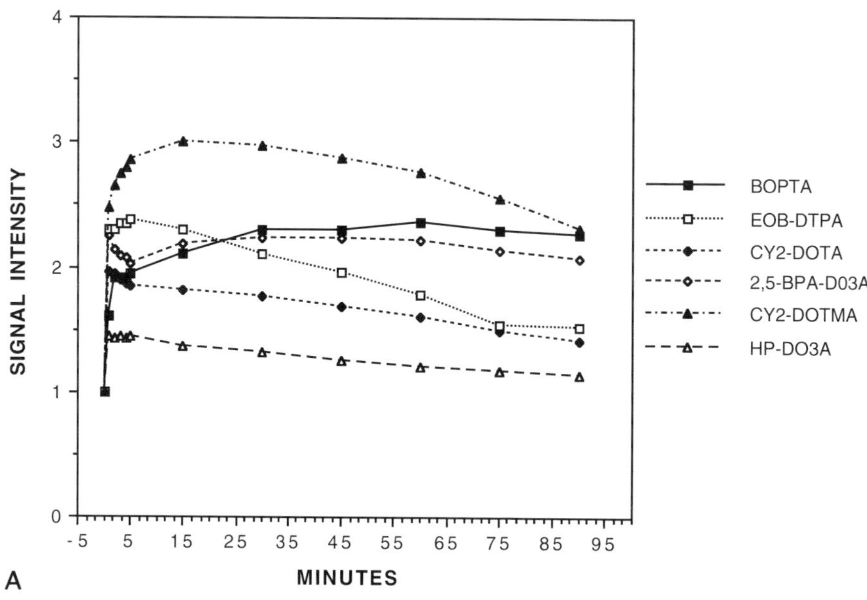

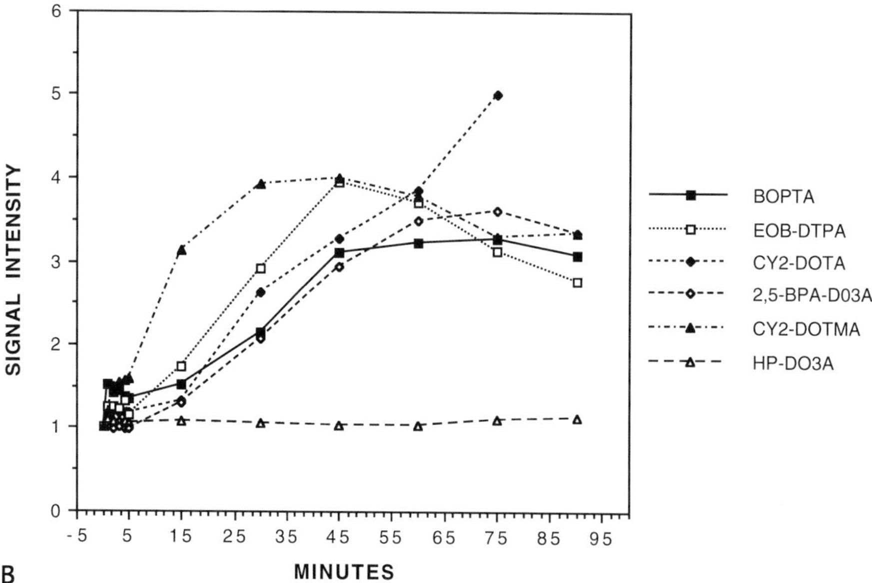

Figure 33. Comparison of enhancement for (A) normal liver parenchyma and (B) gall bladder in the rhesus monkey, using Gd BOPTA, Gd EOB-DTPA, Gd Cy_2-DOTA, Gd 2,5-BPA-DO3A, Gd Cy_2-DOTMA, and Gd HP-DO3A. All agents were supplied by Bracco Research USA. Results are normalized to a baseline value of one pre-contrast. With the exception of Gd HP-DO3A, which is excreted solely by glomerular filtration, the other five agents all demonstrate hepatobiliary uptake and excretion. Agents differ in regard to the magnitude of liver enhancement achieved, and the timing of this peak. Regarding the latter, for some agents, peak liver enhancement is noted immediately post-contrast, while for others this occurs after a delay from 20 to 60 minutes following administration. Caution should be exercised in interpreting the results shown in (B), since the gall bladder can fill at variable rates, given different physiologic conditions. The only firm conclusion that can be drawn from (B) is the grouping of agents into those with and without hepatobiliary excretion.

ated for Gd BOPTA in four tumor models, including both infiltrating and noninfiltrating lesions.[72] Despite differences between models in liver and lesion enhancement, improved tumor conspicuity was noted following Gd BOPTA injection independent of histologic type.

Gd BOPTA has also been evaluated for improved detection of acute myocardial infarction.[73] Using echo-planar technique and imaging during first pass, areas of acute myocardial infarction were well delineated following bolus Gd BOPTA injection. Depending upon the imaging technique chosen, inversion recovery or gradient echo, areas of myocardial infarction were delineated as cold spots (low signal intensity) upon a background of positively enhancing normal myocardium or hot spots (high signal intensity) upon a background of negatively enhancing normal myocardium.

In combination with fast imaging, Gd BOPTA can also be used to detect hypoperfused myocardium in the presence of critical coronary stenosis.[74] Myocardial signal intensity was tracked in dogs with a critical left circumflex coronary artery stenosis. Gd BOPTA was administered as a bolus, both in the basal state with stenosis and after infusion of dipyridamole. In the basal state, normal and hypoperfused myocardium could not be differentiated during first pass. Dipyridamole increased the left anterior descending flow and decreased the left circumflex flow. In this state, first pass studies with Gd BOPTA were able to identify the hypoperfused region.

Evaluation of the use of thrombolytic agents in acute myocardial infarction involves determination of the success of reperfusion. Assessment of the extent of infarction in the reperfused territory is also critical. The use of Gd BOPTA enhanced fast MR in defining the success of reperfusion has been investigated as well in an animal model.[75] Reperfused reversible myocardial injury, reperfused irreversible myocardial injury, and occlusive infarction were examined using echo-planar imaging. Both T1-weighted (IR-EPI) and susceptibility weighted (GR-EPI) imaging techniques were employed. After bolus contrast injection, normal myocardial signal sharply increased on IR-EPI and decreased on GR-EPI, followed by a gradual return towards baseline. In reperfused reversible myocardial injury, normal and previously ischemic areas were indistinguishable on first pass imaging with Gd BOPTA. However, reperfused irreversibly injured myocardium could be identified on both IR-EPI and GR-EPI, as a zone of delayed high signal on the former and a zone of moderate signal loss (but less than normal myocardium) on the latter. In regard specifically to the use of Gd BOPTA in reperfused infarcts, binding by the agent to extravasated proteins has been noted to improve enhancement and thus lesion conspicuity.[76] In occlusive infarction, no change in signal intensity in the ischemic region was noted on either IR-EPI or GR-EPI. In conclusion, the transit of Gd BOPTA monitored by fast MR can be used to differentiate between reperfused reversibly and reperfused irreversibly injured myocardium, as well as between occlusive and reperfused infarction.

Gd EOB-DTPA

In phase I clinical trials in Europe, Gd EOB-DTPA was evaluated at doses of 10, 25, 50, and 100 μmol/kg.[77] Forty-four healthy volunteers were studied in a double-blind, randomized trial, with a placebo as a control. Gd EOB-DTPA was described as well tolerated. Peak enhancement of normal liver parenchyma was noted in humans 20 minutes after contrast injection. As has been shown with Gd BOPTA, the positive contrast enhancement of normal liver with Gd EOB-DTPA is expected to result in relative negative enhancement of parenchymal lesions. However, studies in rats with liver hepatomas have shown that positive lesion enhancement (although rare) can occur after administration of Gd EOB-DTPA.[78] This was seen only in highly differentiated (grade I) hepatocellular carcinomas. Rim enhancement, corresponding to peritumoral malignant infiltration with sequestered normal hepatocytes, was seen in all implanted hepatomas. In sharp distinction to results with Gd EOB-DTPA, more differentiated tumors (specifically hepatocellular carcinomas) consistently demonstrate positive contrast enhancement with Mn DPDP.[79]

In rats, it has been shown that Gd EOB-DTPA is effectively eliminated by either the liver or kidney.[80] Dysfunction of either organ system was fully compensated by the remaining pathway of elimination. Tolerance of the agent has been well studied in the rat.[81] In a chemically induced model of hepatocellular carcinoma (HCC), also using the rat, contrast enhancement with Gd EOB-DTPA was compared to that on nuclear medicine studies with technetium-99m-labeled iminodiacetic acid (IDA).[82] The enhancement pattern of this tumor with Gd EOB-DTPA did not mirror that with Tc-99m-IDA. Lesions enhanced less than the liver with Gd EOB-DTPA, whereas with Tc-99m-IDA uptake in these differentiated HCCs exceeded that of the liver on delayed imaging.

Clinical utility for hepatobiliary gadolinium chelates such as Gd BOPTA and Gd EOB-DTPA has also been suggested in cholestasis, on the basis of animals studies.[83] By contrast administration, the distinction between obstructed and unobstructed liver may be possible on MR. The potential for assessment of excretory function, following liver transplantation, has also been suggested on the basis of animal studies.[84]

Plasma binding of Gd EOB-DTPA is low, despite the resemblance of its pharmacokinetics to that of biliary X-ray contrast media.[85] This may constitute a significant difference, and possible disadvantage, relative to Gd BOPTA. Hepatic uptake of Gd EOB-DTPA appears to take place by the or-

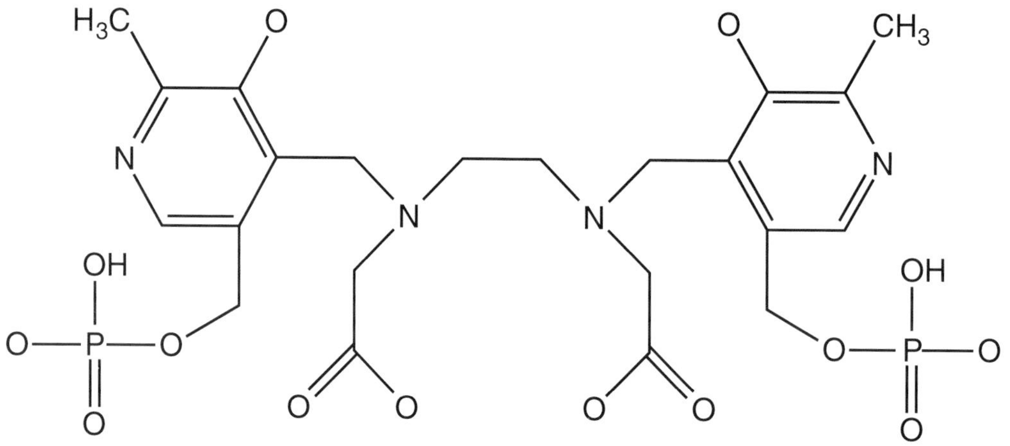

Figure 34. The ligand structure for Mn DPDP (manganese [II] N,N'-dipyridoxylethylenediamine-N,N'-diacetate-5,5'-bis[phosphate]).

ganic anion plasma membrane transport system.[86] Transport of the agent from the cytoplasm to the bile is limited by the capacity of the transport protein glutathione-S-transferase.[87]

Mn DPDP

Although the paramagnetic ion which is responsible for enhancement on MR is different with Mn DPDP (as compared with the gadolinium based hepatobiliary chelates), this agent was also designed to be incorporated into hepatocytes, with partial elimination by the bile (figure 34). Post-contrast, marked enhancement of normal liver parenchyma is seen, improving in some instances lesion conspicuity. In both German[88] and U.S.[89] trials with Mn DPDP, an increase in the number of lesions detected has been shown post-contrast. The presence (or absence) and pattern of enhancement have also been shown to be of value in differentiating hepatocellular from nonhepatocellular tumors.[90] In phase I studies, facial flushing and warmth were observed in 35 of 40 subjects. Dose dependent increases in heart rate and blood pressure were also observed.[91] Subsequent trials have been conducted with lower doses, lower concentrations and slower intravenous administration, with fewer side effects.[92] The high incidence of facial flushing during injection, the enhancement of intestinal mucosa and pancreas and the low thermodynamic stability constant of the complex, when considered together, suggest that substantial release of manganese from the chelate occurs in vivo.[93]

Particulate Compounds

Three major classes of iron particles exist with potential for application as contrast agents in liver MR. These are differentiated by average particle size and bodily distribution. Large superparamagnetic iron oxide particles, as in the formulation for AMI-25, are sequestered by the reticuloendothelial system and thus the Kupffer cells of the liver. When the average particle size is reduced, as in the formulations for AMI-227 and USPIO (ultrasmall superparamagnetic iron oxide), large quantities of the agent remain in the bloodstream for several days, with substantial uptake by the liver within the first few hours. A third class of agents, which includes AG-USPIO and the HS agent, has been created by the application of special surface coats, directing the particle to specific cell receptors. T2-weighted imaging techniques are used for detection of contrast agents in all three classes.

The larger superparamagnetic iron oxide particles contained in the AMI-25 formulation are sequestered following intravenous injection by the reticuloendothelial system (RES). In the initial clinical study with this agent, an improvement in lesion detection was demonstrated, with a greater number of liver lesions seen post-contrast. The size threshold for lesion detection was also reduced following contrast injection.[94] Two of the 15 patients in this trial had adverse reactions to drug administration, specifically transient hypotension and rash, with subsequent trials employing lower doses and slow infusion.[95] In a second study at 0.6 T, post-contrast imaging was shown to be statistically superior to both pre-contrast MR and enhanced CT, with 19% more lesions detected by post- as compared to pre-contrast MR and 36% more lesions as compared to CT.[96] Results at 1.5 T have been mixed, with the benefit of AMI-25 in one study "only marginal when post-contrast images were compared with heavily T2-weighted pre-contrast scans." [97] Marked liver signal reduction has however been observed post-contrast across the range of field strengths employed clinically (figure 35). European clinical trials with super-paramagnetic iron oxide in 467 patients concluded that contrast administration significantly increased the number of lesions visible, as well as the number of liver segments involved, with these results independent of field strength (0.5 to 1.5 T).[98]

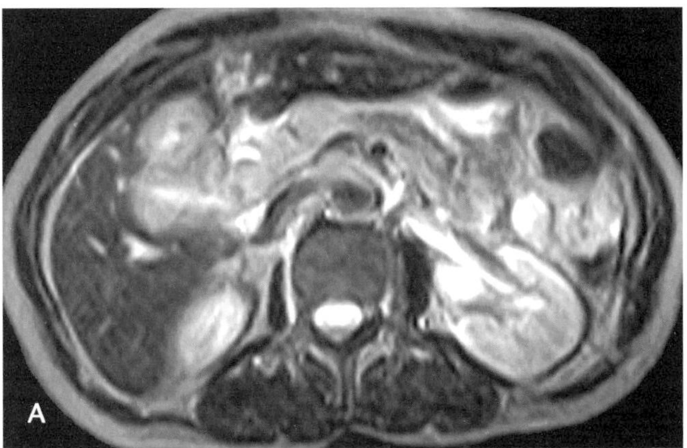

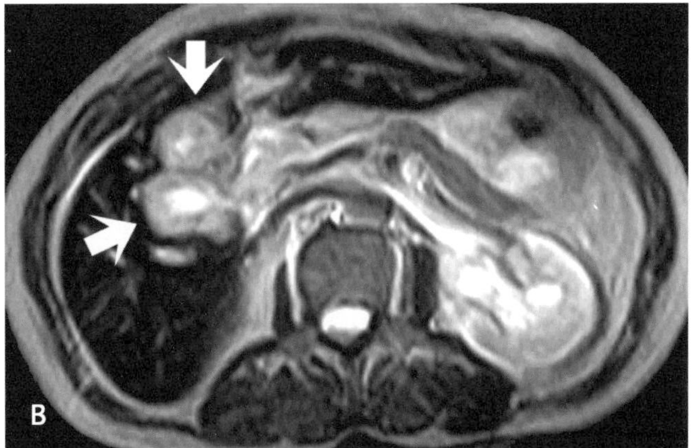

Figure 35. AMI-25, demonstrating improved conspicuity of liver metastases post-contrast. (A) T2-weighted pre-contrast and (B) one hour post-contrast scans at 1.5 T are presented in a patient with metastatic ovarian carcinoma. Following contrast administration, there is a marked reduction in the signal intensity of normal liver. The difference in signal intensity between the lesions (arrows) and normal liver is greatest on the post-contrast exam. The potential exists for detection of additional lesions with AMI-25, due to the marked signal intensity reduction post-contrast of normal liver parenchyma as compared to most lesions. *(From Runge VM, Pels Rijcken TH, Davidoff A, Wells JW, Stark DD. Contrast-enhanced MR imaging of the liver. Journal of Magnetic Resonance Imaging 1994;4:281-289).*

AMI-227 was initially evaluated in animal studies as a potential contrast agent for imaging of lymph nodes and bone marrow. Clinical studies were first initiated for the evaluation of lymph node involvement by metastatic disease (figure 36), and subsequently expanded to the evaluation of intrinsic liver lesions (figure 37). Potential advantages exist in liver imaging due to the blood-pool characteristics of the agent.[99]

Ultrasmall superparamagnetic iron oxide particles can be targeted to the asialoglycoprotein (ASG) receptor (AG-USPIO and the HS agent), providing improved liver enhancement at equivalent doses as compared to AMI-25.[100] Hepatocyte function can also be assessed with such agents. Clinical applications would potentially include improved lesion detectability, differentiation of liver lesions based on content of functional liver tissue,[101] and the evaluation of hepatic function in diffuse cellular diseases — such as hepatitis and cirrhosis.[102] Due to the lack of ASG receptors in the spleen, the agent preferentially effects liver signal intensity, in distinction to AMI-227. Following administration of the latter agent, a marked decrease in signal intensity is seen in both the liver and spleen. To date, no clinical trials have been performed.

Oral Contrast Media

Opacification of the gastrointestinal tract by oral and rectal contrast administration is important on MR to distinguish the bowel from other organs and pathologic lesions.[103] Two general classes of agents exist, those that cause an increase in signal intensity (or positive contrast enhancement), and those that cause a decrease in signal intensity (or negative contrast enhancement). Gadolinium chelates specifically formulated for oral contrast use fall within the first class of agents, and superparamagnetic iron oxides (SPIOs) within the second. Positive enhancement of the bowel contents can lead to image degradation. Motion of high signal intensity bowel contents, due to normal peristalsis, produces ghosting artifacts which can obscure normal structures as well as lesions. This specific problem is not encountered with negative agents. However, delineation of the bowel wall, and disease thereof, is best obtained following the administration of positive agents. Susceptibility artifacts from SPIOs can actually obscure visualization of the bowel wall. In addition to the contrast media described in the following paragraphs, limited studies have been performed with magnetite albumen microspheres[104] and perfluorocarbons.[105] Both of these agents cause a decrease in signal intensity within the bowel. Infant formula is also known to have high signal intensity on both Tl and T2-weighted scans, providing excellent visualization of the gastrointestinal tract in newborns.[106] Certain barium sulfate preparations have also been evaluated as negative agents.[107,108]

Gadolinium Chelates

In an animal study, dilute Gd HP-DO3A (ProHance®) and a mixture of dilute Gd HP-DO3A with Sustacal (Meadjohnson, Evansville, IN), a nutritional drink, were evaluated as potential oral contrast agents.[109] The concentration of Gd HP-DO3A was 2.0 mmolar. Hyperintense, positive enhancement of the gastrointestinal tract was noted following ingestion of each preparation. Medical imaging applications of both for-

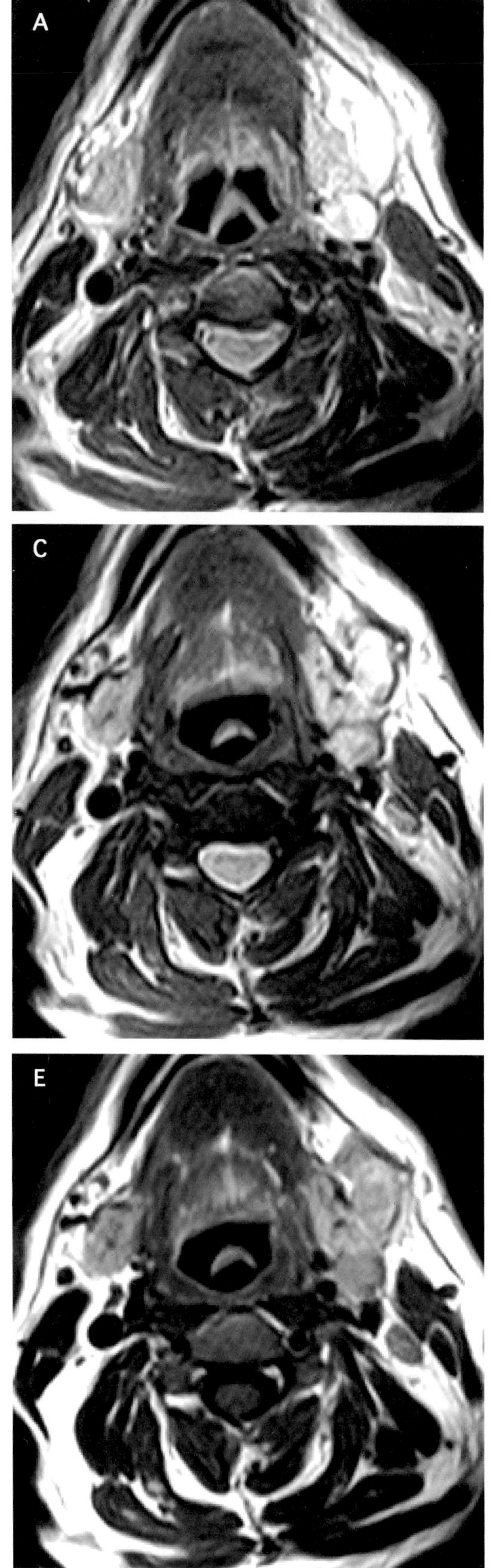

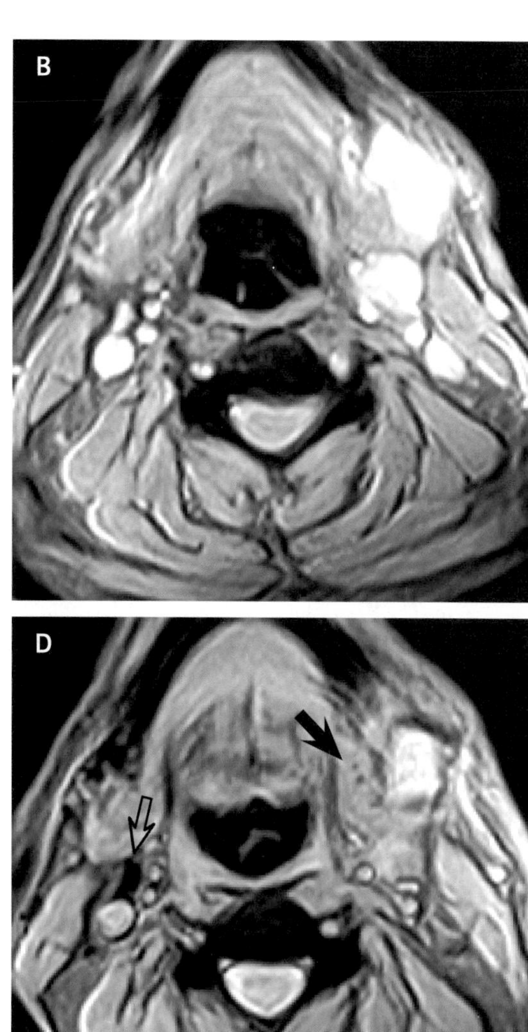

Figure 36. AMI-227, identification of lymph node involvement by neoplastic disease. The patient presents with recurrent squamous cell carcinoma, metastatic to lymph nodes in the neck. (A, B) Pre- and (C, D) post-contrast T2-weighted scans, with (A, C) spin echo and (B, D) gradient echo techniques, are presented. Post-contrast scans were acquired after a 24 hour delay. (E) The pre-contrast T1-weighted scan at the same anatomic level is also shown. A small lymph node (open arrow, D), normal in size and just anterior to the right jugular vein, displays a prominent decrease in signal intensity post-contrast. This indicates normal uniform uptake of the agent by the node. A confluent group of enlarged nodes (arrow, D) on the left does not display a substantial decrease in signal intensity post-contrast, characteristic for tumor involvement. A solitary enlarged node posterior to the jugular vein on the left displays similar features, also consistent with metastatic involvement. The negative enhancement of normal nodes (which appear low signal intensity post-contrast) is more evident on the gradient echo scan, as opposed to the spin echo scan. This is consistent with the higher sensitivity of the gradient echo scan to magnetic susceptibility effects.

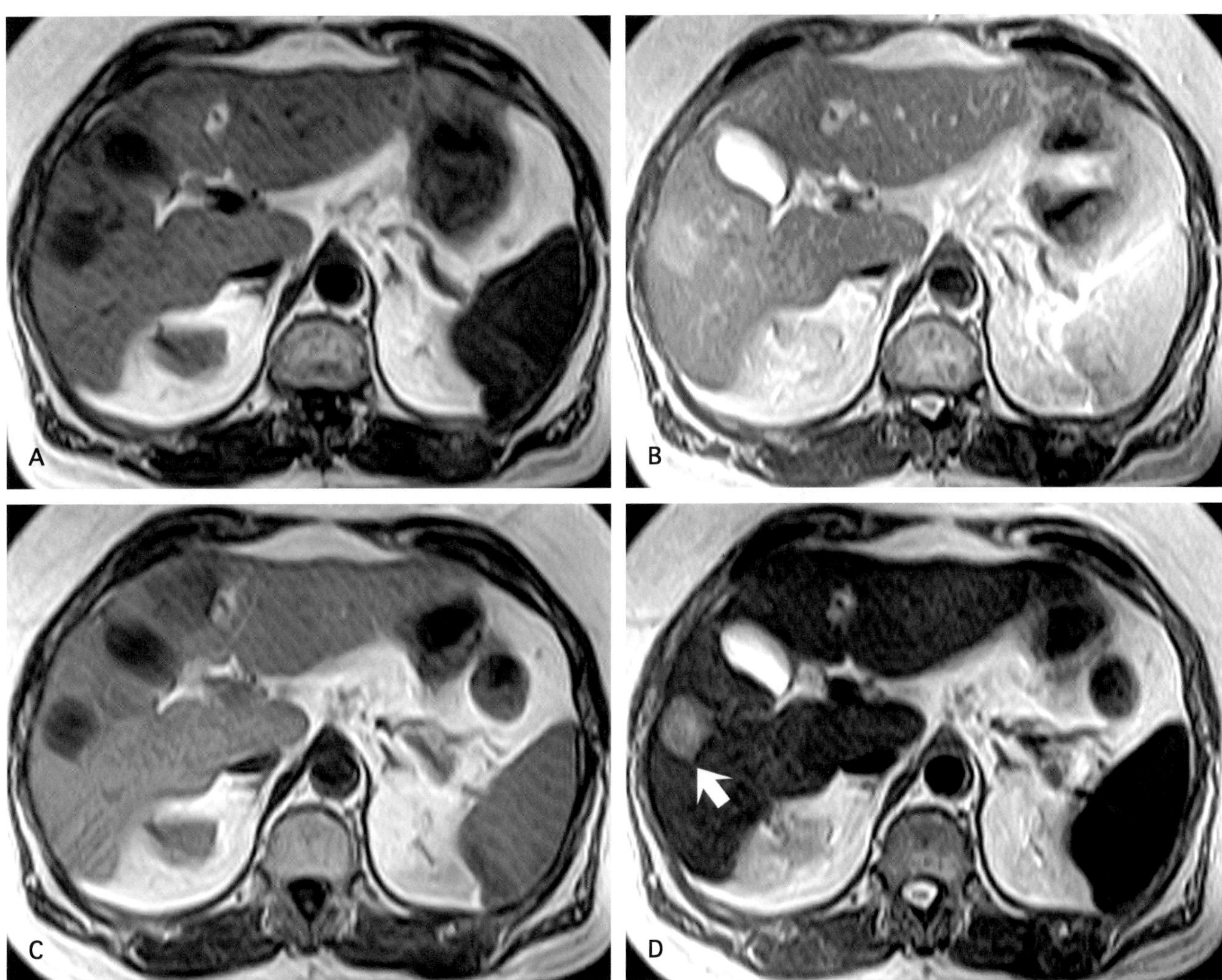

Figure 37. AMI-227, demonstrating improved conspicuity of a liver metastasis post-contrast. T1- and T2-weighted scans are shown from (A, B) prior to and (C, D) one hour following contrast administration. A small lesion with long T1 and T2 relaxation values is noted in the posterior segment of the right lobe. Following contrast injection, there is marked reduction in the signal intensity of normal liver parenchyma on (D) the T2-weighted scan. This improves visualization of the lesion (arrow), which is hyperintense, on the T2-weighted scan. There is a slight increase in signal intensity of the normal liver on the T1-weighted scan following contrast administration, which does not substantially improve lesion visualization. *(From Runge VM, Pels Rijcken TH, Davidoff A, Wells JW, Stark DD. Contrast-enhanced MR imaging of the liver. Journal of Magnetic Resonance Imaging 1994;4:281-289).*

mulations appear feasible. Hypointense, negative enhancement was noted on T2-weighted images.

On occasion, undesirable heterogeneous enhancement of the bowel is noted following oral administration of water soluble gadolinium chelates. To investigate this phenomenon, Gd HP-DO3A (ProHance®) was administered orally to animals at a concentration of 2.0 mmolar.[110] Prominent positive enhancement within the lumen was noted on T1-weighted images. The heterogeneity of signal enhancement was investigated by sampling the gastrointestinal fluid at various times following oral ingestion and at different locations along the gastrointestinal tract. T1 and T2 relaxation times, gadolinium ion concentration, and the viscosity of the bowel contents all contributed to the observed heterogeneity of signal enhancement.

Gd DTPA has been evaluated in clinical trials in Europe[111,112] as an oral contrast agent. The formulation used was a dilution of Gd DTPA in water and mannitol. Bowel opacification permitted ready differentiation between bowel loops and intra-abdominal masses. Pathologic thickening of the bowel wall could also be identified. Prior to contrast use, the bowel and its contents were isointense on T1-weighted images relative to soft tissue and muscle. After Gd DTPA ingestion, the bowel contents were of homogeneous high signal

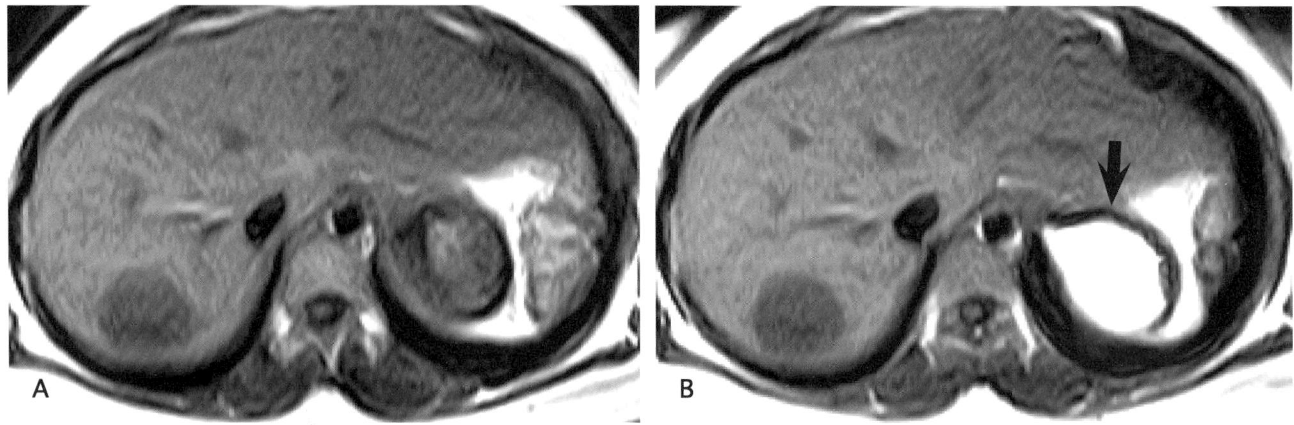

Figure 38. Lumenhance. Breathhold T1-weighted scans, (A) prior to and (B) following oral contrast administration, are presented at the level of the body of the stomach. A large liver lesion is noted, presumed to represent a metastasis from known islet cell pancreatic carcinoma. Following contrast ingestion, there is good opacification of the stomach (arrow) by the agent, which has high signal intensity on T1-weighted imaging.

intensity, and easily differentiated from fecal material (with intermediate signal intensity) and air (with low signal intensity). In one study, the delineation of abdominal abnormalities was improved following oral Gd DTPA ingestion in 19 of 32 MR exams.[113] Diarrhea was reported as a complication, presumably due to the mannitol included in the oral preparation. In a larger series of 150 exams, abdominal distention and diarrhea were noted as side effects in 25% of patients.[114]

Improved delineation of the pancreas has also been noted on exams following oral contrast administration. In 52 patients studied both before and after oral Gd DTPA ingestion, there was improved visualization of the pancreatic head, body, and tail on post-contrast scans in 17, 8, and 6 of 25 patients, respectively, with pancreatic disease.[115] Specifically noted was the improved delineation of pancreatic pseudocysts and bowel wall invasion. In a study of 18 patients with pelvic cancer, improved identification of tumor and differentiation from the intestines was found in 54% after oral contrast administration.[116]

Manganese Based Agents

A manganese chloride-based oral contrast agent (Lumenhance, Bracco Diagnostics, Princeton, NJ) has also been evaluated on MR.[117] Volunteers were studied before and after oral ingestion of 900 ml using three different concentrations (20, 40, and 60 mg/L Mn^{2+}). Opacification was evaluated at three different anatomic sites — the stomach, middle of the small bowel, and the ileocecal region. There were no adverse events. A minimal rise in blood levels of manganese was noted at 6 hours, with a return to baseline by 24 hours. Good-to-excellent hyperintense bowel marking was noted with all three concentrations on T1-weighted images (figure 38). On T2-weighted images, the two higher concentrations provided improved hypointense bowel marking relative to the lower concentration.

Particulate Agents

In a recent clinical study, Gd DTPA was compared with oral magnetic particles (OMP, Nycomed AS, Oslo, Norway) for effectiveness in opacification of the bowel.[118] These agents differ substantially in that Gd DTPA acts as a positive gastrointestinal contrast agent and OMP as a negative agent. The study was conducted in patients referred for MR of the abdomen. The diagnostic accuracy of MR following oral contrast administration was similar to CT in both groups, but substantially higher than plain MR. With OMP, the contrast between the bowel lumen (containing contrast media) and surrounding fat was superior to that with Gd DTPA. Motion artifacts from the bowel contents were absent in the OMP group. The overall accuracy in diagnosis was however higher with Gd DTPA, due to underfilling of the distal bowel with OMP. Gd DTPA was administered both orally and rectally, whereas OMP was administered only orally. Fewer side effects were noted with Gd DTPA, and patients commented that the taste of the formulation was more pleasant (as compared to OMP). Both contrast media were deemed suitable for study of the upper abdomen.

Possible limitations to the use of superparamagnetic particles as oral contrast agents have been noted.[119] Susceptibility induced artifacts have been described since the first imaging evaluations. The concentration of such a negative contrast agent needs to be carefully chosen, so that a signal void is achieved in the desired area without artifacts being induced. If the concentration is too high, artifacts occur in the volume surrounding the contrast agent.

A number of additional clinical trials using OMP have been published in the scientific literature. In two, the dose employed was 0.5 g/l, with the crystals of iron oxide administered in 800 ml as a viscous suspension. This preparation was used in order to obtain uniform distribution of the particles, which is important for effective bowel opacification and minimization of susceptibility artifacts. In studies of 40 patients[120] and 35 patients,[121] respectively, the general contrast effect was described as satisfactory, and an improvement in image quality and diagnostic confidence noted on post-contrast scans. Radiologic diagnosis was only possible following contrast use in one of the two trials in nearly half of the patients. Another small phase III clinical trial (35 patients) further substantiated the utility of OMP.[122] Bowel loops and abdominal organs were more easily recognized after oral contrast ingestion. Also observed was that general image quality improved due to fewer bowel-related artifacts. In regard to scan technique, gradient echo images were not as useful as spin echo images, due to problems with susceptibility artifacts. Evaluation in the future of gradient echo scans with shorter TEs or fast spin echo sequences was suggested.

The most substantial work to date with OMP was reported in 1993, a summary of results from phase II trials in 216 patients in Europe.[123] Various abdominal pathologies were evaluated. Two concentrations were employed, 0.1 g/l for ultralow field and 0.5 g/l for mid/high field. The ingested volume was 300 to 800 ml. The agent was well tolerated. There were no serious adverse events and patient acceptability was good. Use of a viscous formulation proved successful in achieving homogeneous distribution throughout the gastrointestinal tract. Susceptibility artifacts were minimal. Post-contrast diagnostic information was reported as improved in 70% of patients.

A different oral preparation of superparamagnetic iron oxide particles, AMI-121 (Advanced Magnetics Inc, Cambridge, Massachusetts), has also been evaluated. Like OMP, this preparation creates local inhomogeneities in the magnetic field leading to a loss of signal intensity.[124] After oral administration, the bowel lumen appears dark or low signal intensity. The agent is not absorbed by the bowel and is excreted by 24 hours after administration. Phase III clinical trials have been completed.

Conclusion

Four extracellular gadolinium chelates, all with renal excretion, are approved in various countries across the world for clinical use. Within this group, approval for high dose (up to 0.3 mmol/kg) exists in certain instances, for example with Gd HP-DO3A (ProHance®). With linear chelates, including specifically Gd DTPA and Gd DTPA-BMA, the degree to which release of free gadolinium ion occurs is greater due to lower in vivo stability.[17,18] Such data suggests a higher safety margin for macrocyclic (ring) chelates, such as Gd HP-DO3A and Gd DOTA. For bolus injection, nonionic (neutral) chelates are favored, with this group also including Gd HP-DO3A.

Applications of MR contrast media have expanded with the development of new imaging hardware and software. Owing to the emergence of dynamic imaging, the clinical use of MR in the heart, upper abdomen, and for the study of brain perfusion is likely to be much more common in the future. Use of high dose (0.3 mmol/kg) in metastatic disease and other brain pathology is another relatively new expanding area. In addition to the agents described, other compounds exist which are currently undergoing evaluation in both academia and industry.

Hepatobiliary gadolinium chelates, such as Gd BOPTA, are likely to be approved in the not too distant future. Preliminary results in regard to efficacy are quite favorable. In the interim prior to such approval, the use of the extracellular gadolinium chelates, combined with early dynamic breathhold imaging, offers valuable additional diagnostic information in imaging of the upper abdomen. Oral contrast agents are also likely to be approved in the near future. Within this class, both negative and positive agents exist. The former subgroup marks the bowel with high signal intensity, and the latter with low signal intensity.

As with magnetic resonance itself, the development of contrast media has far exceeded expectations. In the future, MR contrast media will continue to play a major role in clinical imaging and future diagnostic advance.[125,126]

Portions of this chapter are reprinted with permission from Runge VM, Pels Rijcken TH, Davidoff A, Wells JW, Stark DD. Contrast enhanced MR imaging of the liver. *J Magn Reson Imaging* 1994;4:281-289.

References

1. Runge VM, Stewart RG, Clanton JA, et al. Potential oral and intravenous paramagnetic NMR contrast agents. Radiology 1983; 147:789-791.

2. Weinmann HJ, Brasch RC, Press WR, Wesbey GE. Characteristics of gadolinium-DTPA complex: a potential NMR contrast agent. AJR 1984;142:619-624.

3. Oksendal AN, Hals PA. Biodistribution and toxicity of MR imaging contrast media. J Magn Reson Imaging 1993;3:157-165.

4. Runge VM. Magnetic resonance imaging contrast agents. Current Opinion in Radiology 1992;4:3-12.

5. Russel EJ, Schiable TF, Dillon W, et al. Multicenter double blind placebo controlled study of gadopentetate dimeglumine as an MR contrast agent: evaluation in patients with cerebral lesions. AJR 1989;152:813-823.

6. Runge VM, Carollo BR, Wolf CR, et al. Gd DTPA: a review of clinical indications in central nervous sytem magnetic resonance imaging. Radiographics 1989;9:929-958.

7. Runge VM, Awh MH, Bittner DF. Neoplastic disease of the spine on MR. MRI Decisions International 1995;2:11-17.
8. Ross JS, Modic MT, Masaryk TJ, et al. Assessment of extradural degenerative disease with Gd DTPA enhanced MR imaging: correlation with surgical and pathologic findings. AJR 1990;154:151-157.
9. Parizel PM, Baleriaux D, Rodesh G, et al. Gd DTPA enhanced MR imaging of spinal tumors. AJR 1989;152:1087-1096.
10. Hudgins PA, Elster AD, Runge VM, et al. Efficacy and safety of gadopentetate dimeglumine in the evaluation of patients with a suspected tumor of the extracranial head and neck. J Magn Reson Imaging 1993;3:345-349.
11. Zoarski GH, Lufkin RB, Bradley WG, et al. Multicenter trial of gadoteridol, a nonionic gadolinium chelate, in patients with suspected head and neck pathology. AJNR 1993;14:955-961.
12. Edelman RR, Mattle HP, Atkinson DJ, et al. Cerebral blood flow: assessment with dynamic contrast enhanced T2* weighted MR imaging at 1.5 T. Radiology 1990;176:211-220.
13. Runge VM, Kirsch JE, Wells JW, et al. Visualization of blood-brain barrier disruption on MR images of cats with acute cerebral infarction: value of administering a high dose of contrast material. AJR 1994;162:431-435.
14. Schubeus P, Schoerner W. Dosing of Gd DTPA in MR imaging of intracranial tumors. In: Workshop on contrast enhanced magnetic resonance imaging. Napa, Calif: Society of Magnetic Resonance in Medicine, 1991:109-123.
15. Tweedle MF. Nonionic or neutral? Radiology 1991;178:891.
16. Cacheris WP, Quay SC, Rocklage SM. The relationship between thermodynamics and the toxicity of gadolinium complexes. Magn Reson Imaging 1990;8:467-481.
17. Wedeking P, Kumar K, Tweedle MF. Dissociation of gadolinium chelates in mice: relationship to chemical characteristics. Magn Reson Imaging 1992;10:641-648.
18. Tweedle MF. Physicochemical properties of gadoteridol and other magnetic resonance contrast agents. Invest Radiol 1992;27S:1-6.
19. Sherry AD. Lanthanide chelates as magnetic resonance imaging contrast agents. J Less Common Metals 1989;149:133-141.
20. Tweedle MF, Hagan JJ, Kumar K, et al. Reaction of gadolinium chelates with endogenously available ions. Magn Reson Imaging 1991;9:409-415.
21. Gennaro MC, Aime S, Santucci E, et al. Complexes of diethylenetriaminepentaacetic acid as contrast agents in NMR image. Computer simulation of equilibria in human blood plasma. Anal Chim Acta 1990;233:85-100.
22. Carr JJ. Magnetic resonance contrast agents for neuroimaging. Safety issues. Neuroimaging Clin N Am 1994;4:43-54.
23. Goldstein HA, Kashanian FK, Blumetti RF, et al. Safety assessment of gadopentetate dimeglumine in U.S. clinical trials. Radiology 1990;174:17-23.
24. Runge VM, Gelblum DY. The role of gadolinium diethylenetriaminepentaacetic acid in the evaluation of the central nervous system. Magn Reson Q 1990;6:85-107.
25. Bydder GM. Clinical use of contrast media in magnetic resonance imaging. Br J Hosp Med 1990;43:149-152.
26. Powers TA, Partain CL, Kessler RM, et al. Central nervous system lesions in pediatric patients: Gd DTPA enhanced MR imaging. Radiology 1988;169:723-726.
27. Niendorf HP, Seifert W. Serum iron and serum bilirubin after administration of Gd DTPA dimeglumine: a pharmacologic study in healthy volunteers. Invest Radiol 1988;23:S275-280.
28. Novak Z, Thurmond AS, Ross PL, et al. Gadolinium DTPA transplacental transfer and distribution in fetal tissue in rabbits. Invest Radiol 1993;28:828-830.
29. Schmeidl U, Maravilla KR, Gerlach R, Dowling CA. Excretion of gadopentetate dimeglumine in human breast milk. AJR 1990;154:1305-1306.
30. Wolf GL. Current status of MR imaging contrast agents: special report. Radiology 1989;172:709-710.
31. Kanal E, Applegate GR, Gillen CP. Review of adverse reactions, including anaphylaxis, in 4,260 intravenous bolus injections. Radiology 1990;177(P):159 (abstract).
32. Weiss KL. Severe anaphylactoid reaction after IV Gd DTPA. Magn Reson Imaging 1990;8:817-818.
33. SMRM Workshop. Contrast enhanced magnetic resonance. Discussion section. Mag Reson Med 1991;22:229-232.
34. Valk J, Algra PR, Hazenberg CJ, et al. A double-blind, comparative study of gadodiamide injection and gadopentetate dimeglumine in MRI of the central nervous system. Neuroradiology 1993;35:173-177.
35. Gibby WA, Puttagunta NR, Smith GT, Clark S. Human comparative studies of zinc and copper transmetallation in serum and urine of MRI contrast agents. Proceedings of the Society of Magnetic Resonance, second meeting, August 1994:389.
36. Sze G, Brant-Zawadzki M, Haughton VM, et al. Multicenter study of gadodiamide injection as a contrast agent in MR imaging of the brain and spine. Radiology 1991;181:693-699.
37. Greco A, McNamara MT, Lanthiez P, et al. Gadodiamide injection: nonionic gadolinium chelate for MR imaging of the brain and spine. Phase II-III clinical trial. Radiology 1990;176:451-456.
38. Cohan RH, Leder RA, Herzberg AJ, et al. Extravascular toxicity of two magnetic resonance contrast agents. Preliminary experience in the rat. Invest Radiol 1991;26:224-226.
39. Runge VM, Kirsch JE, Burke VJ, et al. High-dose gadoteridol in MR imaging of intracranial neoplasms. J Magn Reson Imaging 1992;2:9-18.
40. Yuh WTC, Engelken JD, Muhonen MG, et al. Experience with high dose gadolinium MR imaging in the evaluation of brain metastases. AJNR 1992;13:335-345.
41. Yuh WTC, Fisher DJ, Runge VM, et al. Phase III multicenter trial of high dose gadoteridol in MR evaluation of brain metastases. AJNR 1994;15:1037-1051.
42. Mayr NA, Yuh WTC, Muhonen MG, et al. Cost effectiveness of high dose MR contrast studies in the evaluation of brain metastases. AJNR 1994;15:1053-1061.
43. Brugieres P, Gaston A, Degryse HR, et al. Randomized double blind trial of the safety and efficacy of two gadolinium complexes (Gd DTPA and Gd DOTA). Neuroradiology 1994;36:27-30.
44. Vogl TJ, Friebe CE, Mack MG, et al. MR evaluation of brain metastases: comparison of standard and high-dose Gadobutrol versus standard-dose Gd DTPA. Proceedings of the Society of Magnetic Resonance, second meeting, August 1994:548.
45. Coveney JR, Robison RO, Leese PT. Phase 1 study of Optimark (gadoversetamide injection) in healthy volunteers. Proceedings of the Society of Magnetic Resonance, second meeting, August 1994:905.
46. Vogl TJ, Pegios W, McMahon C, et al. Gadobenate dimeglumine — a new contrast agent for MR imaging: preliminary evaluation in healthy volunteers. AJR 1992;158:887-892.
47. Caramia F, Huang Z, Hamberg LM, et al. Identification of peripheral areas of cerebral flow-volume mismatch in focal transient

ischemia using susceptibility contrast dynamic MRI. Proceedings of the Society of Magnetic Resonance, second meeting, August 1994:1383.
48. Runge VM, Wells JW, Nelson KL, Linville PM. MR imaging detection of cerebral metastases with a single injection of high-dose gadoteridol. J Magn Reson Imaging 1994;4:669-673.
49. Runge VM, Gelblum DY, Pacetti ML, et al. Gd HP-DO3A in clinical MR of the brain. Radiology 1990;177:393-400.
50. Yuh WT, Fisher DJ, Engelken JD, et al. MR evaluation of CNS tumors: dose comparison study with gadopentetate dimeglumine and gadoteridol. Radiology 1991;180:485-491.
51. Yuh WTC, Nguyen HD, Tali ET, et al. Delineation of gliomas with various doses of MR contrast material. AJRN 1994;15:983-989.
52. Vogl TJ, Mack MG, Juergens M, et al. MR diagnosis of tumors of the head and neck: comparison of high dose gadodiamide injection and single dose Gd DTPA in the same patient. Proceedings of the Society of Magnetic Resonance, second meeting, August 1994:1439.
53. Simonson TM, Yuh WTC, Michalson LS, et al. Triple dose contrast studies in evaluation of spinal cord lesions. Proceedings of the Society of Magnetic Resonance, second meeting, August 1994:1447.
54. Mathews VP, King JC, Elster AD, Hamilton CA. Cerebral infarction: effects of dose and magnetization transfer saturation at gadolinium-enhanced MR imaging. Radiology 1994;190:547-552.
55. Runge VM, Kirsch JE, Lee C. Contrast-enhanced MR angiography. J Magn Reson Imaging 1993;3:233-239.
56. Runge VM, Kirsch JE, Wells JW, Woolfolk CE. Assessment of cerebral perfusion by first-pass, dynamic, contrast-enhanced, steady-state free-precession MR imaging: an animal study. AJR 1993;160: 593-600.
57. Kucharczyk J, Vexler ZS, Roberts TP, et al. Echoplanar perfusion sensitive MR imaging of acute cerebral ischemia. Radiology 1993;188:711-717.
58. Runge VM, Wells JW. Choice of metal ion and formulation concentration for first-pass brain perfusion studies with magnetic resonance imaging at 1.5 tesla. Invest Radiol 1996;31(7):395-400.
59. Heiland S, Forsting M, Reith W, et al. Perfusion weighted magnetic resonance imaging of focal cerebral ischemia: use of the new paramagnetic contrast agent gadolinium-butriol. Proceedings of the Society of Magnetic Resonance, second meeting, August 1994:1024.
60. Saeed M, Wendland MF, Tomei E, et al. Demarcation of myocardial ischemia: magnetic susceptibility effect of contrast medium in MR imaging. Radiology 1989;173:763-767.
61. Moseley ME, Kucharczyk J, Mintorovitch J, et al. Diffusion weighted MR imaging of acute stroke: correlation with T2-weighted and magnetic susceptibility enhanced MR imaging in cats. AJNR 1990;11:423-429.
62. Kucharczyk J, Asgari H, Mintorovitch J, et al. Magnetic resonance imaging of brain perfusion using the nonionic contrast agents Dy DTPA-BMA and Gd DTPA-BMA. Invest Radiol 1991;26:S250-252.
63. Moseley ME, Vexler Z, Asgari HS, et al. Comparison of Gd and Dy chelates for T2 contrast enhanced imaging. Magn Reson Med 1991;22:259-264.
64. Schuhmann-Giampieri G. Liver contrast media for magnetic resonance imaging. Interrelations between pharmacokinetics and imaging. Invest Radiol 1993 Aug;28(8):753-761.
65. Runge VM, Kirsch JE, Wells JW, et al. Enhanced liver MR: contrast agents and imaging strategy. Crit Rev Diagn Imaging 1993;34:1-30.
66. Tweedle MF, Zhang X, Pillai R, et al. New Gd chelates with enhanced relaxivity. Contrast Media Research 1993; MRI-13 (abstract).
67. Vittadini G, Felder E, Musu C, Tirone P. Preclinical profile of Gd-BOPTA. A liver-specific MRI contrast agent. Invest Radiol 1990 Sep;25 Suppl 1:S59-60.
68. Cavagna F, Dapra M, Maggioni F, et al. Gd-BOPTA/Dimeg: experimental disease imaging. Magn Reson Med 1991 Dec;22:329-333.
69. Pavone P, Patrizio G, Buoni C, et al. Comparison of Gd-BOPTA with Gd-DTPA in MRI of rat liver. Radiology 1990;176(1):61-64.
70. Rosati G, Pirovano G, Spinazzi A. Interim results of phase II clinical testing of gadobenate dimeglumine. Invest Radiol 1994 Jun;29 Suppl 2:S183-185.
71. Kreft BP, Tanimoto A, Baba Y, et al. Enhanced tumor detection in the presence of fatty liver disease: cell-specific contrast agents. J Magn Reson Imaging 1994 May-Jun;4(3):337-342.
72. Kreft BP, Tanimoto A, Stark DD, et al. Enhancement of tumor-liver contrast-to-noise ratio with gadobenate dimeglumine in MR imaging of rats. J Magn Reson Imaging 1993 Jan-Feb;3(1):41-49.
73. Yu KK, Saeed M, Wendland MF, et al. Real-time dynamics of an extravascular magnetic resonance contrast medium in acutely infarcted myocardium using inversion recovery and gradient-recalled echo-planar imaging. Invest Radiol 1992 27(11):927-934.
74. Saeed M, Wendland MF, Sakuma H, et al. Coronary artery stenosis: detection with contrast-enhanced MR imaging in dogs. Radiology 1995 Jul;196(1):79-84.
75. Saeed M, Wendland MF, Yu KK, et al. Identification of myocardial reperfusion with echo-planar magnetic resonance imaging. Discrimination between occlusive and reperfused infarctions. Circulation 1994 Sep;90(3):1492-1501.
76. Cavagna FM, Marzola P, Dapra M, et al. Binding of gadobenate dimeglumine to proteins extravasated into interstitial space enhances conspicuity of reperfused infarcts. Invest Radiol 1994 Jun;29 Suppl 2:S50-53.
77. Hamm B, Staks T, Muhler A, et al. Phase I clinical evaluation of Gd-EOB-DTPA as a hepatobiliary MR contrast agent: safety, pharmacokinetics, and MR imaging. Radiology 1995 Jun;195(3): 785-792.
78. Ni Y, Marchal G, Yu J, et al. Prolonged positive contrast enhancement with Gd-EOB-DTPA in experimental liver tumors: potential value in tissue characterization. J Magn Reson Imaging 1994 May-Jun;4(3):355-363.
79. Marchal G, Zhang X, Ni Y, et al. Comparison between Gd-DTPA, Gd-EOB-DTPA, and Mn-DPDP in induced HCC in rats: a correlation study of MR imaging, microangiography, and histology. Magn Reson Imaging 1993;11(5):665-674.
80. Muhler A, Heinzelmann I, Weinmann HJ. Elimination of gadolinium-ethoxybenzyl-DTPA in a rat model of severely impaired liver and kidney excretory function. An experimental study in rats. Invest Radiol 1994 Feb;29(2):213-216.
81. Muhler A, Clement O, Saeed M, et al. Gadolinium-ethoxybenzyl-DTPA, a new liver-directed magnetic resonance contrast agent. Absence of acute hepatotoxic, cardiovascular, or immunogenic effects. Invest Radiol 1993 Jan;28(1):26-32.
82. Van Beers BE, Grandin C, Pauwels S, et al. Gd-EOB-DTPA enhancement pattern of hepatocellular carcinomas in rats: comparison with Tc-99m-IDA uptake. J Magn Reson Imaging 1994 May-Jun;4(3):351-354.
83. Ni Y, Marchal G, Lukito G, et al. MR imaging evaluation of liver enhancement by Gd-EOB-DTPA in selective and total bile

duct obstruction in rats: correlation with serologic, micro-cholangiographic, and histologic findings. Radiology 1994 190(3):753-758.
84. Muhler A, Freise CE, Kuwatsuru R, et al. Acute liver rejection: evaluation with cell-directed MR contrast agents in a rat transplantation model. Enhancement patterns with gadolinium. Radiology 1993 Jan;186(1):139-146.
85. Schuhmann-Giampieri G, Frenzel T, Schmitt-Willich H. Pharmacokinetics in rats, dogs and monkeys of a gadolinium chelate used as a liver-specific contrast agent for magnetic resonance imaging. Arzneimittelforschung 1993 Aug;43(8):927-931.
86. Benness G, Khangure M, Morris I, et al. Hepatic kinetics and magnetic resonance imaging of gadolinium ethoxybenzyl diethylenetriaminepentacetic acid (Gd-EOB-DTPA) in dogs. Australas Radiol 1993 Aug;37(3):252-255.
87. Schuhmann-Giampieri G, Schmitt-Willich H, Frenzel T. Biliary excretion and pharmacokinetics of a gadolinium chelate used as a liver-specific contrast agent for magnetic resonance imaging in the rat. J Pharm Sci 1993 Aug;82(8):799-803.
88. Hamm B, Vogl TJ, Branding G, et al. Focal liver lesions: MR imaging with Mn DPDP — initial clinical results in 40 patients. Radiology 1992;182:167-174.
89. Bernardino ME, Young SW, Lee JKT, Weinreb JC. Hepatic MR imaging with Mn DPDP: safety, image quality, and sensitivity. Radiology 1992;183:53-58.
90. Rofsky NM, Weinreb JC, Bernardino ME, et al. Hepatocellular tumors: characterization with Mn DPDP enhanced MR imaging. Radiology 1993;188:53-59.
91. Lim KO, Start DD, Leese PT, et al. Hepatobiliary MR imaging: first human experience with Mn DPDP. Radiology 1991;178:79-82.
92. Kopp AF, Laniado M, Aicher KP, et al. Manganese DPDP as a contrast medium for MR tomography of focal liver lesions. Tolerance and image quality in 20 patients. ROFO 1992;157:539-547.
93. Aicher KP, Laniado M, Kopp AF, et al. Mn DPTP — enhanced MR imaging of malignant liver lesions: efficacy and safety in 20 patients. J Magn Reson Imaging 1993;3:731-737.
94. Stark DD, Weissleder R, Elizondo G, et al. Superparamagnetic iron oxide: clinical application as a contrast agent for MR imaging of the liver. Radiology 1988;168:297-301.
95. Ferrucci JT, Stark DD. Iron oxide enhanced MR imaging of the liver and spleen: review of the first 5 years. AJR 1990;155:943-950.
96. Fretz CJ, Stark DD, Metz CE, et al. Detection of hepatic metastases: comparison of contrast enhanced CT, unenhanced MR imaging, and iron oxide enhanced MR imaging. AJR 1990;155:763-770.
97. Marchal G, Van Hecke P, Demaerel P, et al. Detection of liver metastases with superparamagnetic iron oxide in 15 patients: results of MR imaging at 1.5 T. AJR 1989;152:771-775.
98. Bruel JM, European SPIO Collaborative Study Group. Superparamagnetic iron oxide for the detection of hepatic lesions with MR imaging: results of a phase III trial. Radiology 1993;189(P):273.
99. Reimer P, Kwong KK, Weisskoff R, et al. Dynamic signal intensity changes in liver with superparamagnetic MR contrast agents. J Magn Reson Imaging 1992;2:177-181.
100. Weissleder R, Reimer P, Lee AS, et al. MR receptor imaging: ultrasmall iron oxide particles targeted to asialoglycoprotein receptors. AJR 1990;155:1161-1167.
101. Reimer P, Weissleder R, Lee AS, et al. Receptor imaging: application to MR imaging of liver cancer. Radiology 1990;177:729-734.
102. Reimer P, Weissleder R, Lee AS, et al. Asialoglycoprotein receptor function in benign liver disease: evaluation with MR imaging. Radiology 1991;178:769-774.
103. Hamm B, Laniado M, Saini S. Contrast enhanced MR imaging of the abdomen and pelvis. Magn Reson Q 1990;6:108-135.
104. Widder DJ, Edelman RR, Grief WI, Monda L. Magnetite albumin suspension: a superparamagnetic oral MR contrast agent. AJR 1987;149:839-843.
105. Mattrey RF, Hajek PC, Gylys-Morin VM, et al. Perfluorochemicals as gastrointestinal contrast agents for MRI: preliminary studies in rats and humans. AJR 1987;148:1259-1263.
106. Gerscovich EO, McGahan JP, Buonocore MH, et al. The rediscovery of infant feeding formula with magnetic resonance imaging. Pediatr Radiol 1990;20:147-151.
107. King CPL, Tart RP, Fitzsimmons JR, et al. Barium sulfate suspension as a negative oral MRI contrast agent: in vitro and human optimization studies. Magn Reson Imaging 1991;9:141-150.
108. Marti-Bonmati L, Vilar J, Paniagua JC, Talens A. High density barium sulphate as an MRI oral contrast. Magn Reson Imaging 1991;19:259-261.
109. Wan X, Wedeking P, Tweedle MF. MRI evaluation of potential GI contrast media. Magn Reson Imaging 1995;13(2):215-218.
110. Wan X, Wedeking P, Tweedle MF. Sources of heterogeneous contrast enhancement in the gastrointestinal tract. Magn Reson Imaging 1994;12(7):1009-1012.
111. Laniado M, Kornmesser W, Hamm B, et al. MR imaging of the gastrointestinal tract: value of Gd-DTPA. AJR 1988;150:817-821.
112. Kaminsky S, Laniado M, Gogoll M, et al. Gadopentetate dimeglumine as a bowel contrast agent: safety and efficacy. Radiology 1991;178:503-508.
113. Claussen C, Kornmesser W, Laniado M, et al. Oral contrast media for magnetic resonance tomography of the abdomen: III. Initial patient research with gadolinium DTPA. ROFO 1988;148:683-689.
114. Krahe T, Dolken W, Lackner K, et al. Gadolinium DTPA as an oral contrast medium for MR tomography of the abdomen. ROFO 1990;153:167-173.
115. Neumann K, Kaminsky S, Gogoll M, et al. Gadolinium DTPA as an oral contrast medium for magnetic resonance tomography of the pancreas. ROFO 1991;154:262-268.
116. Hotzinger H, Salbeck R, Toedt C, Beyer HK. Initial experience with the use of oral gadolinium DTPA in nuclear magnetic resonance tomography of the pelvis. Digitale Bilddiagn 1990;10:42-45.
117. Bernardino ME, Weinreb JC, Mitchell DG, et al. Safety and optimum concentration of a manganese chloride-based oral MR contrast agent. J Magn Reson Imaging 1994 Nov-Dec;4(6):872-876.
118. Vlahos L, Gouliamos A, Athanasopoulou A, et al. A comparative study between Gd-DTPA and oral magnetic particles (OMP) as gastrointestinal (GI) contrast agents for MRI of the abdomen. Magn Reson Imaging 1994;12(5):719-726.
119. Bach-Gansmo T. Ferrimagnetic susceptibility contrast agents. Acta Radiol Suppl 1993;387:1-30.
120. Bach-Gansmo T, Dupas B, Gayet-Delacroix M, Lambrechts M. Abdominal MRI using a negative contrast agent. Br J Radiol 1993 May;66(785):420-425.
121. MacVicar D, Jacobsen TF, Guy R, Husband JE. Phase III trial of oral magnetic particles in MRI of abdomen and pelvis. Clin Radiol 1993 Mar;47(3):183-188.
122. Boudghene FP, Bach-Gansmo T, Grange JD, et al. Contribution of oral magnetic particles in MR imaging of the abdomen with spin-echo and gradient-echo sequences. J Magn Reson Imaging 1993 Jan-Feb;3(1):107-112.

123. Oksendal AN, Bach-Gansmo T, Jacobsen TF, et al. Oral magnetic particles. Results from clinical phase II trials in 216 patients. Acta Radiol 1993 Mar;34(2):187-193.
124. Erquiaga E, Ros PR, Torres GM, et al. Oral superparamagnetic iron oxide: use in pancreatic magnetic resonance imaging [abstract]. Radiology 1990;177:377.
125. Saini S, Modic MT, Hamm B, Hahn PF. Advances in contrast enhanced MR imaging. AJR 1991;156:235-254.
126. Runge VM, Wells JW. Update: safety, new applications, new MR agents. Top Magn Reson Imag 1995;7(3):181-195.

Index

Page numbers for illustrations are in italic typeface.